PAIN MANAGEMENT SECRETS

SECRETS

FOURTH EDITION

PAIN MANAGEMENT SECRETS

FOURTH EDITION

CHARLES E. ARGOFF, MD
Professor of Neurology, Albany Medical College; Director, Comprehensive
Pain Program, Albany Medical Center, Albany, NY, USA

ANDREW DUBIN, MD, MS
Professor of PM&R, Albany Medical College; Chief of PM&R, Samuel
Stratton VA Medical Center Hospital, Albany, NY, USA

JULIE G. PILITSIS, MD, PhD
Chair, Department of Neuroscience and Experimental Therapeutics;
Professor, Neurosurgery and Department of Neuroscience and
Experimental Therapeutics, Albany Medical College, Albany, NY, USA

ELSEVIER

ELSEVIER

ISBN: 978-0-323-27791-4
E-ISBN: 978-0-323-41386-2

First edition 1997
Second edition 2003
Third edition 2009

Content Strategist: James Merritt
Content Development Manager: Joanne Scott
Project Manager: Beula Christopher
Designer: Bridget Hoette
Illustration Manager: Amy Faith Heyden
Illustrator: Best Set; Marie Dean
Marketing Manager: Melissa Darling

Printed in the United States of America

Last digit is the print number: 9 8 7 6 5 4 3 2

Working together
to grow libraries in
developing countries

www.elsevier.com • www.bookaid.org

CONTENTS

VI   SPECIAL PATIENT POPULATIONS

VII   PHARMACOLOGIC MANAGEMENT

VIII   NONPHARMACOLOGIC MANAGEMENT

PREFACE

Inspection of the "pain" section of any bookstore will reveal a wide and diverse range of texts that address everything from the basic science that underpins our understanding of pain, all the way through to the clinical treatment of specific conditions. We are spoiled with choices. These books largely use scientific evidence to validate the propositions that they make, and provide an invaluable resource for anyone interested in pain and its treatment, although deciding which book best fits the individual's requirement can be problematical.

The fourth edition of *Pain Secrets* differs from most of these books. It contains a refreshing mixture of scientifically robust information combined with a more anecdotal nature. It has become fashionable to discredit opinion unless it is based on the results of rigorously performed studies, and yet by ignoring the combined wealth of knowledge possessed by experienced practitioners based on years of involvement in their field, we risk having a less complete knowledge of our field of interest than would otherwise be the case. *Pain Secrets* is liberally seeded with little "pearls of wisdom," which many will find interesting, thought provoking, and hopefully useful. Some of these you may know already, but almost certainly others will be new. They have the potential for transforming the practitioner from being knowledgeable and widely read to being even more effective in his or her practice than before. These useful pieces of knowledge have a value that is timeless, and they are not a representation of a current fashion in our thinking about pain. As such, they can provide the reader with an insight that normally is acquired only by long years of practical experience.

Perhaps one of the other distinguishing features of *Pain Secrets* is that it can be used when a specific answer to a specific question is needed. Each chapter concentrates on one facet of pain management. Contained in each chapter are a series of individual questions for which an answer is provided. Alternatively, the book can be read chapter by chapter to give a more comprehensive insight into the subject being considered. Given the style used and the content of each chapter, this book should be of interest, indeed value, to anyone involved in pain management, whether they are fully qualified or still in training. It should also be of use to those in whom pain management is an incidental requirement rather than a primary focus of interest.

I am so fortunate to have two of my colleagues at Albany Medical College, Dr. Julie Pilitsis, a neurosurgeon and neuroscientist, and Dr. Andrew Dubin, a physical medicine and rehabilitation specialist and electrodiagnostician, join me as editors of this edition. Both Dr. Pilitsis and Dr. Dubin are internationally recognized for their innovative contributions to pain management. We are also fortunate that so many new chapters have been added to this edition, each written by internationally recognized contributors. Pain management as a medical specialty has grown significantly and is in an active state of maturation. We now have the ability to evaluate and treat our patients with more medical, nonmedical, invasive, complimentary, regenerative approaches than ever before. These are indeed exciting times in pain management, with an explosion of new information that itself might appear daunting to the providers who are not pain specialists. This is why we have included the preface to the 3rd edition of *Pain Management Secrets*. The fourth edition holds true to the third edition in how it is organized and how it is intended to be used by all, regardless of their level of training. Thank you to all who have contributed to this edition, and I am confident that this edition will be of immense value to all interested in pain management.

Charles E. Argoff, MD
Andrew Dubin, MD, MS
Julie G. Pilitsis, MD, PhD

CONTRIBUTORS

The editor(s) would like to acknowledge and offer grateful thanks for the input of all previous editions' contributors, without whom this new edition would not have been possible.

Adedamola Adepoju, MD
Neurosurgery Resident, Department of Neurosurgery, Albany Medical College, Albany NY, USA

Charles E. Argoff, MD
Professor of Neurology, Albany Medical College; Director, Comprehensive Pain Program, Albany Medical Center, Albany, NY, USA

Maya A. Babu, MD, MBA
Department of Neurologic Surgery, Mayo Clinic, Rochester, MN, USA

Miroslav "Misha" Backonja, MD
Professor Emeritus, University of Wisconsin-Madison; Senior Medical Director, Worldwide Clinical Trials, NC, USA

Allan I. Basbaum, PhD
Professor and Chair, Department of Anatomy and William Keck Foundation Center for Integrative Neuroscience, University of California, San Francisco, CA, USA

Abigail Bemis
Albany Medical Center, Neurosurgery, Albany, NY, USA

Anisha Bhangav, MD
Chief Resident, Department of Neurology, University of Minnesota, Minneapolis, MN, USA

Alan S. Boulos, MD
Department of Neurosurgery, Albany Medical Center, Albany, NY, USA

Darren Brenner, MD, AGAF
Associate Professor of Medicine and Surgery, Director of Functional Bowel Program and Motts Tonelli GI Physiology Laboratory, Division of Gastroenterology, Northwestern University, Feinberg School of Medicine, Chicago, IL, USA

Michael A. Bushey MD, PhD
Chief Resident, Department of Psychiatry and Behavioral Sciences, Johns Hopkins University School of Medicine, Baltimore, MD, USA

Kevin S. Chen, MD
Resident Physician, Department of Neurosurgery, University of Michigan Health System, Ann Arbor, MI, USA

Nita Chen, BS, MD
Physician, Neurology, University of California, Irvine, CA, USA

Michael R. Clark, MD, MPH, MBA
Vice Chair, Clinical Affairs, Director, Pain Treatment Program, Department of Psychiatry and Behavioral Sciences, Johns Hopkins University School of Medicine, Baltimore, MD, USA

Jacqueline H. Cleary, BS, PharmD, BCACP
Assistant Professor of Pharmacy Practice, Albany College of Pharmacy and Health Sciences, Albany, NY, USA

Claire Collison, MS
Medical Student Researcher, Department of Neuroscience and Experimental Therapeutics, Albany Medical College, Albany, NY, USA

Robert A. Duarte, MD
Director, Pain Center, Northwell Neuroscience Institute; Assistant Professor, Hofstra Northwell School of Medicine, Great Neck, NY, USA

Andrew Dubin, MD, MS
Professor of PM&R, Albany Medical College; Chief of PM&R, Samuel Stratton VA Medical Center Hospital, Albany, NY, USA

Grace Forde, MD
Director of Neurological Services, North American Partners in Pain Management, Lake Success, NY, USA

Jeffrey Fudin, BS, PharmD, DAIPM, FCCP, FASHP
Clinical Pharmacy Specialist and Director, PGY2 Pharmacy Pain and Palliative Care Residency (WOC), Adjunct Associate Professor Pharmacy Practice, Samuel Stratton VA Medical Center, Albany College of Pharmacy and Health Sciences, Albany, NY, USA

Katherine Galluzzi, DO
Professor and Chair, Department of Geriatrics, Philadelphia College of Osteopathic Medicine, Philadelphia, PA, USA

Sara Gannon
Department of Neurosurgery, Albany Medical College, Albany, NY, USA

Fady Girgis, BSc Pharm, MD, EdM, FRCSC
Assistant Professor, Department of Neurological Surgery, UC Davis School of Medicine, Sacramento, CA, USA

Eric Gruenthal, MD
Department of Neurosurgery, Albany Medical College, Albany, NY, USA

Salim Hayek, MD, PhD
Professor, Department of Anesthesiology, Case Western Reserve University; Chief, Division of Pain Medicine, University Hospitals of Cleveland, Cleveland, OH, USA

Marilyn S. Jacobs, PhD, ABPP
Assistant Clinical Professor, Department of Psychiatry and Biobehavioral Sciences, David Geffen School of Medicine at UCLA, Los Angeles, CA, USA

R. Carter W. Jones III, MD PhD
Assistant Professor of Anesthesiology, Department of Anesthesiology, University of California San Diego, San Diego, CA, USA

Tyler J. Kenning, MD, FAANS
Director, Pituitary and Cranial Base Surgery, Department of Neurosurgery, Albany Medical Center, Albany, NY, USA

Vignessh Kumar, BS
Department of Neurosurgery, Albany Medical College, Albany, NY, USA

Steven Lange, MD
Department of Neurosurgery, Albany Medical College, Albany, NY, USA

Andras Laufer, MD
Anesthesiologist, Assistant Professor, Department of Anesthesiology, Albany Medical Center, Albany Medical College, Albany, NY, USA

Kenneth R. Lofland, PhD
President, Northshore Integrative Healthcare, Adjunct Associate Professor, Department of Anesthesiology, Northwestern University Feinberg School of Medicine, Chicago, IL, USA

Renee C.B. Manworren, PhD, RN-BC, APRN, PCNS-BC, AP-PMN, FAAN
Posy and Fred Love Chair in Nursing Research; Director of Nursing Research and Professional Practice, Ann & Robert H. Lurie Children's Hospital of Chicago; Associate Professor, Department of Pediatrics, Northwestern University, Feinberg School of Medicine, Chicago, IL, USA

David McLain, MD, FACP, FACR
Rheumatologist, McLain Medical Associates PC; Symposium Director, Annual Congress of Clinical Rheumatology; Executive Director, Alabama Society for the Rheumatic Diseases, Birmingham, AL, USA

Jonathan Miller, MD, FAANS, FACS
Director, Functional and Restorative Neurosurgery Center; Associate Professor and Vice Chair, Department of Neurological Surgery, Case Western Reserve University School of Medicine/UH Cleveland Medical Center, Cleveland, OH, USA

Alon Y. Mogilner, MD, PhD
Associate Professor of Neurosurgery and Anesthesiology, Director, Center for Neuromodulation, Department of Neurosurgery, NYU Langone Medical Center, New York, NY, USA

Karin M. Muraszko, MD
Chair and Julian T. Hoff Professor, Department of Neurosurgery; Professor, Plastic Surgery, and Pediatrics, University of Michigan, Ann Arbor, MI, USA

Sarah Narayan, MD
Assistant Professor, Department of Physical Medicine and Rehabilitation, Albany Medical College; Pain Specialist, Comprehensive Spine Center, Albany Medical Center, Albany, NY, USA

Gaetano Pastena, MD/MBA
Assistant Professor, Section Head, Neuroradiology, Department of Radiology, Albany Medical Center, Community Care Physicians, PC, Albany, NY, USA

Parag G. Patil, MD, PhD
Associate Professor, Departments of Neurosurgery, Neurology, Anesthesiology, and Biomedical Engineering, University of Michigan Medical School, Ann Arbor, MI, USA

Alexandra R. Paul, MD
Department of Neurosurgery, Albany Medical Center, Albany, NY, USA

Katherin Peperzak, MD
Acting Assistant Professor, Department of Anesthesiology and Pain Medicine, University of Washington School of Medicine, Seattle, WA, USA

Julie G. Pilitsis, MD, PhD
Chair, Department of Neuroscience and Experimental Therapeutics; Professor, Neurosurgery and Department of Neuroscience and Experimental Therapeutics, Albany Medical College, Albany, NY, USA

Julia Prusik, BS
Department of Neurosurgery, Department of
Neuroscience and Experimental Therapeutics,
Albany Medical College, Albany, NY, USA

Nataly Raviv, MD
Neurosurgery Resident, Department of
Neurosurgery, Albany Medical College, Albany
NY, USA

Gaddum Duemani Reddy, MD, PhD
Department of Neurosurgery, Toronto Western
Hospital, University of Toronto, Toronto, ON,
Canada

Alycia Reppel, MD
Interventional Pain Management Physiatrist, St.
Mary's Physiatry Services, Auburn, ME, USA

Joshua M. Rosenow, MD, FAANS, FACS
Director of Functional Neurosurgery; Associate
Professor of Neurosurgery, Neurology and
Physical Medicine and Rehabilitation,
Northwestern University Feinberg School of
Medicine, Chicago, IL, USA

Noah Rosen, MD FAHS FANA
Co-Director, Northwell Pain and Headache Center;
Associate Professor, Neurology and Psychiatry,
Hofstra Northwell; Health Adjunct Assistant
Professor, Albert Einstein School of Medicine,
New York City, NY, USA

Nidhi Sondhi, DO
Resident Physician, Department of Anesthesiology
and Perioperative Medicine, Case Western
Reserve University, University Hospitals
Cleveland Medical Center, Cleveland, OH, USA

Steven Sparkes, PharmD, BCPS
Clinical Pharmacist, Samuel Stratton VA Medical
Center, Albany, NY, USA

Brett R. Stacey, MD
Medical Director, UW Center for Pain Relief,
Professor, Anesthesiology and Pain Medicine,
University of Washington, Seattle, WA, USA

Emily K. Stern, MD
Gastroenterology Fellow, Division of
Gastroenterology, Northwestern University,
Feinberg School of Medicine, Chicago, IL, USA

Lekeisha A. Sumner, PhD, ABPP
Director of Health Psychology, Department of
Psychiatry and Behavioral Sciences, Cedars-
Sinai Medical Center, Los Angeles, CA, USA

Ashwin Viswanathan, MD
Department of Neurosurgery, Baylor College of
Medicine, Houston, TX, USA

David Walk, MD
Associate Professor, University of Minnesota
Department of Neurology, Minneapolis, MN,
USA

Mark S. Wallace, MD
Professor of Clinical Anesthesiology, Department of
Anesthesiology, University of California, San
Diego, La Jolla, CA, USA

Ian Walling, BS
Research Assistant, Department of Neuroscience
and Experimental Therapeutics, Albany Medical
College, Albany, NY, USA

Meghan Wilock, PA-C
Physician Assistant, Neurosurgery, Albany Medical
Center, Albany, NY, USA

Benjamin Yim, MD
Neurosurgery Resident, Department of
Neurosurgery, Albany Medical College, Albany
NY, USA

Youngwon Youn, BA
Department of Neurosurgery, Department of
Neuroscience and Experimental Therapeutics,
Albany Medical College, Albany, NY, USA

ACKNOWLEDGMENTS

To Julie Pilitsis, Andrew Dubin, Pya Seidner and to all contributing authors- your hard work and collaboration is what has allowed this project to be completed.

Charles E. Argoff

A special thank you to Pya Seidner who aided considerably with editing and communicating with the authors, editors and publishers.

Julie G. Pilitsis

DEDICATION

To my wife Pat and out children David, Melanie and Emily. Your love and our family make everything possible.
Charles E. Argoff

I would like to dedicate this book to my residents. Their inquisitiveness and curiosity are my inspiration to teach and educate.
Andrew Dubin

To Tim, Ryan, Lauren and my mother, whose undying support makes all my work possible. To my clinical and basic science team, thank you for all you do to care for existing patients and improve treatment for future patients.
Julie G. Pilitsis

TOP SECRETS

1. **What are the chronic pain syndromes that involve muscle and fascia?**
   Myofascial pain syndrome and fibromyalgia are chronic pain syndromes that are associated with muscle and soft tissue pain. Myofascial pain syndrome is regional in distribution, whereas fibromyalgia involves the entire body. These diagnoses may represent two points in a spectrum of disease, as subgroups of fibromyalgia have been identified based on differing clinical findings and prognoses.

2. **Describe the myofascial pain syndrome.**
   The myofascial pain syndrome is a chronic, regional pain syndrome that involves muscle and soft tissues. It is characterized by trigger points and taut bands (see Questions 7 and 8). Originally described by Travell and later elaborated on by Travell and Simons, myofascial pain syndrome occurs in most body areas, most commonly in the cervical and lumbar regions.

3. **What is fibromyalgia?**
   Fibromyalgia is a clinical syndrome characterized by chronic, diffuse pain and multiple tender points at defined points in muscle and other soft tissues. Periosteal tender points are frequently present. Widespread pain can be felt both above and below the waist and bilaterally. Other characteristic features of the syndrome include fatigue, sleep disturbance, irritable bowel syndrome (IBS), interstitial cystitis, stiffness, paresthesias, headaches, depression, anxiety, and decreased memory and vocabulary.

4. **What are the latest criteria for the diagnosis of fibromyalgia?**
   The latest criteria are 2016 revisions to the 2010/2011 fibromyalgia diagnostic criteria.
   * Generalized pain, defined as pain in at least four of five regions, is present.
   * Symptoms have been present at a similar level for at least 3 months.
   * Widespread pain index (WPI) ≥7 and symptom severity scale (SSS) score ≥5 OR WPI of 4–6 and SSS score ≥9.
   * A diagnosis of fibromyalgia is valid irrespective of other diagnoses. A diagnosis of fibromyalgia does not exclude the presence of other clinically important illnesses.
   * The tender point examinations were removed in the 2010/2011 criteria. They were part of the 1990 criteria.

5. **How do you determine a score using the WPI?**
   * WPI definition: note the number of areas in which the patient has had pain over the last week. In how many areas has the patient had pain? The score will be between 0 and 19.

Left upper region (Region 1)	Right uper region (Region 2)	Axial region (Region 5)
Jaw, left	Jaw, right	Neck
Shoulder girdle, left	Shoulder girdle, right	Upper back
Upper arm, left	Upper arm, right	Lower back
Lower arm, left	Lower arm, right	Chest
		Abdomen

Left lower region (region 3)
Hip (buttock, trochanter), left
Upper leg, left
Lower leg, left

Right lower region (Region 4)
Hip (buttock, trochanter), right
Upper leg, right
Lower leg, right

Symptom severity scale (SSS) score
Fatigue
Waking unrefreshed
Cognitive symptoms
Forthe each of the 3 symptoms above, indicate the level of severity over the past week using
   the following scale:
0 = No problem
1 = Slight or mild problems, generally mild or intermittent
2 = Moderate, considerable problems, often present and/or at a moderate level
3 = Severe: perasive, continuous, life-disturbing problems

The symptom severity scale (SSS) score: is the sum of the severity scores of the 3
   symptoms (fatigue, waking unrefreshed, nd cognitive symptoms) (0–9) plus the sum (0–3) of
   the number of the following symptoms the patient has been bothered by that occurred during
   the previous 6 months:
(1) Headaches (0–1)
(2) Pain or cramps in lower abdomen (0–1)
(3) And depression (0–1)

The final symptom severity score is between 0 and 12
The fibromyalgia severity (FS) scale is the sum of the WPI and SSS

- From Wolfe F, Clauw DJ, Fitzcharles MA et al. 2016 Revisions to the 2010/2011
  fibromyalgia diagnostic criteria. Semin Arthritis Rheum. 2016 Dec;46(3):319–329.

6. Do all fibromyalgia patients have the same symptoms?
   No. There is a high degree of variability in the presentation of fibromyalgia. Subgroups
   of the syndrome have been identified based on the number of active tender points,
   sleep quality, and cold pain threshold. These subgroups have different prognoses.
   Patients may also be grouped according to related disease. Of patients with IBS,
   20% demonstrate findings consistent with fibromyalgia. Fibromyalgia is more common
   in diabetics than in the general population, and the severity of pain correlates
   with the duration of diabetes. These may constitute additional subgroups of
   fibromyalgia. Fibromyalgia is also common in autoimmune diseases, such as Sjögren's
   syndrome, systemic lupus erythematosus, Hashimoto's thyroiditis, and rheumatoid
   arthritis.

7. Name syndromes that are associated with fibromyalgia.
   - Chronic fatigue syndrome
   - IBS
   - Restless leg syndrome
   - Interstitial cystitis
   - Temporomandibular joint dysfunction
   - Sicca syndrome
   - Raynaud's phenomenon
   - Autonomic dysregulation with orthostatic hypotension
   - Mood disorder
   - Hypermobility syndrome

8. What are trigger points?
   Trigger points are sites in muscle or tendon that, when palpated, produce pain at a
   distant site. These occur in consistent locations with predictable patterns of pain
   referral. Trigger points are often associated with prior trauma, "near falls," or
   degenerative osteoarthritis.

9. What are "taut bands"? How are they associated with trigger points?
   In patients with myofascial pain, deep palpation of muscle may reveal areas that feel
   tight and bandlike. Stretching this band of muscle produces pain. This is a taut band.

Trigger points are characteristically found within taut bands of muscle. Despite the muscle tension, taut bands are electrophysiologically silent (i.e., the electromyogram [EMG] is normal). Rolling the taut band under the fingertip at the trigger point (snapping palpation) may produce a local "twitch" response. This shortening of the band of muscle is one of the cardinal signs of fibromyalgia.

10. Describe the prevalence and typical demographics of the fibromyalgia patient.
    In most reported series, 80% to 90% of patients with fibromyalgia are female, with a peak incidence in middle age and a prevalence of 0.5% to 5% of the general population.

11. What laboratory investigations are useful in fibromyalgia?
    All laboratory values in fibromyalgia are used for exclusionary purposes. There are no characteristic chemical, electrical, or radiographic laboratory abnormalities. However, several consistent investigational serum markers of the disease have been reported in the literature. An increase in cytokines, with a direct relationship between pain intensity and interleukin-8, has been reported. Other investigational findings include a decrease in circulating cortisol (this may play a role in decreased exercise tolerance), a decrease in branched-chain amino acids (perhaps correlating with muscle fatigue), and decreased lymphocyte Gi protein and cAMP concentrations. Four studies have shown an increase in substance P in the cerebrospinal fluid (CSF) in fibromyalgia. At present, these findings are not clinically useful for the diagnosis, prognosis, or monitoring of the treatment response of fibromyalgia patients. Elevation of spinal fluid substance P has been seen in many disease states including sickle cell crisis, inflammatory bowel disease, rheumatoid arthritis, spina bifida, major depression, and post traumatic stress disorder (PTSD). Sleep studies are often abnormal ("alpha-delta," nonrestorative sleep), but the abnormalities are also seen in other chronic painful conditions. Functional magnetic resonance imaging studies have shown augmented responses in the insula and anterior lingual gyrus to nonpainful sensory stimuli in fibromyalgia patients but not in controls.

12. What is the relationship of small fiber polyneuropathy (SFPN) to fibromyalgia?
    Recent studies have discovered SFPN in up to 50% of patients with fibromyalgia. This has suggested that perhaps patients diagnosed with "fibromyalgia" have SFPN, a condition that can be objectively tested for and sometimes treated. This is an area of controversy in present fibromyalgia research. For example, many patients with fibromyalgia experience the burning pain or nerve tingling characteristic of SFPN, but most patients with SFPN do not experience the symptom of widespread deep tissue pain, a hallmark of fibromyalgia. Moreover, even if these small fibers in the skin are somehow contributing to pain, how are these findings responsible for the fatigue, memory, sleep, and mood problems that often are a bigger problem for patients with fibromyalgia than the pain?

13. What treatments are commonly used for fibromyalgia and for myofascial pain?
    A combination of physical, anesthesiologic, and pharmacologic techniques are employed. Some of the most common treatments involve lidocaine injection or dry-needling of trigger points. These approaches are based on the concept that trigger points represent areas of local muscle spasm. However, the efficacy of trigger point injections has never been fully substantiated, although they do offer transient relief to some patients. Physical techniques, such as stretching, spray and stretch (see Question 19), massage, and heat and cold application, have all been advocated, but none are fully validated by well-controlled studies.

14. Describe the role of physical therapy modalities in the treatment of myofascial pain.
    Most studies documenting the efficacy of physical therapy modalities are anecdotal and include relatively small subject numbers. They suggest the efficacy of transcutaneous electrical nerve stimulation (TENS), balneotherapy, ice, massage, ischemic compression (acupressure), and biofeedback in the treatment of myofascial pain. Low-power laser has been studied for its effect on myofascial pain associated with fibromyalgia. This modality seems to significantly reduce pain, muscle spasm, stiffness, and number of tender points.

15. Which medications are commonly used in the treatment of fibromyalgia and myofascial pain syndrome?

Tricyclic antidepressants are widely used drugs for these disorders. They are used because they have the potential to regularize sleep patterns, decrease pain and muscle spasms, and because of their mood-enhancing properties. However, many tricyclic antidepressants are on the Beers List of drugs that are potentially inappropriate for the elderly and not allowed by Medicare. Selective serotonin-reuptake inhibitors (SSRIs) are used to elevate mood but have little analgesic effect. Serotonin-norepinephrine reuptake inhibitors (SNRIs), such as duloxetine and milnacipran, have recently been shown to have pain-reducing properties in patients with fibromyalgia and can also improve mood. Pregabalin, milnacipran, and duloxetine have received an indication for the treatment of fibromyalgia in the United States. Nonsteroidal antiinflammatory drugs (NSAIDs), opioids, and nonnarcotic analgesics are also frequently used, but their role is also unclear and not evidence based. Many medications, such as cyclobenzaprine, baclofen, tizanidine, and chlorzoxazone, have been used to achieve symptom relief. However, a treatment effect has not been consistently supported. Medications that target associated symptoms are often employed. Among the most common of these are sleep medications such as zolpidem and fludrocortisone to treat postural hypotension and adynamia.

16. What are some other interventions that have been studied for the treatment of fibromyalgia?

There is a large series investigating the role of diet in treating fibromyalgia. Some studies promote a raw vegetarian diet, which others tout *Chlorella pyrenoides* (algae) as a dietary supplement. Monosodium glutamate and aspartame have both been implicated in producing symptoms common to fibromyalgia and may play a role in pathogenesis for certain fibromyalgia subgroups.

Botulinum toxin injection and acupuncture have also been studied. They appear to be helpful in certain instances, but the consistent efficacy has not been proven.

17. Is exercise useful in the treatment of fibromyalgia and myofascial pain syndrome?

Yes! The most consistent improvement in fibromyalgia and myofascial pain syndrome occurs with exercise. The exercise hormonal response is abnormal in patients with fibromyalgia (increase in growth hormone concentration, the opposite of normal response), so the frequency and intensity of exercise need to be carefully adjusted to the patient's tolerance. Although strengthening (progressive resistive or isokinetic) exercise can be helpful, the best outcome appears to result from conditioning, or aerobic, exercise.

18. What are the proposed pathophysiologic mechanisms for fibromyalgia?

Fibromyalgia is associated with an augmentation of sensation. Pathophysiologic explanations for fibromyalgia have ranged from primarily central to a combination of central and peripheral and to primarily peripheral. Examples:
- Fibromyalgia is a variation of an affective disorder. This idea was based on its common association with depression, IBS, and chronic fatigue syndrome.
- A sleep abnormality is the main disturbance, leading to altered pain perception.
- Peripheral factors, especially musculoskeletal derangements, are most important, along with the depression resulting from chronic pain.
- Travell and Simons believed that the muscle problem was primary.

19. What are the current systemic hypotheses of fibromyalgia under investigation?

It remains unclear whether there is one pathological mechanism for fibromyalgia or a variety of etiologic factors. Nevertheless, current hypotheses under investigation hold some promise that the pathogenesis and pathophysiology of fibromyalgia may soon be clarified:
- The cause is neuroendocrine in origin. This concept is largely based on the observation of decreased circulating cortisol levels and abnormal 5-HT metabolism.
- Peripheral C-fiber and central nociceptive sensitization occurs following a painful stimulus (windup). This sensitization is ameliorated by N-methyl-D-aspartate (NMDA)

receptor blockade. NMDA activation causes the release of substance P that has been found to be elevated in the CSF in fibromyalgia patients. Consequently, fibromyalgia represents "central sensitization."
- Association with infection: High levels of circulating immunoglobulin M (IgM) in response to an enteroviral infection have been demonstrated in some fibromyalgia patients. Hepatitis C has been associated with fibromyalgia.

20. What are the current hypothesis involving the brain that are under investigation for etiology of fibromyalgia?
- A Chiari I malformation, with brainstem compression, leads to an altered autonomic response, orthostasis, and fibromyalgia syndrome.
- Glial cell activation which includes neuroinflammation, glial cell dysfunction (GCD), cellular destruction, hyperarousal of the sympathetic nervous system, and stimulation of the hypothalamic-pituitary complex. Neurogenic neuroinflammation due to glial cell activation leads to production of proinflammatory cytokines, nitric oxide, prostaglandin E2, and reactive oxygen and nitrogen species. This is an active area of current fibromyalgia research.

21. How is sleep disturbance related to fibromyalgia?
Sleep disturbance is one of the most common complaints of patients with fibromyalgia. It was initially described as "nonrestorative sleep." Some patients were shown to have an intrusion of alpha rhythms into their stage-IV sleep ("alpha-delta" sleep). However, the same electroencephalographic pattern is often seen in other chronically painful conditions. Moreover, other disorders frequently found in association with fibromyalgia, such as the restless leg syndrome, can contribute to a sleep disorder. The incidence of sleep disturbance seems more related to the duration of chronic pain than to the specific diagnosis of fibromyalgia.

22. What is the "spray and stretch" technique?
The spray and stretch technique is based on the theory that trigger points located in taut muscle bands are the principal cause of pain in fibromyalgia and in myofascial pain syndrome. A taut band in the muscle is identified, and then a vapo-coolant spray (ethylchloride or fluoromethane) is applied directly along the muscle band. Once cooled, the muscle is stretched along its long axis. This helps to relax muscle tension (via muscle spindle and Golgi tendon organ stimulation), improve local circulation, decrease the number of active trigger points, and reduce the amount of pain.

23. True or false: There are a number of controlled studies that demonstrate the efficacy of the various treatments used for fibromyalgia.
False. There is a paucity of controlled studies with adequate outcome measures. Most studies have small cohorts and are largely anecdotal. Studies have been performed using tricyclic antidepressants, EMG biofeedback, education, physical training, hypnotherapy, a variety of drug combinations, and many other treatment strategies. In 145 reports of outcome measures, only 55 could differentiate the active treatment from placebo.
The treatment of fibromyalgia and myofascial pain syndrome remains a significant challenge to the practice of evidence-based medicine.

24. Are there any factors that can precipitate the onset of fibromyalgia?
Fibromyalgia can occur without any identifiable precipitating factors. However, it seems that it can also be initiated by trauma (e.g., surgery, childbirth, accident, severe infection, severe emotional strain, sexual abuse) and can then be classified as "posttraumatic fibromyalgia."

25. What drugs have recently been added to the list of medications used in the symptomatic treatment of fibromyalgia?
Although only Pregabalin, milnacipran, and duloxetine have received a specific indication for use in the treatment of fibromyalgia, a number of others have recently been used in increasing volumes. These include SNRIs, muscle relaxants such as tizanidine, and the 5-HT3 antagonists such as ondansetron, granisetron, and

tropisetron. Low-dose naltrexone (LDN) has been shown in a small double-blind study to be effective in fibromyalgia. It is a microglial modulator and must be compounded.

26. Are there any alternative therapeutic options for the treatment of myofascial syndrome?
Pregabalin and duloxetine are examples of oral drugs, indicated for other disease states, which can be used with benefit in the treatment of myofascial syndrome. A number of topical options also exist. These include topical capsaicin, glyceryl trinitrate (which has a localized antiinflammatory effect), lidocaine (Lidoderm patch), and doxepin (a tricyclic antidepressant with localized analgesic effects). Injection of local anesthetic into tender points can be used, as well as injection with corticosteroid. Corticosteroids stabilize nerve membranes, reduce ectopic neural discharge, and have a specific effect on dorsal horn cells and their well-known anti-inflammatory effects.

27. Are there any acute treatments that can be used to lessen the pain of fibromyalgia during a flare-up of this condition?
It has recently been shown that parenteral injection of the 5-HT3 antagonist tropisetron can reduce the pain of fibromyalgia.

28. High-pressure headaches are positional; they are worse when lying flat and improved when upright. Low-pressure headaches are also positional; they are worse when upright and improved by lying flat.

29. Treatment of idiopathic intracranial hypertension (IIH) is chiefly directed at preserving visual function.

30. Headache can be the only symptom of a brain tumor. Brain tumor headaches, however, are often commonly associated with other neurologic signs including focal neurologic deficit, evidence of increased intracranial pressure, and/or seizures.

31. The complaint of "the worst headache of my life" or "thunderclap headache" should prompt evaluation for subarachnoid hemorrhage.

32. Further workup of back pain with advanced imaging early in the evaluation process is often indicated by findings indicating concern for neoplasm, infection, trauma/fracture, and/or severe neurologic impairment.

33. A formal evaluation by a psychologist skilled in the evaluation of patients with chronic pain is important to the development of an overall plan of care.

34. Topical analgesics exert their effect via a local mechanism and do not have any systemic activity in contrast to transdermal agents that require a systemic concentration of analgesic.

35. Specific pain syndromes may be more likely to occur in the older population; this should be considered when evaluating the older patient in pain.

36. Neuropathic pain may be caused by peripheral or central nervous system pathologies.

37. Surgery predictably will result in pain, and untreated postoperative pain negatively influences the surgical outcome.

38. Postoperative pain is influenced by not only the nature of the surgery, but also the patient age, gender, and medical, psychological, and social history.

39. GPN shares similar triggers with that of trigeminal neuralgia, such as talking and chewing, but swallowing is a trigger that is often specific to glossopharyngeal headache (GPN).

40. The differential diagnosis of facial pain should include trigeminal neuralgia, geniculate neuralgia, occipital neuralgia, Ramsay-Hunt syndrome, Tolosa-Hunt syndrome, superior laryngeal neuralgia, sphenopalatine neuralgia, dental or periodontal disease, and temporomandibular joint pain.

41. Pain is best understood according to the biopsychosocial model, i.e., it is a perceptual experience that involves sensation (tissue damage due to illness or injury), emotion (feelings), and cognition (thoughts).

42. It is important to consider sociocultural factors when assessing pain patients.

43. Pain is most effectively treated with the approach of a multidisciplinary team.

44. Cordotomy is ideal for unilateral pain below the C5 dermatome.

45. Midline myelotomy can be performed open or percutaneously to allow sicker patients to be treated.

46. Prior to permanent spinal cord stimulator implantation, pain relief should be demonstrated with a temporary externalized trial.

47. Food and Drug Administration approved intrathecal medications in the United States for pain include morphine and ziconotide.

48. There is no consensus on which trialing method is most appropriate or accurate, and all have advantages and disadvantages. Furthermore, a negative trial does not necessarily predict a negative treatment response to intrathecal drug delivery, while, conversely, placebo effect may produce a false positive trial.

49. Practitioners should have a high clinical suspicion for granuloma formation if patients report diminished efficacy of intrathecal therapy especially with escalation of therapy and/or if they report new neurologic signs and symptoms.

50. Opioids are classified from Schedule I through V according to their medical use and their potential to be abused. Drugs, substances, or chemicals that are Schedule I have little medical use and very high potential to be abused compared to those that are Schedule V, which are useful medically and have little to no potential to be abused.

51. The regulation of opioid use begins on both a state and federal level by requiring proper evaluation of patients and physician certification before treatment approval. If the physicians do not abide by federal and state law, there are legal consequences.

52. When diagnosed and treated within 6 months, patients with complex regional pain syndrome (CRPS) are highly responsive to treatments such as physical therapy, neuropathic medication, stellate ganglion blocks, and spinal cord stimulation. Thus, it is urgent that patients be diagnosed and treated early.

53. Status migrainosus is defined as a severe headache that lasts longer than 72 hours.

54. Trigeminal neuralgia is defined by intense localized pain resulting from nonpainful stimuli to the face. It is most commonly caused by vascular compression of a nerve.

55. Medications, specifically anticonvulsants, are the first line of defense against trigeminal neuralgia.

56. Best estimates are that misuse occurs in nearly 25% of patients and addiction occurs in around 10% of patients treated with opioids for chronic pain.

57. Long-term opioid treatment is not first-line treatment of chronic pain.

58. 50%–70% of patients experience short-term relief with spinal cord stimulation (SCS). At 2 years, SCS was shown to provide superior pain relief, improve quality of life, and improve functional capacity as compared to conventional medical management alone.

59. Complementary and alternative medicine, while differing greatly in method of implementation, generally share the ideas of focusing on the body's ability for self-recovery and the importance of preventative measures in healthcare.

60. A broad range of complementary and alternative medicine are currently implemented with varying degrees of evidence to back up their efficacy for treating different conditions, and as studies improve in quantity and quality, these practices will either be further refined and introduced into mainstream medicine or fall into disuse if shown inefficacious.

61. Due to the potential for drug-herb/supplement interactions having potential deleterious consequences, it is crucial that practitioners, both mainstream and alternative, conduct thorough medication history checks to prevent such interactions.

62. Understand that peripheral nerve blocks can be used for diagnostic and therapeutic purposes.

63. Understand the potential complication of increasing pain post procedure and its management.

64. Understand where peripheral nerve blocks fit into the armamentarium of pain management and evaluation.

65. Members of a multidisciplinary pain management clinic should share a common philosophy.

66. It is desirable for pain management clinics to be certified by, for example, the Committee of Accreditation of Rehabilitation Facilities or the American Academy of Pain Medicine.

67. The aim of pain clinic treatment is reduction in suffering, which may be physical, mental, or more often both.

68. Taking an appropriate history is essential for the assessment and treatment of patients with acute and chronic pain.

69. Detailed history taking of non–pain-related issues may lead to more effective treatment of the pain by identifying potential adverse treatment interactions prior to their prescription.

70. Detailed history taking may also lead to improved functional outcome in patients with chronic pain by identifying more completely the true needs of the patient.

71. Pain scales are of limited utility in patients with chronic pain and poorly correlate with function.

72. The presence of auto antibodies in rheumatoid arthritis (RA) is a marker of disease severity.
There are no true diagnostic criteria for RA.

73. A combination of aerobic conditioning and light strength training can be helpful in the management of RA patients and their associated pain.

74. The pathogenesis of osteoarthritis is a combination of wear and tear and inflammation

75. The primary pathology of osteoarthritis is at the level of the articular cartilage.

76. The primary initial pathology of RA is at the level of the synovium.

77. Chronic pelvic pain may result from a variety of etiologies, including intrapelvic sources and pain that is referred from nonpelvic sources.

78. Numerous medications may contribute to chronic lower abdominal pain; thus, this needs to be considered when evaluating a patient with chronic pelvic pain.

79. Chronic pelvic pain does not only occur in women.

80. Electrodiagnostic testing (EDX) specifically needle EMG of the anal sphincter is highly sensitive for evaluation of S2–S4 nerve function.

81. Physical examination of the pelvic pain patient must include assessment of lower extremity strength and reflexes.

82. Multiple NSAIDs, including both nonselective agents and one selective agent, are commercially available. Unlike opioid analgesics, these medications appear to have a ceiling effect.

83. The risk for nephrotoxic effects appear to be increased when different NSAIDs are used in combination with each other or with acetaminophen.

84. If an adequate trial of one type of NSAID does not result in adequate pain relief, the clinician should consider switching the patient to a different type of NSAID.

85. The clinician should prescribe these drugs cautiously, especially based on the potential for cardiovascular, gastrointestinal, and renal adverse effects.

86. Changing from one class of NSAID to another can result in improved efficacy as patient metabolism and response can vary from one class to another.

I. OVERVIEW

GENERAL PAIN DEFINITIONS

Charles E. Argoff, MD

1. What is pain?

   Some dictionaries define pain as "An unpleasant sensation, occurring in varying degrees of severity as a consequence of injury, disease, or emotional disorder." The International Association for the Study of Pain defines pain as "An unpleasant sensory and emotional experience associated with actual or potential tissue damage, or described in terms of such damage." Inherent to either of these definitions is the recognition that pain always has both a physical and emotional component. It is both a physiologic sensation and an emotional reaction to that sensation. In certain instances, pain may be experienced in the absence of obvious tissue injury; yet the pain is no less "real." New information emphasizes how important it is to view the experience of pain as a complex neurobiological experience that is influenced by multiple factors occurring at multiple areas of the peripheral and central nervous system. Some of these factors are easily identifiable, while others are not as of yet.

2. What is suffering?

   Suffering is the state of undergoing pain, distress, or hardship. Both physical and psychological issues are actively part of the suffering, and the pain itself may be only a small component. In some instances, pain may be an expression of suffering as has been described in somatoform disorders.

3. What is the difference between impairment and disability?

   Impairment is any loss or abnormality of psychological, physiologic, or anatomic structure or function (e.g., impairment of vision). According to the World Health Organization (WHO) definition, disability results from impairment; it is any restriction or lack of ability to perform an activity in the manner or within the range considered normal for a human. In governmental terms, disability is sometimes called a functional limitation. Another definition of disability is a disadvantage (resulting from an impairment or functional limitation) that limits or prevents the fulfillment of a role that is normal for an individual (depending on age, sex, and social and cultural factors). This definition corresponds to the WHO classification of handicap. Importantly, the presence of an impairment (e.g., visual impairment) does not necessarily have to lead to disability—individuals with visual impairment such as myopia can be assisted with corrective lenses to limit any disability associated with myopia.

4. What is meant by "inferred pathophysiology"?

   Even for well-recognized pain syndromes (e.g., migraine headache or painful diabetic neuropathy), we can rarely define with certainty the pathophysiologic mechanisms underlying a specific pain syndrome. This hinders our ability to specifically target and treat such mechanisms directly. However, a specific set of symptoms may lead us to believe that a pain syndrome is more likely due to nerve injury (neuropathic pain), lesions of muscle or bone (somatic nociceptive pain), or disease of the internal organs (visceral nociceptive pain). This "inferred pathophysiology" implies that we understand some of the basic mechanisms underlying a pain syndrome, and leads to the pathophysiologic classification of pain syndromes (see Chapter 2, Classification of Pain). However, this pathophysiologic classification is limited, because we can only infer, and rarely verify, the true mechanism.

5. What is the definition of *nociception*?

   Nociception is the activation of a nociceptor by a perception of a potentially tissue-damaging (noxious) stimulus. It is the first step in the pain pathway.

6. **What is a nociceptor?**
A nociceptor is a specialized, neurologic receptor that is capable of differentiating between innocuous and noxious stimuli. In humans, nociceptors are the undifferentiated terminals of a-delta and c-fibers, which are the thinnest myelinated and unmyelinated fibers, respectively. A-delta fibers are also called high-threshold mechanoreceptors. They respond primarily to mechanical stimuli of noxious intensity.

7. **What is the difference between pain threshold and pain tolerance?**
Pain threshold refers to the lowest intensity at which a given stimulus (mechanical, thermal) is perceived as painful; it is relatively constant across subjects for a given stimulus. Similarly, barring disease states, mechanical pressure produces pain at approximately the same amount of pressure across subjects. Specific devices have been developed to specifically measure thermal and mechanical pain thresholds, for example.
   In contrast, pain tolerance is the greatest level of pain that a person is able to endure. Tolerance varies much more widely across individuals and depends on a variety of medical and nonmedical factors. Clinically, pain tolerance is of much more importance than pain threshold. (More detailed discussions of threshold and tolerance are found in Chapter 6, Specific Pain Measurement Tools.)

8. **What is allodynia?**
Allodynia refers to the state in which an innocuous (e.g., normally nonpainful) stimulus is perceived as painful. *It is not normal!* It is common in many neuropathic pain conditions, such as postherpetic neuralgia, diabetic neuropathy complex regional pain syndrome, and other peripheral neuropathies. In thermal allodynia, the innocuous warm or cold sensation may be perceived as painful. With mechanical allodynia, a very light touch, such as the clothes rubbing against the skin or bed sheets placed on the lower extremities, may be extremely painful, while firmer pressure is not.
   When allodynia occurs in a person experiencing a neuropathic painful disorder, the skin surface may appear normal. Allodynia is also present in skin sensitized by a burn or inflammation (ankle sprain), but in these situations the affected skin is visibly abnormal.

9. **What is analgesia?**
Analgesia is the absence of pain in response to a normally noxious stimulus. Analgesia can be produced peripherally (at the site of tissue damage, receptor, or nerve) or centrally (in the spinal cord or brain). Different analgesic agents may target all or primarily one of these regions.

10. **What is the difference between analgesia and anesthesia?**
Anesthesia implies loss of many sensory modalities, leaving the area "insensate." Analgesia refers specifically to the easing of painful sensation.

11. **What is meant by paresthesia?**
A paresthesia is *any* abnormal sensation. It may be spontaneous or evoked by a specific event. The most common paresthesia is the sense of "pins and needles" when a nerve in a limb is compressed (e.g., the limb "falls asleep"). Paresthesias are not always painful.

12. **What is a dysesthesia?**
A dysesthesia is a painful paresthesia. By definition, the sensation is unpleasant. Examples include the burning feet that may be felt in various peripheral neuropathies, or the spontaneous pain in certain types of diabetic neuropathy.

13. **What is hypoesthesia?**
Hypoesthesia is decreased sensitivity to stimulation. Essentially, it is an area of relative numbness and may be the consequence of any kind of nerve injury. Areas of hypoesthesia are often created intentionally (e.g., by local infiltrations of anesthetics).

14. **What is formication?**
Formication is a form of paresthesia in which the patient feels as though bugs are crawling on his or her body.

15. **What is anesthesia dolorosa?**
Anesthesia dolorosa is a syndrome in which pain is felt in an area that is otherwise numb or desensitized. It commonly occurs after partial nerve lesions and may be a complication of radiofrequency coagulation of the trigeminal nerve.

In a certain percentage of patients, the original trigeminal neuralgia pain is replaced by spontaneous pain in a now denervated area. The paradox is that an otherwise insensitive area is painful.

16. **What is meant by neuralgia?**
Neuralgia is a clinically descriptive term, meaning intermittent pain in the distribution of a nerve or nerves. The condition described as "sciatica" may be due to the injury of the sciatic nerve, but is more commonly due to spinal nerve root compression (L5 or S1); pain is felt in the distribution of the sciatic nerve (radiating down the posterior aspect of leg). Trigeminal neuralgia, one of the most common primary neuralgias, is characterized by a jabbing pain in one or more of the distributions of the trigeminal nerve. Postherpetic neuralgia may occur after an outbreak of acute herpes zoster (shingles). Neuralgias are characteristically associated with an electrical, shock-like pain.

17. **What is hyperpathia?**
Hyperpathia refers to a symptom in which nociceptive stimuli result in greater than expected or exaggerated levels of pain. The term hyperpathia also refers to an abnormally intense pain response to repetitive stimuli not sensitive to a simple stimulus, but over-responds to multiple stimuli. For example, a single pinprick may not be felt, but repetitive pinpricks produce intense pain. Hyperpathia is sometimes called summation dysesthesia.

18. **What are algogenic substances?**
Algogenic substances, when released from injured tissues or injected subcutaneously, activate or sensitize nociceptors (algos = pain). Histamines, substance P, glutamate, potassium, and prostaglandins are a few examples of algogenic substances.

19. **What is meant by sensitization?**
Sensitization is a state in which a peripheral receptor or a central neuron either responds to stimuli in a more intense fashion than it would under baseline conditions, or responds to a stimulus to which it is normally insensitive. Sensitization occurs both at the level of the nociceptor in the periphery and at the level of the second-order neuron in the spinal cord (see Chapter 3, Basic Mechanisms).
    In the periphery, tissue injury may convert a high-threshold mechanoreceptor (which normally would respond only to noxious mechanical stimuli) into a receptor that responds to gentle stimuli as though they were noxious. Centrally, the second-order neurons (those on which the primary afferents synapse) also may become hyper-excitable. When spinal cord neurons are hyper-excitable, they may fire spontaneously, giving rise to spontaneous pain. This is typically the case after deafferentation.

20. **What is a "lancinating" pain? What does its presence imply?**
Lancinating literally means "cutting." It is a sharp, stabbing pain that is often associated with neuropathic syndromes. The word is virtually never used by patients, but is frequently used by pain specialists who are writing about a patient's complaint of "jabbing" pain.

21. **Define *deafferentation*.**
Deafferentation implies the loss of normal input from primary sensory neurons. It may occur after any type of peripheral nerve injury. Deafferentation is particularly common in postherpetic neuralgia and in traumatic nerve injuries. The central neuron on which the primary afferent was to synapse may become hyper-excitable.

22. **Describe the gate control theory of pain.**
The basic premises of the gate control theory of pain are that activity in large (nonnociceptive) fibers can inhibit the perception of activity in small (nociceptive) fibers, and that descending activity from the brain also can inhibit that perception. Given this construct, it is easy to understand why deafferentation may cause pain. If the large fibers are preferentially injured, the normal inhibition of pain perception does not occur.

23. **What is meant by "breakthrough" pain?**
If a patient has acceptable baseline pain control on a stable analgesic regimen and suddenly develops an acute exacerbation of pain, this is referred to as breakthrough pain. It often occurs toward the end of a dosing interval, because of a drop in analgesic levels (end-of-dose breakthrough pain). "Incident" pain is a type of breakthrough pain that occurs either with a maneuver that would

normally exacerbate pain (weight bearing on an extremity with a bone metastasis) or with sudden disease exacerbation (hemorrhage, fracture, or expansion of a hollow viscus). Breakthrough pain can occur in an idiopathic fashion as well. The concept of breakthrough is generally accepted for cancer-related pain but is more controversial for non-cancer-related pain.

Recognizing the type(s) of breakthrough pain is important for treatment purposes. Pain consequent to decreasing analgesic levels may be controlled by increasing the dose or shortening the intervals between doses (if not otherwise contraindicated). Incident pain may be addressed by administering a dose of an appropriate analgesic before the exacerbating activity.

24. True or false: Central pain arises only when the original insult was central.
    False. The term *central pain* is applied when the generator of the pain is believed to be in the spinal cord or the brain. The original insult may have been peripheral (nerve injury or postherpetic neuralgia), but the pain is sustained by central mechanisms. The basic process may be central sensitization. Central pain also may occur after central injuries, such as strokes or spinal cord injuries. The pain tends to be poorly localized and of a burning nature.

25. What is meant by *referred pain*?
    Pain in an area removed from the site of tissue injury is called *referred pain*. The most common examples are pain in the shoulder from myocardial infarction, pain in the back from pancreatic disease, and pain in the right shoulder from gallbladder disease. The presumed mechanism is that afferent fibers from the site of tissue injury enter the spinal cord at a similar level to afferents from the point to which the pain is referred. This conjoint area in the spinal cord results in the mistaken perception that the pain arises from the referral site.

26. What is phantom pain?
    Phantom pain is pain felt in a part of the body that has been surgically or otherwise removed. It is common for patients to have phantom sensation postoperatively; that is, after limb amputation, the patient feels as though the limb is still present. This sensation occurs in nearly all patients undergoing amputation. It usually subsides over days to weeks. A small percentage of patients develop true phantom limb pain, which may be extraordinarily persistent and resistant to conventional medical treatment.

27. What is meralgia paresthetica?
    Meralgia paresthetica is a syndrome of tingling discomfort (dysesthesias) in an area of nerve injury, most commonly the lateral femoral cutaneous nerve. It is characterized by a patch of decreased sensation over the lateral thigh; this area is dysesthetic. Meralgia paresthetica may be due to more proximal nerve compression. A change in weight is commonly associated with the onset of meralgia paresthetica.

28. What is the difference between primary and secondary pain syndromes?
    In primary pain syndromes, the pain itself is the disease. Examples include migraine, trigeminal neuralgia, and cluster headache. A secondary pain syndrome is due to an underlying (often structural) cause—for example, trigeminal neuralgia due to a tumor pressing on the cranial nerve. One of the major issues in any primary pain syndrome is to exclude an underlying destructive cause (tumor or infection).

29. What is palliative care?
    The World Health Organization defines palliative care as "The active total care of patients, controlling pain and minimizing emotional, social, and spiritual problems at a time when disease is not responsive to active treatment." In a broader sense, it is usually taken to mean the alleviation of symptoms when the primary disease cannot be controlled. The concept is now being extended to include symptom management at earlier stages of terminal diseases.

30. What is meant by the term *addiction*?
    Addiction has been defined as a primary, chronic neurobiologic disease, with genetic, psychosocial, and environmental factors influencing its development and manifestations. It is characterized by behaviors that include one or more of the following: impaired control over drug use, compulsive use, continued use despite harm, and craving. Tolerance may or may not be present. Physical dependence may occur in a person experiencing addiction; however, physical dependence is not synonymous with addiction and may occur in people who do not suffer from addiction, as well as with nonanalgesic medications (discussed later).

31. What is the definition of *physical dependence*?

Physical dependence is a state of adaptation that is manifested by a drug class–specific withdrawal syndrome that can be produced by abrupt cessation, rapid dose reduction, decreasing blood level of the drug, and/or administration of an antagonist. The term applies to non-opioid medications as well.

32. What is the definition of *drug tolerance*?

Drug tolerance is a state of adaptation in which exposure to a drug induces changes that result in a diminution of one or more of the drug's effects (positive or negative) over time.

33. What is the definition of *pseudoaddiction*?

The term *pseudoaddiction* refers to an iatrogenic syndrome of abnormal behavior developing as a direct consequence of inadequate pain management. Treatment strategies include establishing trust between the patient and the health care team and providing appropriate and timely analgesics to control the patient's level of pain.

KEY POINTS

1. The experience of pain by definition involves an emotional response; therefore assessment and treatment of pain must address *all* components of the painful experience.
2. The clinician should be familiar with the various types of abnormal sensations that can result in pain (e.g., allodynia) in order to optimally assess and treat painful conditions.
3. Treatment of both baseline pain and breakthrough pain are both important so that a patient can be as comfortable as possible.
4. Understanding the difference among addiction, pseudoaddiction, physical dependence, and tolerance is essential to effectively prescribing analgesics to patients with chronic pain.

BIBLIOGRAPHY

1. Merskey N, Bogduk N, eds. *Classification of Chronic Pain. Task Force on Taxonomy.* 2nd ed. Seattle: International Association for the Study of Pain Press; 1994.
2. Nicholson B. Taxonomy of pain. *Clin J Pain.* 2000;16:S114-S117.
3. Portenoy RK, Kanner RM. Definition and assessment of pain. In: Portenoy RK, Kanner RM, eds. *Pain Management: Theory and Practice.* Philadelphia: F.A. Davis; 1996:3-18.
4. Turner JA, Franklin G, Heagerty PJ, et al. The association between pain and disability. *Pain.* 2004;112(3):307-314.
5. Heit HA. Addiction, physical dependence, and tolerance: precise definitions to help clinicians evaluate and treat chronic pain patients. *J Pain Palliat Care Pharmacother.* 2003;17(1):15-29.

CHAPTER 2

CLASSIFICATION OF PAIN

Robert A. Duarte and Charles E. Argoff

1. **List the bases for the most widely used classifications of pain.**
   Pain is a subjective experience that does not lend itself to the usual classifications for a variety of reasons. For example, although many mechanisms of pain have been hypothesized, unlike our ability to determine that a urinary tract infection is caused by a specific pathogen, it is rarely if ever possible to link a specific pain mechanism to the etiology of a person's pain experience. On a practical basis, pain classifications depend on the following:
   - Inferred pathophysiology (nociceptive vs. non-nociceptive)
   - Time course (acute vs. subacute vs. chronic)
   - Location (localized painful region vs. generalized)
   - Etiology (e.g., cancer, arthritis, nerve injury or a combination of these)

2. **What is the neurophysiologic classification of pain?**
   The neurophysiologic classification is based on the inferred mechanism for pain. There are essentially two types: (1) nociceptive, which is due to injury in pain-sensitive structures, and (2) non-nociceptive, which is neuropathic and psychogenic. Nociceptive pain can be subdivided into somatic and visceral (depending on which set of nociceptors is activated). Neuropathic pain can be subdivided into peripheral and central (depending on the site of injury in the nervous system believed responsible for maintaining the pain). Although the term has been used for many years, psychogenic pain is a very vague term that should be reserved for only those instances in which one has conclusively excluded all nonpsychogenic causes—that being stated, it is rare for a person to be experiencing psychogenic pain alone. Too often, we have seen underevaluated patients with chronic pain being diagnosed with psychogenic pain when in fact, there was a clear etiology for their pain that had been overlooked due to suboptimal diagnostic evaluation.

3. **What is nociceptive pain?**
   Nociceptive pain results from the activation of nociceptors (A delta fibers and C fibers) by noxious stimuli that may be mechanical, thermal, or chemical. Nociceptors may be sensitized by endogenous chemical stimuli (algogenic substances), such as serotonin, substance P, bradykinin, prostaglandin, and histamine. Somatic pain is transmitted along sensory fibers. In comparison, visceral pain is transmitted along autonomic fibers; the nervous system is intact and perceives noxious stimuli appropriately.

4. **How do patients describe pain of somatic nociceptive origin?**
   Somatic nociceptive pain may be sharp or dull and is often aching in nature. It is a type of pain that is familiar to the patient, much like a toothache. It may be exacerbated by movement (incident pain) and relieved upon rest. It is well localized and consonant with the underlying lesion. Examples of somatic nociceptive pain include metastatic bone pain, postsurgical pain, musculoskeletal pain, and arthritic pain. These pains tend to respond well to the primary analgesics, such as nonsteroidal antiinflammatory drugs (NSAIDs) and opioids.

5. **How do patients describe pain of visceral nociceptive origin?**
   Visceral nociceptive pain arises from distention of a hollow organ. This type of pain is usually poorly localized, deep, squeezing, and crampy. It is often associated with autonomic sensations including nausea, vomiting, and diaphoresis. There are often cutaneous referral sites (e.g., heart to the shoulder or jaw, gallbladder to the scapula, and pancreas to the back). Examples of visceral nociceptive pain include pancreatic cancer, intestinal obstruction, and intraperitoneal metastasis.

6. **How do patients describe pain of neuropathic origin?**
   Patients often have difficulty describing pain of neuropathic origin because it is an unfamiliar sensation. Words used include *burning*, *electrical*, and *numbing*. Innocuous stimuli may be perceived as painful (allodynia). Patients often complain of paroxysms of electrical sensations (lancinating or

lightning pains). Examples of neuropathic pain include trigeminal neuralgia, postherpetic neuralgia, and painful peripheral neuropathy.

7. **Clinically, how do you distinguish between paresthesia and dysesthesia?**
Paresthesia is described simply as a nonpainful altered sensation (e.g., numbness). Dysesthesia is an altered sensation that is painful (e.g., painful numbness).

8. **What are examples of deafferentation pain?**
Deafferentation pain is a subdivision of neuropathic pain that may complicate virtually any type of injury to the somatosensory system at any point along its course. Examples include well-defined syndromes precipitated by peripheral (phantom limb) or central (thalamic pain) lesions. In all of these conditions, pain usually occurs in a region of clinical sensory loss. With phantom-limb pain, the pain is actually felt in an area that no longer exists. Patients with thalamic pain, also known as Dejerine-Roussy syndrome, report pain in all or part of the region of clinical sensory loss.

9. **What is the difference between complex regional pain syndromes I and II?**
According to the International Association for the Study of Pain (IASP), complex regional pain syndrome I (CRPS I; formerly known as reflex sympathetic dystrophy) is defined as "continuous pain in a portion of an extremity after trauma, which may include fracture but does not involve a major nerve, associated with sympathetic hyperactivity." The IASP defines CRPS II (formerly known as causalgia) as "burning pain, allodynia, and hyperpathia, usually in the foot or hand, after partial injury of a nerve or one of its major branches."

10. **Describe "phantom limb" phenomena.**
A phantom limb sensation is a nonpainful perception of the continued presence of an amputated limb. It is part of a deafferentation syndrome, in which there is loss of sensory input secondary to amputation. Phantom limb pain describes painful sensations that are perceived in the missing limb. Phantom limb sensation is more frequent than phantom limb pain, occurring in nearly all patients who undergo amputation. However, the sensation is time limited and usually dissipates over days to weeks. On occasion, these sensations may be confused with stump pain, which is pain at the site of the amputation. Thoroughly examine the stump of any patient complaining of persistent phantom limb pain to rule out infection and neuroma.

11. **How is the Multidimensional Pain Inventory used to classify chronic pain patients?**
The Multidimensional Pain Inventory is a self-report questionnaire designed to assess chronic pain patients' adaptation to their symptoms and behavioral responses by significant others. Section 1 includes five scales that describe pain severity and cognitive-affective responses to pain. Section 2 assesses the patient's perceptions of how his or her significant others respond to pain complaints. Section 3 examines various activities, such as those undertaken in the household, in society, and outdoors.

12. **What is meant by psychogenic pain?**
Psychogenic pain is presumed to exist when no nociceptive or neuropathic mechanism can be identified and there are sufficient psychologic symptoms to meet criteria for somatoform pain disorder, depression, or another *Diagnostic and Statistical Manual of Mental Disorders (DSM-IV)* diagnostic category commonly associated with complaints of pain. As mentioned previously, psychogenic pain is rarely pure. More commonly, psychological issues complicate a chronic pain syndrome or vice versa.

13. **What is the World Health Organization ladder?**
In the 1980s the World Health Organization (WHO) published guidelines for the control of pain in cancer patients. These guidelines correlate intensity of pain to pharmacologic intervention: Mild pain (step 1) requires non-opioid analgesics with or without adjuvant medications. If the patient does not respond to treatment or the pain increases, the guideline suggests moving to step 2 by adding a mild opioid to the previous therapy. If the pain continues or increases in severity, then the clinician goes to step 3 and adds a strong opioid to the prior therapy. This algorithm has also been used in patients with non-cancer-related pain. It is unclear what its value is in clinical practice especially in developed countries.

14. **What is myofascial pain syndrome?**
Myofascial pain syndrome is defined as a regional pain syndrome characterized by the presence of trigger points and localized areas of deep muscle tenderness in a taut band of muscle. Pressure on a trigger point reproduces the pain. In comparison, fibromyalgia is a systemic pain disorder associated with tender points in all four quadrants of the body for at least 3 months' duration, often with associated sleep disturbance, irritable bowel syndrome, and depression. In myofascial pain syndrome, these associated features are significantly less frequent.

15. **What is the advantage of classifying pain?**
Classification provides the clinician with invaluable information about the possible origin of the pain, as well as possible mechanisms underlying it. More importantly, it directs the health care practitioner toward a proper treatment plan in general; this is especially relevant when considering pharmacologic approaches. For example, neuropathic pain syndromes generally respond to adjuvant medications, such as tricyclic antidepressants, and to anticonvulsants. In nociceptive pain states, the implementation of NSAIDs alone or in combination with opioids is the mainstay of treatment.

16. **Describe the temporal classification of pain. What is its shortcoming?**
The temporal classification of pain is based on the time course of symptoms and is usually divided into acute, chronic, and recurrent. The major shortcoming is that the division between acute and chronic is arbitrary and the period in between, sometimes referred to as subacute pain, is often overlooked.

17. **How is acute pain defined?**
Acute pain is temporally related to injury and resolves during the appropriate healing period. There is usually no secondary gain on the patient's part, but social, cultural, and personality factors may play some role. Acute pain often responds to treatment with analgesic medications and treatment of the precipitating cause. Delay or improper therapy can lead to chronic pain.

18. **How is chronic pain defined?**
Chronic pain is often defined as pain that persists for more than 3 months or that outlasts the usual healing process. However, the cognitive-behavioral aspect, not duration, is probably the essential criterion of the chronic nonmalignant pain syndrome. Chronic non-cancer-related pain serves no useful biologic purpose.

19. **How is chronic pain classified in patients with cancer?**
Chronic pain in patients with cancer is categorized according to whether it is tumor related, treatment related, or unrelated to the cancer. Tumor-related pain may occur at the site of the primary tumor or at a site of metastasis. Treatment-related pain can be secondary to the use of chemotherapeutic agents (peripheral neuropathy), radiation therapy (radiation plexitis, myelopathy, or secondary tumors), or surgery (postmastectomy syndrome, radical neck syndrome, postthoracotomy syndrome). Approximately 10%–15% of the pain syndromes that occur in cancer patients are unrelated to the underlying cancer and cancer treatment.

20. **What is meant by an etiologic classification?**
An etiologic classification pays more attention to the primary disease process in which pain occurs, rather than to the pathophysiology or temporal pattern. Examples include cancer pain, arthritis pain, and pain in sickle cell disease. Therapeutically, it is less useful than a pathophysiologic classification.

21. **What is the basis of the regional classification of pain?**
The regional classification of pain is strictly topographic and does not infer pathophysiology or etiology. It is defined by the part of the body affected then subdivided into acute and chronic.

KEY POINTS

1. Pain can be classified according to inferred pathophysiology, time course, location, or etiology.
2. Proper pain classification may aid in the proper treatment of the pain problem.
3. Chronic non-cancer-related pain significantly differs from acute pain in that chronic non-cancer-related pain serves no useful biologic purpose.

BIBLIOGRAPHY

1. Bruehl S, Harden RN, Galer BS, et al. External validation of IASP diagnostic criteria for complex regional pain syndrome and proposed research diagnostic criteria. *Pain.* 1999;81:147-154.
2. Donaldson CC, Sella GE, Mueller HH. The neural plasticity model of fibromyalgia. *Pract Pain Manag.* 2001;1(6):12-16.
3. Merskey H, Bogduk N, eds. *Classification of Chronic Pain: Task Force on Taxonomy 2.* Seattle: International Association for the Study of Pain Press; 1994.
4. Nicholson B. Taxonomy of pain. *Clin J Pain.* 2000;16:S114-S117.
5. Okifuji A, Turk DC, Eveleight DJ. Improving the rate of classification of patients with the Multidimensional Pain Inventory: classifying the meaning of "significant other." *Clin J Pain.* 1999;15:290-296.
6. Simons DG, Travell JG. Myofascial origins of low back pain. Part 1 and Part 2. Principles of diagnosis and treatment. *Postgrad Med.* 1983;73:66-108.
7. Twycross R. Cancer pain classification. Part 1 of 2. *Acta Anesthesiol Scand.* 1997;41:141-145.
8. World Health Organization. *Cancer Pain Relief 2.* Geneva: WHO; 1996.

CHAPTER 3

BASIC MECHANISMS

Allan I. Basbaum

1. **What are nociceptors?**
   Nociceptors are sensory neurons that respond to noxious thermal, mechanical, or chemical stimulation. The term is used for both peripheral and central neurons; however, because the receptor is located in the periphery, the term is best associated with small myelinated (A delta) and unmyelinated (C) fiber primary afferent neurons. In the central nervous system, neurons that respond to noxious stimulation are considered nociresponsive. These are the "higher order" neurons.

2. **What properties characterize A delta and C fibers?**
   A delta fibers are small-diameter (1 to 6 μm), myelinated primary afferent fibers; C fibers are smaller-diameter (1.0 μm) unmyelinated primary afferents. The A delta fibers conduct at velocities between 5 and 25 milliseconds; C fibers conduct at 1.0 μm/sec. Many C fiber nociceptors are polymodal and respond to thermal, mechanical, and chemical noxious stimulation. Other primary afferent nociceptors respond more selectively to noxious thermal or mechanical stimulation. It is unclear whether there are specific neurotransmitters associated with the modality subtypes of A delta and C fibers.

3. **Distinguish between first and second pain.**
   First and second pain refers to the immediate and delayed pain responses to noxious stimulation. Other terms that denote these pains are fast and slow pain or sharp/pricking and dull/burning pain. The stimuli that generate first pain are transmitted by A delta, small, myelinated afferents. Second pain results from activation of C fibers, which conduct impulses much more slowly, thus accounting for the time difference.

4. **What are some of the molecules that are unique to the nociceptor?**
   All nociceptors use glutamate as their primary excitatory neurotransmitter. However, several other transmitters coexist with glutamate, and the differences in transmitters define the two major classes of nociceptors: The peptidergic class expresses calcitonin gene-related peptide (CGRP) and substance P. The non-peptide class is characterized by its binding of a unique lectin (IB4) and the fact that many of these neurons express the P2X3 purinergic receptor, which responds to adenosine triphosphate (ATP). Whether these classes mediate different types of pain remains to be determined; however, recent tracing studies indicate that the different subsets of nociceptors engage different circuits in the spinal cord and different ascending pathways.

   A molecule that is present only in C fiber nociceptors and that is relevant to the transmission of nociceptive messages is a possible therapeutic drug target. This is because the side effect profile of such a drug would be limited by the fact that it is less likely to bind to unwanted sites in the central or peripheral nervous system. The cell bodies of small-diameter neurons in the dorsal root ganglion (which are the cell bodies of C fibers) contain several unique molecules, including the following:
   - A tetrodotoxin-resistant Na channel (TTX-R)
   - The vanilloid receptor (TRPV1), which is targeted by capsaicin, the active ingredient in hot peppers (See TRP channels, below)
   - TRPM8, which responds to cool temperatures and to menthol
   - The P2X3 subtype of purinergic receptor, which is targeted by ATP
   - A special type of dorsal root ganglion specific acid-sensing ion channel (DRASIC)

5. **What is NaV1.7?**
   There are 9 different subtypes of voltage-gated Na channels. Of particular interest is the selective expression of a tetrodotoxin-sensitive voltage-gated Na channel, namely NaV1.7, in sensory neurons. Loss of function of this channel is associated with the condition of congenital insensitivity/indifference to pain. Conversely, gain of function of the channel underlies the clinical condition of

erythromelalgia, which is characterized by severe ongoing, burning pain of the distal extremities. Lidocaine and other local anesthetics block all voltage-gated Na channels. Ideally, a selective NaV1.7 antagonist could provide pain relief with a much better therapeutic window.

6. What are TRP channels?

TRP channels are a large family of transient receptor potential channels that allow ions to flow in response to a variety of stimuli, including temperature, many plant-derived compounds, and endogenous molecules. Different TRP channels cover the range of temperatures sensed by afferent fibers. For example, the threshold for TRPV1 is approximately 43 to 45 °C, which is close to the threshold for evoking heat pain. TRPV3 responds to warm temperatures. TRPM8 responds to cooling. TRPA1 responds to irritants.

Capsaicin is the exogenous stimulus that binds TRPV1. Camphor binds TRPV3; wasabi, mustard oil, garlic, and cinnamaldehyde bind TRPA1. We have little information about the endogenous chemical ligands that activate these channels. However, there is evidence that bradykinin, via an action at the B2 subtype of G protein–coupled receptor, regulates the properties of the TRPV1 and TRPA1 receptors.

Importantly, the properties of the channels are altered in the setting of injury. For example, TRPV1 not only responds to capsaicin and noxious heat but also is regulated by pH. In the setting of tissue injury, where pH is lowered, the threshold for opening the channel is reduced sufficiently so that normally innocuous temperatures can evoke action potentials in nociceptors that express TRPV1. Studies in animals indicate that the pain of bone metastasis is significantly attenuated in animals in which TRPV1 is deleted genetically.

7. How are nociceptors altered by tissue injury?

When there is tissue injury (e.g., an arthritic joint), the nociceptor is exposed to an inflammatory "soup" containing a host of molecules that influence the properties of the nociceptor. These molecules include prostaglandin products of arachidonic acid metabolism, bradykinin, cytokines, serotonin, and growth factors (notably nerve growth factor). This all occurs in the setting of lowered pH. Together these molecules contribute to peripheral sensitization, a process through which the threshold for firing of the nociceptor is lowered. The most direct way to treat peripheral sensitization is with nonsteroidal anti-inflammatory drugs, (NSAIDS), which block the cyclooxygenase enzyme. In clinical development are antibodies that target NGF for the management of osteoarthritis pain.

8. Where do nociceptive fibers enter the spinal cord?

Nociceptive primary afferent fibers have their cell bodies in dorsal root ganglia (or trigeminal ganglia for the face). The central branches of these afferents enter the spinal cord through the dorsal root and ascend or descend a few segments in the tract of Lissauer. The central branches terminate predominantly in the superficial laminae of the dorsal horn, including lamina I, the marginal zone, and lamina II, the substantia gelatinosa. Some A delta primary afferent nociceptors also terminate more ventrally in the region of lamina V and around the central canal.

The fact that the level of analgesia observed after anterolateral cordotomy may be up to two segments below the segment at which the cordotomy was performed is presumed to reflect the anatomic course of axons in Lissauer tract. Some small-diameter primary afferents ascend the spinal cord one to two segments in the Lissauer tract, ipsilaterally, before entering the spinal cord and synapsing upon dorsal horn neurons, including cells at the origin of the spinothalamic, spinoreticular and spinoparabrachial pathways (See below).

9. Where is the first synapse in the spinal cord?

There is a differential projection of small-diameter and large-diameter primary afferent fibers to the spinal cord dorsal horn. The largest diameter Ia primary afferents arise from muscle spindles and make monosynaptic connection with motoneurons in the ventral horn. Large-diameter, non-nociceptive primary afferents synapse on neurons in lamina III and lamina IV that are at the origin of the spinocervical tract and on wide dynamic range neurons (see Question 7) in lamina V. Small-diameter nociceptive A delta and C fibers arborize most densely in the superficial dorsal horn. The C fibers predominantly synapse with neurons in lamina I; they also synapse upon dorsally directed dendrites of neurons located more ventrally (e.g., in lamina V). In addition, there are connections with interneurons in the substantia gelatinosa. Many A delta nociceptors terminate in lamina V.

10. **What is meant by a second-order neuron?**
    Second order refers to all of the spinal cord neurons that receive input from the primary afferent fibers, including interneurons and projection neurons. Second-order neurons are also located in the dorsal column nuclei; these receive input from large, non-nociceptive, primary afferent fibers that ascend to the medulla via the posterior columns. Note that many second-order neurons in the dorsal horn receive convergent input from small-diameter nociceptive and from large-diameter non-nociceptive primary afferent fibers.

11. **What is a wide dynamic range neuron?**
    Wide dynamic range refers to neurons in the spinal cord that respond to a broad range of intensity of stimulation. For example, there are neurons in lamina V that respond to non-noxious brushing of the cell's receptive field, as well as to intense mechanical stimulation and to noxious heat. Many wide dynamic range neurons also receive a visceral afferent input. By contrast, nociceptive-specific neurons respond exclusively to stimulus intensities in the noxious range.

    Importantly, all primary afferent fibers are excitatory. Thus any inhibitory effect that results from stimulation of large-diameter fibers (e.g., by vibration) results from an indirect mechanism involving inhibitory interneurons that influence the firing of the wide dynamic range neuron.

12. **Describe the major ascending pathways that transmit nociceptive information.**
    The three major pathways of nociceptive information are the spinothalamic, spinoparabrachial and spinoreticular tracts. The cell origin of the spinothalamic tract is in the dorsal horn and intermediate gray matter of the spinal cord. Axons of these neurons cross to the anterolateral quadrant and ascend to the thalamus, where they synapse on neurons in the lateral thalamus and in the intralaminar nuclei, located more medially. An additional ascending pathway, recently described, arises from neurons in the most superficial lamina of the dorsal horn, lamina I. These neurons project to the rostral brainstem, particularly to the parabrachial nuclei of the dorosolateral pons. This pathway has now been strongly implicated in generating the emotional component of the pain experience as parabrachial neurons project to the amygdala, as well as to the insular and anterior cingulate cortex, namely to limbic areas the process emotions.

    The spinoreticular pathway parallels the spinothalamic tract. Neurons at the origin of the spinoreticular pathway are abundant in the deeper parts of the dorsal horn and in the ventral horn (laminae VII and VIII). The axons of these neurons project bilaterally to reticular formations at all levels of the brainstem. The output of the reticular neurons is predominantly to intralaminar thalamic nuclei and to the hypothalamus, thus the origin of the term *spinoreticulothalamic pathway*.

    There are other ascending pathways, including one that projects directly from the spinal cord to the hypothalamus. Also, a visceral "pain" pathway that courses in the dorsal columns of the spinal cord has been described.

13. **What are the major neurotransmitters involved in nociception?**
    Primary afferent nociceptors contain a variety of neurotransmitters, including the excitatory amino acid glutamate and a variety of neuropeptides, such as substance P and CGRP. Glutamate acts upon several subtypes of receptors, including AMPA receptors that mediate a rapid depolarization of dorsal horn neurons, via influx of sodium and efflux of potassium. The *N*-methyl-D-aspartate (NMDA) receptor, which gates calcium, in addition to sodium and potassium, is involved in noxious stimulus induced long-term changes in dorsal horn processing. Substance P activates subpopulations of dorsal horn neurons and also contributes to some of the long-term changes produced by persistent injury.

14. **What are the major neurotransmitters involved in antinociceptive functions?**
    Dorsal horn nociception can be regulated by both local inhibitory interneurons and descending inhibitory pathways that arise in the brainstem. The majority of inhibitory interneurons use the neurotransmitters, gamma-aminobutyric acid (GABA) or glycine. These neurotransmitters inhibit the firing of dorsal horn nociceptive neurons by both presynaptic and postsynaptic controls. Other interneurons contain one of the endorphin peptides: enkephalin or dynorphin. These increase potassium conductance, thereby hyperpolarizing neurons. In some cases, they presynaptically block the release of neurotransmitters from primary afferent fibers by decreasing calcium conductance. The major descending inhibitory pathways use either serotonin or norepinephrine. Consistent with the presence of these diverse inhibitory neurotransmitter mechanisms, intrathecal injection of a variety of compounds (e.g., opioids, clonidine) produces profound antinociceptive effects.

Another major approach to regulating nociceptive processing is to influence $Ca^{2\pm}$ channel function on primary afferents. Reduction of voltage-gated $Ca^{2\pm}$ channels will result in decreased transmitter release. This can be generated directly, via drugs that act on the channel. For example, gabapentin binds to the $\alpha\delta2$ subunit of a variety of $Ca^{2\pm}$ channels. Ziconotide, a cone snail–derived peptide approved for intrathecal use in the treatment of pain in patients who already carry an intrathecal pump, blocks the N-type calcium channel. Morphine and other opioids reduce $Ca^{2\pm}$ channel activity as well as increase K channel activity, producing presynaptic and postsynaptic inhibition, respectively of dorsal horn "pain" transmission neurons.

15. What are the clinical and investigational roles of capsaicin?

Capsaicin, the algogenic substance in hot peppers, selectively stimulates primary afferent C fibers. These C fibers express TRV1, capsaicin receptors that nonselectively gate cations, including sodium and calcium, which depolarize axons. Selective antagonists to capsaicin have been developed. These may reduce the contribution of this channel in conditions in which the environment of injury (e.g., low pH) results in prolonged opening of the channel.

Capsaicin itself may help as an analgesic. When administered to neonatal animals, capsaicin destroys C fibers; when administered to adults, it produces a long-term desensitization of the C fibers, possibly by depletion of their peptide neurotransmitters, such as substance P, or by transient ablation of the nociceptor terminals. The desensitization is associated with a decreased response to noxious stimulation, which provides a rational basis for the therapeutic use of capsaicin in patients. To date, topical application of capsaicin has shown some promise in the treatment of postherpetic neuralgia pain and postmastectomy intercostal neuralgia.

16. What is the laminar organization of the dorsal horn of the spinal cord?

The dorsal horn of the spinal cord can be divided into distinct laminae based on cytoarchitectural grounds, using traditional cell (Nissl) stains. This anatomic organization is paralleled by a physiologic laminar organization. Neurons in laminae I and II, the substantia gelatinosa, respond either exclusively to noxious stimulation or to both noxious and nonnoxious stimuli. Neurons in laminae III and IV, the nucleus proprius, predominantly respond to nonnoxious stimuli. The majority of neurons in lamina V are of the wide dynamic range type (i.e., they respond to both nonnoxious and noxious stimuli and have visceral afferent inputs). Neurons in lamina VI respond predominantly to nonnoxious manipulation of joints.

17. What is substance P-saporin, and how might it be used to treat chronic pain?

When substance P is released from primary afferent nociceptors, it binds to the neurokinin-1 (NK1) receptor that is located on large numbers of "pain" transmission neurons, many of which are located in lamina I of the superficial dorsal horn. Although antagonists of the NK1 receptors failed in clinical trials, perhaps because selective blockade of the contribution of substance P is insufficient, another approach that targets the NK1 receptor is showing promise. The idea is to ablate the neurons that receive the substance P input. To this end, substance P is conjugated to the plant-derived toxin saporin. When saporin enters cells, it blocks protein synthesis, leading to the death of the cells. By itself saporin cannot enter cells. It requires a carrier, which in this case is substance P. The substance P-saporin conjugate binds to the NK1 receptor, which is then internalized into the neuron, carrying the toxin with it. Intrathecal injection of the conjugate in animals produces a significant reduction of tissue and nerve injury-induced pain (allodynia and hyperalgesia), but it does not interfere significantly with acute pain processing. The molecule is undergoing studies in larger animals with a view to eventual use in patients. This is an irreversible ablative procedure, but it is much more selective compared with, for example, anterolateral cordotomy.

18. How is the spinal cord influenced by peripheral nerve injury?

Peripheral nerve injury was originally thought to only functionally disconnect the periphery from the spinal cord. Because the dorsal root ganglion is not injured when the peripheral nerve is damaged, neither anatomical nor biochemical changes in the proximal limb of the dorsal root or in the dorsal horn were expected. In fact, we now know that there are changes in the dorsal root ganglia and in the spinal cord neurons with which they are connected.

Among the changes is a significant decrease in the concentration of substance P message and substance P peptide in neurons of the dorsal root ganglia. In addition, substance P levels are decreased in the terminals of primary afferent fibers in the dorsal horn. Significant changes also in postsynaptic dorsal horn neurons.

The electrophysiological consequences of peripheral nerve injury are also profound. A massive release of glutamate acts on NMDA receptors to produce long-term changes in the properties of the dorsal horn neurons. Central sensitization (i.e., hyperexcitability) of dorsal horn neurons in the setting of injury is particularly common and may contribute to postinjury pain states. Peripheral nerve injury also induces a loss of inhibitory controls, by reducing the action of GABAergic inhibitory interneurons. This produces an epileptic-like condition that likely contribute to the ongoing burning pain and the allodynia and hyperalgesia in neuropathic pain conditions. It is not surprising, therefore, that anticonvulsants, such as gabapentinoids, are the first-line therapy for neuropathic pain. Most recently preclinical studies have demonstrated that dorsal horn transplantation of embryonic precursors of cortical GABAergic interneurons can ameliorate mechanical hypersensitivity produced by peripheral nerve injury.

19. **Provide a plausible explanation for the phenomenon of referred pain.**
A very likely explanation for the phenomenon of referred pain relates to the convergence of visceral and somatic afferent input to wide dynamic range neurons of lamina V. As a result of the convergence, injury-induce increased activity of visceral afferent nociceptors is interpreted by the brain as having arisen from the source of the convergent somatic input. It is thus "referred" to the somatic site. Indeed, local anesthetic injection of the site of reference can reduce referred pain even though the site of injury is clearly in the viscera.

20. **What is neurogenic inflammation?**
Neurogenic inflammation refers to the inflammation that is produced by the peripheral release of substances from the nervous system—in particular, from small-diameter primary afferent fibers. Although most studies emphasize the contribution of the primary afferent C fibers, there is also evidence for a contribution of sympathetic postganglionic terminals. The primary afferents release peptides that act on postcapillary venules. These become leaky, resulting in plasma extravasation and vasodilatation. Electrical stimulation of peripheral nerves that have been disconnected from the central nervous system can evoke neurogenic inflammation by antidromic activation of C fibers and the resultant release of neuropeptides in the periphery.

21. **How are substance P and calcitonin gene-related peptide implicated in the phenomenon of neurogenic inflammation?**
Cell bodies in the dorsal root ganglion synthesize substance P and CGRP and transport these peptides by axoplasmic transport both to the central and peripheral terminals of the primary afferents. The peptides are stored in the periphery and can be released when the terminals are depolarized as a result of injury. The targets of substance P in the periphery include mast cells, blood vessels, and a variety of immunocompetent cells. In concert with CGRP, which produces a profound vasodilatation, substance P significantly increases plasma extravasation from postcapillary venules. The extravasation of protein from vessels is accompanied by fluid, producing the characteristic swelling (tumor) of inflammation. The heat and redness (calor and rubor) of inflammation can be accounted for by the neurogenic vasodilatation.

There is considerable evidence that neurogenic inflammation contributes to the pain of migraine. Indeed, triptans block neurogenic inflammation, via an action on 5HT-1B/D receptors located on the terminals of primary afferent nociceptors. Although antagonists of the NK1 receptor failed as a treatment for migraines in clinical trials, antibody-mediated blockade of CGRP shows significant promise as a migraine treatment.

22. **Differentiate primary and secondary hyperalgesia**
Primary hyperalgesia refers to the sensitization process that enhances "pain" transmission via a peripheral mechanism. For example, in the setting of inflammation, there is synthesis of arachidonic acid, which is acted upon to produce prostaglandins. These lipid mediators in turn act on the terminals of primary afferent nociceptors and lower their threshold for firing. The nociceptors are sensitized. All of this occurs via a peripheral mechanism.

Secondary hyperalgesia refers to the sensitization that occurs because of changes in spinal cord processing. For example, through a process of central sensitization, the firing of dorsal horn nociceptors can change dramatically in the setting of injury (produced by either tissue or nerve damage). The threshold for activation of dorsal horn "pain" transmission neurons drops, their receptive field size increases, and they may become spontaneously active. Pain can now be produced by activation of uninjured, low threshold mechanoreceptive (A beta) afferents.

23. What is the contribution of the NMDA receptor to the production of pain?

Glutamate that is released from primary afferent fibers acts upon two major receptor types in the dorsal horn: the AMPA and the NMDA receptors. Under normal conditions, the NMDA receptor is blocked by the presence of a magnesium ion in the channel. When neurons are depolarized via glutamate action at the AMPA receptor, the magnesium block is relieved, and glutamate action at the NMDA receptor is effective. This results in entry of calcium into the postsynaptic neuron, which in turn activates a variety of second messenger systems that produce long-term biochemical and molecular changes in these neurons.

The physiological consequence of these changes is a hyperexcitability of the dorsal horn neuron (i.e., central sensitization). This is manifest as an increase in the size of the receptive field of nociresponsive neurons, a decreased threshold, and a potential for spontaneous activity of the neuron. The allodynia (pain produced by nonnoxious stimuli) and hyperalgesia (exacerbated pain produced by noxious stimuli) associated with nerve injury may reflect NMDA-mediated long-term changes in dorsal horn neuronal processing.

24. Describe the regions of the thalamus that have been implicated in the processing of nociceptive information.

Two major regions of thalamus have been implicated in the processing of nociceptive information: (1) the lateral thalamus, including the ventral posterolateral (VPL) and ventral posteromedial nuclei (VPM), and (2) the intralaminar nuclei of the medial thalamus. The VPL receives input via the spinothalamic tract, as well as a major input from non-nociceptive lemniscal pathways originating in the dorsal column nuclei. The VPM receives input via the nucleus caudalis and the principal trigeminal nucleus. Stimulation of the lateral thalamus in patients who are not experiencing pain does not produce significant pain. By contrast, in patients who have ongoing pain, electrical stimulation can reproduce pain, suggesting a reorganization of the nociceptive input to the thalamus under conditions of persistent injury.

The output of the lateral thalamus is largely to the somatosensory cortex. Neurons in this circuit code for the sensory-discriminative features of pain, namely intensity and location. In contrast, connections with the anterior cingulate and insular cortex process information that underlies the affective components of pain. As noted earlier, "pain" inputs engage the limbic system via connections from the spinal cord to the amygdala via the spinoparabrachio-amygdala pathway. The medial thalamus, including the intralaminar nuclei, receives direct spinothalamic and spinoreticular thalamic projections. Cells in this region have larger receptive fields and are thought to contribute to the diffuse character of pain perception. The cortical connections of the more medial regions of the thalamus, notably the anterior cingulate gyrus, are involved in the affective component of the pain perception.

25. Is there a cortical representation of pain?

Yes, there is a cortical representation of pain. Traditional teaching suggested that the cortex was not necessary for the experience of pain. This was based on clinical studies wherein stimulation rarely produced pain and large lesions did not completely disrupt the pain experience. However, imaging studies with positron emission tomography (PET) or functional magnetic resonance imaging have identified several cortical regions that are activated when humans experience pain. Among these are the somatosensory cortex, the anterior cingulate gyrus, and the insular cortex. This distributed processing in the cortex clearly reflects the complex nature of the pain experience, which includes sensory discriminative, affective, and cognitive aspects. Lesions of any single region may thus not be sufficient to eliminate pain.

26. What do we know about the cortical mechanism underlying the sensory and emotional components of the pain experience?

PET studies mentioned in Question 25 also examined what occurs during hypnotic analgesia. When subjects were hypnotized so as to decrease the unpleasantness generated by a heat stimulus, the "activity" generated in the anterior cingulate gyrus was dramatically decreased, but without significant change in activity in the somatosensory cortex. These studies illustrate that under hypnotic analgesia, the information about the stimulus does access the cortex, but that the nature of the perception reported is altered. These results also provide strong evidence that the anterior cingulate gyrus processes information more related to the affective component of the pain experience than to the sensory discriminative component. Consistent with these findings, ablation of the anterior cingulate gyrus, in animal studies, reduces behavior indicate of the affective impact of noxious stimuli.

27. **What information do we have on the mechanism of placebo analgesia?**
Several years ago it was reported that the opiate antagonist naloxone can reverse the analgesia produced by a placebo. This led to the hypothesis that placebo analgesia involves release of endorphins and activation of an endogenous pain control circuit. This striking finding has received considerable support in recent studies in which regulators of endorphin processing have been shown to enhance the effect of a placebo. The new studies followed upon basic experimental evidence that the neuropeptide cholecystokinin (CCK) counteracts the effect of endogenous opioids. The new studies demonstrated that injection of a CCK receptor antagonist significantly increased the analgesic effect of a placebo. Furthermore, the enhancing effect of the original placebo effect were both blocked by naloxone, indicating that the circuit involves release of endogenous opioids, which act at opioid receptors. Recent imaging studies demonstrated that placebo analgesia is associated with activation of areas involved in the endorphin-mediated descending control of pain processing (e.g., the periaqueductal gray region of the midbrain).

KEY POINTS

1. Nociceptors are neurons that respond to noxious thermal, mechanical, or chemical stimulation.
2. All nociceptors use glutamate as their primary excitatory neurotransmitter; however, several other transmitters coexist with glutamate and the differences in transmitters define the two major classes of nociceptors. The first major class of nociceptors synthesize and release peptide neurotransmitters, notably substance P and CGRP. The second major class is the nonpeptide class, characterized by its binding of a unique lectin and the fact that many of these neurons express the P2X3, purinergic receptor, which responds to ATP.
3. Glutamate that is released from primary afferent fibers acts upon two major receptor types in the dorsal horn: the AMPA and NMDA receptors. The subsequent increased neuronal excitability that can follow such glutamate activity produces central sensitization.

BIBLIOGRAPHY

1. Apkarian AV, Bushnell MC, Treede RD, Zubieta JK. Human brain mechanisms of pain perception and regulation in health and disease. *Eur J Pain.* 2005;9:463-484.
2. Basbaum AI, Bautista DM, Scherrer G, Julius D. Cellular and molecular mechanisms of pain. *Cell.* 2009;139:267-284.
3. Basbaum AI, Jessel T. The perception of pain. In: Kandel ER, Schwartz J, Jessel T, Siegelbaum SA, Hudspeth AJ, eds. *Principles of Neuroscience.* New York: McGraw-Hill; 2013:530-555.
4. Braz JM, Etlin A, Juarez-Salinas D, Llewellyn-Smith IJ, Basbaum AI. Rebuilding CNS inhibitory circuits to control chronic neuropathic pain and itch. *Prog Brain Res.* 2017;231:87-105.
5. Braz J, Solorzano C, Wang X, Basbaum AI. Transmitting pain and itch messages: A contemporary view of the spinal cord circuits that generate Gate Control. *Neuron.* 2014;82:522-536.
6. Craig AD, Bushnell MC, Zhang ET, Blomqvist A. A thalamic nucleus specific for pain and temperature sensation. *Nature.* 1994;372:770-773.
7. Denk F, McMahon SB, Tracey I. Pain vulnerability: a neurobiological perspective. *Nat Neurosci.* 2014;17:192-200.
8. Hoeijmakers JG, Faber CG, Merkies IS, Waxman SG. Painful peripheral neuropathy and sodium channel mutations. *Neurosci Lett.* 2015;596:51-59.
9. Hökfelt T, Zhang X, Wiesenfeld HZ. Messenger plasticity in primary sensory neurons following axotomy and its functional implications. *Trends Neurosci.* 1994;17:22-30.
10. Ji RR, Chamessian A, Zhang YQ. Pain regulation by non-neuronal cells and inflammation. *Science.* 2016;354:572-577.
11. Julius D. TRP channels and pain. *Annu Rev Cell Dev Biol.* 2013;29:355-384.
12. Julius D, Basbaum AI. Molecular mechanisms of nociception. *Nature.* 2001;413:203-210.
13. Nichols ML, Allen BJ, Rogers SD, et al. Transmission of chronic nociception by spinal neurons expressing the substance P receptor. *Science.* 1999;286:1558-1561.
14. Xu Q, Yaksh TL. A brief comparison of the pathophysiology of inflammatory versus neuropathic pain. *Curr Opin Anaesthesiol.* 2011;24:400-407.
15. Woolf CJ. Central sensitization: implications for the diagnosis and treatment of pain. *Pain.* 2011;152(suppl 3):S2-S15.
16. Woolf CJ, Salter MW. Neuronal plasticity: increasing the gain in pain. *Science.* 2000;288:1765-1769.

HISTORY TAKING IN THE PATIENT WITH PAIN

Andrew Dubin

1. **What are the key elements in taking the clinical history of a patient with a complaint of pain?**

   The first step in taking the clinical history of a patient with a complaint of pain is to evaluate the pain complaint. Important factors are location; radiation; intensity; characteristics and quality; temporal aspects; exacerbating, triggering, and relieving factors; circumstances surrounding the onset of pain; and potential mechanisms of injury. In addition, the clinician should ascertain if the pain is constant and steady, intermittent or sporadic, or constant with exacerbating circumstances, by gathering information regarding the occurrence and characteristics of any breakthrough pain. Furthermore, one should ascertain the patient's perception of why he or she has persistent pain, the duration of the pain, and changes in pain since its onset (e.g., any gradual or rapid progression in intensity or "spread" of location).

   The patient should specifically be asked about any perceived exacerbation of pain with innocuous light touch, with sheets or clothes on the painful body part(s), with the wind blowing on the pain, and with external temperature changes (e.g., Is the pain worse in winter?). Patients should be asked about any specific clothing they wear, aides they use, or behaviors or activities they engage in to function optimally with the pain.

   The patient should be questioned about the function of the specific painful area and resultant changes in global physical functioning. Information should also be obtained regarding perceived restriction of range of motion; stiffness; swelling; muscle aches, cramps, or spasms; color or temperature changes; changes in sweating; changes in skin; changes in hair; nail growth; perceived changes in muscle strength; perceived positive (dysesthesias/itching) or negative (numbness) changes in sensation—including what may trigger these changes (if they are not constant) and when they are likely to occur.

   Many aspects of the patient's current life and perceived quality of life, along with how this has changed because of pain, should be questioned. Include the following:
   - Social functioning
   - Recreational functioning (e.g., how often the patient goes out to the movies, spectator sports, concerts, to play cards)
   - Emotional functioning
   - Mood/affect, anxiety
   - Identification of family members/significant others/friends and their relationships with the patient
   - Occupation (if any)—last time worked and why stopped

2. **If pain is a purely subjective phenomenon, how can its intensity be measured?**

   The only reliable measure of pain's intensity is the patient's report. Measures of pain intensity are not meant to compare one person's pain with another's; rather, they compare the intensity of one patient's pain at any given time with its intensity at another given time. Thus physicians and patients can judge whether pain intensity is increasing or decreasing with time and treatment. It is sometimes helpful to have the patient compare the intensity of the current pain experience with prior experiences. Realize that pain is a highly unique experience, and as such the intensity of the perceived pain is as well a highly unique experience. This in turn can limit the utility of pain scales such as the visual analog scale (VAS).

3. **How should pain intensity be recorded?**

   There are a number of different measurements for pain intensity (see Chapter 6), and it is not clear that any particular scale is universally better than any other. Some patients have greater ease with a verbal scale, some with a numerical, and some with a VAS. However, it is a good idea to use the same measure across time. Thus verbal descriptors, such as "no pain, mild pain, moderate pain, severe pain, unbearable pain," or numerical scales can be graded on each visit.

4. **Can pain intensity be measured in children, the older person, and the cognitively impaired?**

   After children reach an age of verbal skills, pain intensity can usually be quantified on a verbal scale. However, a number of scales work even for preverbal children (see Chapter 34). After children reach the preteen years, the same tools used in adults can be applied.

   The older person may present more difficult problems. If the patient is cognitively impaired, it is often difficult to assess pain intensity on a precise scale, and it becomes more valuable to judge the functional impairments resulting from pain. Furthermore, medications used to treat pain may increase cognitive impairment and make assessment even more difficult. Older patients may tend to be more stoic about pain and are reluctant to report high intensities. One of the most helpful factors when assessing pain in children, older patients, and/or cognitively impaired patients is eliciting from the caregivers any changes from the patient's baseline behavior.

5. **What information can be gathered from the character of the pain?**

   The McGill Pain Questionnaire contains numerous descriptors for pain. Certain words that patients choose may help to infer a specific pathophysiology. For example, a burning, dysesthetic, or electric shock–like pain usually implies neuropathic pain. An aching, cramping, waxing and waning pain in the abdomen usually indicates visceral, nociceptive pain.

6. **Why are the temporal characteristics of pain important?**

   The onset of pain is extremely important. The approach to pain of relatively recent onset should follow more closely the medical model (i.e., a search for underlying cause). Acute pain usually indicates a new pathologic process, correction of which will relieve the pain. Chronic pain of long duration is less likely to be amenable to a standard medical model and requires a biopsychosocial approach (see Chapter 51). Chronic pain often outlives the initial cause and develops a life of its own; however, the events that initially resulted in the onset of pain may help to guide potential therapeutic approaches to chronic pain.

7. **Why is the temporal course of the pain important?**

   Certain pain syndromes have classic temporal patterns. For example, cluster headaches may occur at the same time of the day, every day, during only certain months of the year. Rheumatoid arthritis is characteristically worse early in the morning on rising (morning stiffness). Similarly, chronic, daily abdominal pain that has persisted in an unchanging way for years is unlikely to have a clear medical cure, whereas episodic abdominal pain that allows long pain-free intervals punctured by severe bouts of pain is more likely to be due to focal pathology. The intensity of pain over time is also of significance. Acute, severe back pain that gradually improves probably should be followed expectantly, assuming that there are no signs of tumor or infection. On the other hand, pain that increases over days to weeks is of more concern.

8. **What is the best way to elicit the time course of a pain syndrome if the patient is having difficulty being specific?**

   For the onset, ask the patient what he or she was doing when the pain started. If the patient can give a specific act or time of day, it is likely that the pain was of acute onset. To judge whether the pain is worsening or improving, look for functional signs; for example, ask the patient what he or she cannot do that he or she could do a few months ago. Also ask what can they do. If functional ability is decreasing, the pain probably is increasing. The patient and clinician should attempt to construct a timeline of the pain, as well as precisely what interventions the patient attempted to help the pain and any treatment designed by clinicians, including pharmacologic, interventional, neurophysical medicine techniques and modalities, behavioral medicine techniques, and neuromodulation techniques.

9. **What is the importance of ascertaining exacerbating and relieving factors?**

   Specific pain syndromes have specific exacerbating and relieving factors. For example, tension headache is often relieved by alcohol, whereas cluster headache is characteristically exacerbated by alcohol intake. Back pain from a herniated disc is usually relieved by recumbency, whereas back pain from tumor or infection is either unrelieved or exacerbated by recumbency.

10. **A patient complains of back and leg pain but has trouble describing the exact distribution. What can you do to clarify the matter?**
Pain maps (body maps) are often useful for patients who have difficulty with verbal expression. A front and rear view of the body is presented on paper, and the patient simply pencils in the location of the pain. The patient may use different colors or different types of lines to describe different types of pain. This technique helps to define whether pain is in a nerve distribution or simply somatic. In addition, having patients map out the pain distribution on their own body may be helpful for determining somatic versus nerve distributions.

11. **A patient has a rather nondescript headache that is getting worse over days to weeks. What should you consider?**
This patient's pain—a temporal pattern of vague onset with rapid acceleration in symptoms—should raise suspicion that a space-occupying lesion could be present. Even in patients with back pain, one should consider tumor or infection as a possibility.

12. **An 80-year-old woman complains of severe pain in the chest wall after having a rash in that area. You made the diagnosis of postherpetic neuralgia and plan to use a tricyclic antidepressant. What questions should you ask in the history?**
Before prescribing any medication, a careful history of prior medication use and prior medical illnesses is imperative. Particularly in an older person in whom we consider using a tricyclic antidepressant, these matters are of maximal importance. Tricyclic antidepressants have anticholinergic properties. Therefore they can exacerbate glaucoma, cause urinary retention, and increase confusion (factors that are fairly common in the older person). Orthostatic hypotension and other anticholinergic side effects are also more common in older patients than in young patients. This combination of side effects could markedly increase the risk to fall with associated orthopedic trauma and the attendant morbidity and mortality associated with hip fracture in older adults.

13. **What specific questions should be asked about the medical history in patients with complaint of pain?**
Questions should be directed at ascertaining comorbid medical conditions, including at least the following three major factors: (1) Has the patient had other painful illnesses? The response to these illnesses helps to guide current therapy. (2) How has the patient responded to medications or treatments in the past? This information should include the following: how long it was tried and at what level/dose (e.g., celecoxib 400 mg for 3 weeks and then celecoxib 200 mg for 6 weeks); perceived effectiveness; perceived adverse side effects at various doses; and all testing/imaging and visits/evaluation by any health care professionals (with clinician addresses and phone numbers). Attempts should be made to obtain all records from clinician offices, hospitals, imaging centers/laboratories, pharmacies, etc. The patient's current primary care physician and other involved health care specialists, along with current pharmacy/pharmacies, medication list (including complementary and alternative medications [e.g., herbal vitamins and over-the-counter agents]), and diet should be recorded. This information may limit the drugs that can be prescribed. For example, in patients with a history of hypersensitivity to a given medication, any medication in the same group should be avoided. If the patient has an aspirin allergy, nonsteroidal antiinflammatory drugs (NSAIDs) cannot be used without great caution. If patients tend to develop orthostatic hypotension or confusion easily, the tricyclics probably should be avoided. (3) Medical conditions that may limit treatment should be investigated. For example, glaucoma, benign prostatic hypertrophy, and cognitive impairment are relative contraindications to the use of tricyclic antidepressants because their anticholinergic properties may precipitate crises. In patients with a history of opioid abuse, the opioids may be used with great caution. In patients with active peptic ulcer disease, aspirin and NSAIDs may have limited utility. In patients with renal disease, NSAIDs and gabapentin may need to be "dose adjusted" and used with caution. In patients with significant hepatic dysfunction, acetaminophen, NSAIDs, antiepileptic medications, antidepressants, opioids, and muscle relaxants should be used with caution.

14. **How does the family history affect a patient with pain?**
Aside from the obvious issue of familial diseases, role models are often found in the family. A careful history should be taken to determine whether either parent or older siblings have suffered from a chronic pain syndrome. In addition, the family's reaction to the pain syndrome should be noted.

15. Is history of disability benefits of any importance?

The issue has caused a great deal of argument in the literature, but there is no clear resolution. The general wisdom is that patients receiving significant compensation for illness are reinforced in their chronic pain. This has been called compensation neurosis. However, the evidence is somewhat tenuous at best, and such patients are probably best treated in the rehabilitative fashion.

16. Are there any helpful clues in the history taking of a patient with ischial bursitis—"weaver's bottom"—that help to support the diagnosis?

The following clues, if uncovered during history taking, will help to point to an ischial bursitis diagnosis: In patients with this condition (known as "weaver's bottom"), pain invariably occurs when they sit and always goes away when they stand up or lie on their side. However, when the patient resumes a seated position, the pain returns. They can point to the spot where it hurts and pressure reproduces their pain. In addition, most patients with weaver's bottom are able to say "it hurts right here" and consistently point with their finger to the precise location of the painful spot.

17. What are some elements that could help to determine residual function?

- Is the patient ambulatory? If yes, do they need an assist device? (e.g., cane, brace, walker, crutch)
- How far can the patient ambulate?
  - Room distances
  - House distances
  - Limited community distances (150 to 200 feet)—able to walk length of driveway to mailbox
  - Community distances (e.g., mall walking)
- How fast can the patient walk? (e.g., How long does it take the patient to get from the parking lot to your office? Compare this with your own time.) In general, community velocity ambulation is taken to mean 3 mph or a 20-min mile. From a functional standpoint, asking the patient if he or she can walk without shortness of breath can be a very practical easy question for the patient to respond to.
- What capacity do the patients have to mobilize themselves in the community? (Know the environmental barriers they will encounter coming from parking lot to your office.)
- Is the patient able to dress himself/herself? Ask the following questions:
  - Can you put your own shoes and socks on with assist devices?
  - Do you use slip-on shoes?
  - Can you put a shirt on yourself?
  - Can you put on a pullover by yourself?
- For women with shoulder injuries:
  - If you wear a bra, are you able to put it on by yourself?
  - Do you fasten it in the back or do you fasten it in the front and then rotate it around?
- Are you able to do activities of daily living such as household duties and chores? (Can you brush your teeth? comb your hair?)
- Are you able to drive a car?
  - Can you get in and out of a car with relative ease in a reasonable time period?
- Are you able to get up and down from sitting on the toilet?
  - Do you have a sitting or standing or lying intolerance?
  - Are you able to bathe yourself?
  - Are you able to toilet yourself?

Acknowledgment

Dr. Howard S. Smith, MD FACP, was instrumental in writing this original chapter, and his insights and expertise in the field of pain management will be missed. The pain management community not only lost a prolific writer and expert, but we all lost a near and dear friend.

KEY POINTS

1. Taking an appropriate history is essential for the assessment and treatment of patients with acute and chronic pain.
2. Detailed history taking of non-pain-related issues may lead to more effective treatment of the pain by identifying potential adverse treatment interactions prior to their prescription.
3. Detailed history taking may also lead to improved functional outcome in patients with chronic pain by identifying more completely the true needs of the patient.

BIBLIOGRAPHY

1. Fields HL, ed. *Core Curriculum for Professional Education in Pain*. Seattle: International Association for the Study of Pain Press; 1995.
2. Pappagallo M, ed. *The Neurological Basis of Pain*. New York: McGraw-Hill; 2005.
3. Portenoy RK, Kanner RM. Definition and assessment of pain. In: Portenoy RK, Kanner RM, eds. *Pain Management: Theory and Practice*. Philadelphia: F.A. Davis; 1996:3-18.

SUGGESTED READINGS

1. Hord ED, Haythornwaite JA, Raja SN. Comprehensive evaluation of the patient with chronic pain. In: Pappagallo M, ed. *The Neurological Basis of Pain*. New York: McGraw-Hill; 2005.
2. Horowitz SH. The diagnostic workup of patients with neuropathic pain. In: Smith HS, ed. *The Medical Clinics of North America: Pain Management*. Vol 91. Philadelphia: Elsevier; 2007:21-30.

CHAPTER 5

PHYSICAL EXAMINATION OF THE PATIENT WITH PAIN

Miroslav "Misha" Backonja

1. **Why does a physician, nurse practitioner, physician assistant, or other person directly evaluating and caring for patients need to do physical examination when evaluating a patient who presents with pain?**

   With advancing medical technologies, especially laboratory and imaging, most of the diagnostic decision making is based on ordering tests and less on physical examination. However, patients with pain may or may not have abnormalities on any tests, but what they have are findings on physical examination that should lead to more specific diagnosis, or most commonly to a few diagnoses because the majority of patients have more than one pain diagnosis. The physical exam should include examination of musculoskeletal and neurologic systems in all patients and then selective examinations of head and neck, chest and abdomen, as dictated by history. The musculoskeletal exam should be performed to document findings for what is the most common source of pain: joints, from knees and low back as most common sources of pain, and muscles and ligaments as the sources of myofascial pain. The neurologic exam is done to demonstrate presence of neuropathic pain.

   So in conclusion, the simple answer is to make a pain diagnosis because the physical exam is the only way to make that diagnosis, together with history. In many areas of medicine, performing tests leads to diagnosis, such as bleeding disorder, and perhaps the exam could be skipped, but in pain medicine the physical exam is essential.

2. **What is the medial hamstring reflex, and what are its implications?**

   When testing the medial hamstring reflex, the examiner has the patient sit on the examination table with knee flexed to 90 degrees. Then using outstretched fingers, the examiner compresses and stretches the medial hamstring tendons. Percussion over the fingers with the reflex hammer elicits the normal response of knee flexion. This is useful in determining whether the patient has an L5 radiculopathy. In case of L5 radiculopathy the patient has normal patellar tendon and Achilles tendon reflexes but an absent medial hamstring reflex.

3. **What are the elements of testing lateral neck range of motion, and what is the significance of limited neck range of motion?**

   The patient is asked to extend neck and then to look to one side and then to the other side. In case of normal anatomy, patient should be able to look directly over each shoulder (i.e., range is 90% to each side). In case that range of motions is limited, the examiner should record degree of limitation. The examiner then can place the one hand on top of the head and the other at the chin and gently move to the point when head stops: if the stop is bouncy, the limitation is due to muscle spasms, and if it is a hard stop, then it is due to bony abnormalities. Report of pain on range of motion should certainly be recorded.

4. **What is a Spurling test, and what are the implications of a positive test?**

   A Spurling test is conducted on examination of cervical spine: neck is slightly extended, rotated, and tilted toward one side. In a positive test, pain radiates distally, usually in a radicular distribution, indicating nerve root compression in the mid to lower cervical region. The nerve root compression is ipsilateral to the side that the neck is tilted.

5. **Under what circumstances is the chest expansion test used?**

   The chest expansion test may be used if ankylosing spondylitis is suspected. In normal subjects, the difference between the totally deflated and totally inflated chest is usually more than 4 cm. In ankylosing spondylitis, it is almost invariably less than 4 cm. The patient is asked to exhale fully, and the chest is measured. The patient is then asked to inhale fully, and the chest is measured again. The difference between the two measurements is the chest expansion and if less than 4 cm may indicate ankylosing spondylitis.

6. **What is the straight leg raising test, and what are its implications?**
Straight leg raising (SLR) is used to demonstrate lower lumbar root irritation (radiculitis) or radiculopathy. In a supine position, the patient's leg is passively elevated from the ankle. The knee is kept straight. Normal patients can reach nearly 90 degrees without pain. In patients with lower lumbar nerve root irritation, SLR is relatively sensitive and produces pain radiating distally in a radicular distribution. Somewhat less sensitive but more specific is contralateral SLR. In this case, the pain-free leg is elevated; in a positive test, pain is felt on the affected side (e.g., the side of the nerve root's involvement).

   The straight leg raise is usually positive for pain related to nerve root stretch going below the knee at 30 to 45 degrees, except in flexible dancers and athletes. Pain from tight hamstrings is localized to the muscle and tendons and may limit range of motion. If true radicular pain radiating down the leg in a radicular distribution is experienced by the patient, then the examiner should bring down the leg 10 degrees until the pain subsides and perform dorsiflexion of the foot, asking "Does this make the pain worse?" If it does, this indicates the stretch of the nerve root again which worsens the pain of root irritation or impingement. If the examiner brings the leg down to where the pain gets better and then externally rotates the leg (hip), this should make the pain better, and internal rotation of the leg may make it worse. A more central herniation may yield pain in the affected leg on raising of the well leg.

7. **What is a sitting root test?**
A sitting root test (SRT) is essentially the same as the SLR test, but the patient is sitting rather than supine. The implications are the same. Findings on straight leg raise and SRT should correlate. A positive SLR but negative SRT may indicate enhanced pain behaviors. In the Lasegue test, after the leg is extended from a sitting or supine position, the foot is dorsiflexed, which further stretches the root and causes or exacerbates pain.

8. **What is the FABER test, and how is it different from the Patrick maneuver?**
FABER is an acronym for flexion, abduction, and external rotation of both hips. When it reproduces low back pain on one side, it is indicative of sacroiliac (SI) joint dysfunction. When the same maneuver produces groin pain, it is called the Patrick maneuver and is indicative of hip joint pathology. The Patrick maneuver may be performed unilaterally, but the FABER test must be done bilaterally to avoid pelvic rotation.

9. **What is the tipped can test, and what are its implications?**
In the tipped can test, patients attempt to assume the posture of holding a full cup in the hand with the shoulder abducted at 90 degrees and then horizontally adducted 45 degrees. They are then instructed to turn their hand over to empty out the cup. A positive test that correlates with a rotator cuff tear (or partial tear) would be pain and the arm dropping or inability to assume the test position secondary to pain and weakness. Minimal force applied by the examiners to the test arm may elicit a positive test in equivocal situations.

10. **How is the iliopsoas muscle evaluated?**
The iliopsoas muscle originates from the transverse processes of vertebrae L2-L4 (or L1-3) and inserts into the lesser trochanteric tubercle. Iliopsoas pathology may present with paraspinal pain just off of midline and radiating to SI regions in the lower abdomen, groin, and/or medial thigh. With the patient sitting on the table, resistive hip flexion reproduces the back and groin pain, and stretching the hip flexor will also reproduce the back pain and the groin pain. Iliopsoas spasm commonly occurs in patients with degenerative disc and/or joint disease.

11. **What is the scarf test, and what are its implications?**
The patient abducts the affected upper extremity to 90 degrees at the shoulder and then horizontally adducts (actively or passively) the upper extremity across the chest to reach for the opposite shoulder. A positive test reproduces focal sharp pain at the acromioclavicular (AC) joint and may result in the patient dropping his or her arm to the side with abrupt complaint of pain. This may indicate AC pathology (e.g., arthritis) or AC joint separation.

12. **How is the piriformis syndrome evaluated?**
There are many approaches to evaluate the piriformis syndrome. With the patient sitting, the piriformis muscle is stretched by the examiner passively moving the hip into internal rotation with reproduction of radiating pain. The pain is relieved by the examiner passively moving the hip into external rotation. The patient then actively externally rotates the hip against resistance; reproduction of buttock pain may be indicative of piriformis pathology. If groin pain is experienced, this may be more indicative of hip pathology. In addition, there is generally point tenderness on point palpation of the piriformis muscle.

13. **What is involved in the evaluation of chronic leg pain in the athlete?**
The patient with a recurring dull ache in the distal third of the tibia posteromedial aspect along with palpable tenderness in that area may have medial tibial stress syndrome ("shin splints"). Pain and tenderness (usually located above the distal third of the tibia but not necessarily) occasionally associated with erythema and/or localized swelling may be more indicative of a stress fracture. Using a tuning fork over the fracture site aids diagnosis of vibratory pain and is also common with stress fractures. Nerve entrapments may also cause leg pain over the distribution/location of the nerve(s) involved, which may be associated with Tinel sign. Pain associated with common peroneal entrapment is often referred to the lateral aspect of the leg and foot. Pain associated with superficial peroneal nerve entrapment often involves the lateral calf or dorsum of the foot. Pain associated with saphenous nerve entrapment usually occurs just above the medial malleolus but may be referred to the medial aspect of the dorsum of the foot.

14. **What are the examination differences between tender and trigger points when examining musculoskeletal system?**
Manual examination consisting of applying light pressure with fingers along the muscles, tendons, and ligaments. Frequent findings are pain and tenderness that are described in nondescript terms such as "that hurts" or "that is tender," and those are then designated as tender points. In contrast, when areas of muscle, tendons, or ligaments are described as reproducing patient's original pain and reproducing also radiation of pain, then we are dealing with trigger points. In addition, trigger points are characterized by positive finding of taut bands that twitch if a finger is moved across (positive twitch sign, which is that muscle under the finger that snaps) and positive jump sign (patient jumps when trigger point is slightly pressed). Tender points are signs of recent injury to the affected area, which is most likely to improve with minimal intervention, whereas findings of trigger points are indications of chronic pain that is treated with physical therapy modalities.

15. **What are the components of the abdominal examination, and what are their implications?**
Abdominal and visceral pain are frequent presenting symptoms either as the sole or primary reason for visit to a pain clinic or as a coexisting comorbidity of other pain syndromes. History can guide how abdominal exam is conducted, but in all cases, a systematic approach is needed. After observation and noticing scars and their status of healing, next asymmetry of abdomen is noted. Gentle palpation follows and starts in one quadrant, moving to/from side to side and up or down, covering all four quadrants. Attention is paid to areas that elicit tenderness and guarding, and they are noted, keeping in mind which organs are in the abdominal and visceral areas that are being examined (such as liver and gallbladder in the right upper quadrant). While performing palpation, the examiner is to also notice any masses or enlargement of organs in that area. To differentiate whether pain and tenderness are from the visceral organs or from the abdominalis muscles, the patient is requested to tighten abdominal muscles and palpation is performed along all abdominal wall muscles and, if patient's original pain is reproduced, then this is a positive finding for myofascial pain rather than pain from abdominal visceral pathology, requiring physical therapy modalities rather than therapy focusing on visceral organs.

16. **How is the sensory examination conducted to demonstrate the presence or absence of painful neuropathy (i.e., of neuropathic pain)?**
There are two aspects of conducting a sensory exam: the first one is to demonstrate evidence of nerve injury or neuropathy, which consists of systematically applying a battery of sensory stimuli, including light touch, punctate, deep pressure, vibration, cold, and warm, based on the concept that each of those sensory modalities is conveyed by specific components of the nervous system; and the second one is to determine whether in the area of neuropathy the predominant finding is a

negative finding, such as loss of sensory function (i.e., deficits) or positive findings, such as hyperalgesia (patient reports that evoked pain is more intense than in the site that is not affected by neuropathy [i.e., control site]). It should be noted that patients with neuropathic pain have coexisting negative and positive sensory findings in the same area, and this is the pathognomonic sign of neuropathic pain.

17. **How can you differentiate between an L4 and an L5 radiculopathy on physical exam?**
An L4 radiculopathy may manifest with an absent or attenuated patellar tendon reflex with weakness of quadriceps and tibialis anterior (TA) and maintained extensor hallucis longus (EHL) function because both the quadriceps and TA share L4 innervation and the EHL is L5 innervation. An attenuated or absent medial hamstring reflex with weakness in EHL with maintained patellar tendon reflex and TA function would be consistent with an L5 radiculopathy.

18. **What is the most sensitive muscle on manual muscle testing to assess for an S1 radiculopathy?**
The flexor hallicus longus (FHL) is the most sensitive muscle on manual muscle testing (MMT) for S1 radiculopathy because it allows for more discrete grading of S1 motor function than does the gastrocnemius. The MMT of the FHL is performed by having the patient flex the great toe and the examiner tries to overpower the muscle using his or her hand.

KEY POINTS

1. Performing a comprehensive physical examination is vital for the assessment and the basis for the pain diagnosis (or more likely to multiple pain diagnoses) of the patient with pain. This skill is attained with practice.
2. The examiner should be familiar with the anatomic localization information of every system examined and the range of physiologic and pathophysiologic manifestation that can be obtained during a physical examination.
3. Gaining skills and accumulating experience in conducting comprehensive physical examination becomes the basis for the appreciation of the range with which all of the physical examination findings present and how they lead to individualized pain diagnosis.

BIBLIOGRAPHY

1. Argoff CE, Backonja MM, Belgrade MJ, et al. Consensus guidelines: treatment planning and options—diabetic peripheral neuropathic pain. *Mayo Clin Proc.* 2006;81(suppl 4):S12-S25.
2. Buckup K. *Clinical Tests for the Musculoskeletal System.* Stuttgart, New York: Thieme; 2004.
3. Ebraheim N. Shoulder Examination: Subacromial and Cuff Pathologies. Video by University of Toledo; 2016. https://www.youtube.com/watch?v=xn-c2goYzLE. Accessed 14 December 2016.
4. Wassner G, Binder A, Baron R. Definitions, anatomic localization and signs and symptoms of neuropathic pain. In: Simpson DM, Macarthur JC, Dworkin RH, eds. *Neuropathic Pain: Mechanisms, Diagnosis and Treatment.* Oxford: Oxford Press; 2012:58-75.

CHAPTER 6

SPECIFIC PAIN MEASUREMENT TOOLS

Miroslav "Misha" Backonja

1. **Which major aspects or dimensions of pain and suffering must be considered when assessing pain?**

   Melzack and Casey argue for the following three dimensions of pain: (1) The sensory-discriminative dimension comprises the sensory aspects of pain, including intensity, location, and temporal aspects. (2) The affective-motivational dimension reflects the emotional and aversive aspects of pain and suffering. (3) The cognitive-evaluative dimension reflects the patient's evaluation of the meaning and possible consequences of the pain and illness or injury, including impact on quality of life and even death itself. This three-dimensional model is widely accepted because it integrates much of what is known about the physiology and psychology of pain and suffering.

2. **Describe the analog, numerical, and category scales. Which is most suitable for use with patients?**

   Visual analog scales (VAS) are 10-cm lines anchored at the ends by words that define the bounds of various pain dimensions. The patient is asked to place a vertical mark on the scale to indicate the level of intensity of his or her pain, anxiety, depression, etc. The anchors for assessment of pain would be on the left end "no pain at all" and on the other end "the worst pain imaginable," and for anxiety it would be "no anxiety at all" and on the other end "the worst anxiety imaginable."

   Numerical rating scales are similar to analog scales except that numbers (e.g., 0 to 10, where 0 is "no pain at all" and 10 is "the worst pain imaginable") are entered for what they experience at that moment.

   With category scales, the patient is asked to circle the word that best describes his or her condition (e.g., for pain intensity: none, moderate, severe, unbearable).

   Each of the presented scales are appropriate for patients and could be modified depending on needs.

3. **What does a score obtained from the overall pain rating mean?**

   The overall pain rating score is supposed to reflect the intensity of the patient's physical (sensory) pain. However, it has been demonstrated that the score on a pain rating scale is not, as one might expect, related only to the intensity of somatosensory aspects of physical pain but also to the intensity of cognitive and emotional aspects of pain. More specifically it is reflection of the patient's assigning meaning of pain rather than any specific somatic sensation.

4. **What is the difference between a rating scale and a questionnaire?**

   A rating scale represents a single dimension related to some aspect of pain or suffering; a questionnaire contains a large number of rating scales that encompass many dimensions of pain and related emotions.

5. **What is the Brief Pain Inventory?**

   The Brief Pain Inventory (BPI) measures both the intensity of the pain (sensory component) and the interference of the pain in the patient's life. Originally developed by a group focusing on cancer pain, the BPI is now one of the most commonly used pain assessment tools for all types of pain for both clinical and research purposes. It helps to better understand the impact of the reported pain intensity on various common activities in a person's life.

6. **How is pain assessed in patients who cannot communicate verbally, such as infants and cognitively impaired or aphasic adults?**

   Pain in cognitively impaired patients and young children can be estimated by their responses to a scale consisting of a series of faces whose expressions range from smiling to discomfort to desperate crying. Patients indicate their pain by pointing to one of the faces. The Iowa Pain Thermometer has been developed to assess pain in younger patients, as well as in older adults. This scale is being increasingly used in practice.

7. What is the effect on the physician-patient relationship when giving the patient a psychologic status questionnaire?
Many patients resent being given a questionnaire that was obviously designed for psychiatric patients because it gives the impression that the physician does not believe that their pain is "real."

8. Are there assessment tools that would assist in measurement of different components of neuropathic pain?
Yes, there are a number of neuropathic pain assessment tools. They could be divided between tools that assist in differentiating neuropathic from non-neuropathic pain and those that could be used to monitor neuropathic pain over time, and a few that can do both. Tools that differentiate neuropathic pain from non-neuropathic pain are Douleur Neuropathique 4 (DN4), a self-report version of the Leeds Assessment of Neuropathic Symptoms and Signs pain scale (LANSS-S Scale), Neuropathic Pain Questionnaire, Pain Detect, and ID Pain. Quantitative scales used to monitor neuropathic pain over time are Neuropathic Pain Scale and Neuropathic Pain Symptoms Inventory. Tools that can serve for both functions are Neuropathic Pain Questionnaire and Pain Detect.

9. What are the two essential characteristics of a rating scale or questionnaire?
The two essential characteristics of a rating scale or questionnaire are reliability and validity.

10. What is a reliable measure? Name three types of reliability tests.
A reliable measure has the property of yielding consistent results. The following are the most common ways to assess reliability: by test-retest reliability; and by inter-rater reliability. Test-retest reliability indexes the consistency of the questionnaire. Patients should give the same answer to the same question if their medical status has not changed.
For questionnaires that may be answered by an outside observer (e.g., those concerning behavioral symptoms), inter-rater reliability is assessed by comparing the evaluations of the same patient by two or more raters.

11. What is meant by the validity of a questionnaire?
Validity means that the test measures what it is supposed to measure. To determine this, the scores on the measure are compared with various kinds of external standards; for example, the test score on a pain scale should be high in response to postoperative pain or to calibrated noxious stimuli.

12. What have brain imaging studies revealed about the dimensions of pain?
Brain imaging studies have demonstrated that noxious calibrated stimuli activate not only the primary and secondary somatosensory cortex, but many other regions of the brain including the anterior cingulate gyrus (which mediates emotions) and the prefrontal cortex (associated with cognitive processes). Other regions that respond to the intensity of noxious stimulation include the cerebellum, putamen, thalamus, and insula. These structures mediate the affective, motoric, attentional, and autonomic responses to pain and respond to gradations in the intensity of noxious stimuli. These regions are, of course, not solely pain-processing areas. Studies of patients suffering chronic pain and hypnotized subjects have revealed altered brain activity. The promise is there, but much work needs to be done before these complex brain activities can be fully understood and related to a patient's report of pain.

KEY POINTS

1. A number of pain assessment tools are available to assist in the measurement and more specifically characterizing of pain.
2. Pain assessment is a multidimensional approach to the evaluation of pain attributes that assists in the development of the most appropriate diagnosis and by extension more appropriate treatment plan for an individual patient.
3. Specialized pain assessment tools are available and are to be considered based on the particular condition, age, and abilities of the patient being evaluated.

BIBLIOGRAPHY

1. Cleeland CS, Ryan KM. Pain assessment: global use of the Brief Pain Inventory. *Ann Acad Med Singapore*. 1994;23(2):129-138.
2. Herr K, Spratt KF, Garand L, Li L. Evaluation of the Iowa pain thermometer and other selected pain intensity scales in younger and older adult cohorts using controlled clinical pain: a preliminary study. *Pain Med*. 2007;8(7):585-600.
3. Jones RC, Backonja MM. Review of neuropathic pain screening and assessment tools. *Curr Pain Headache Rep*. 2013;17(9):363. doi:10.1007/s11916-013-0363-6.
4. Linton SJ, Shaw WS. Impact of psychological factors in the experience of pain. *Phys Ther*. 2011;91:700-711.
5. Williams A, Davies HTO, Chadury Y. Simple pain rating scales hide complex idiosyncratic meanings. *Pain*. 2000;85:457-463.

CHAPTER 7

BEHAVIORAL ASSESSMENT OF PATIENTS WITH CHRONIC PAIN

Joshua M. Rosenow and Kenneth R. Lofland

1. Why are psychological factors important in the evaluation of a patient experiencing pain?

   It is exceedingly difficult to completely separate the physical and emotional components of pain, and this is almost impossible to accomplish for those patients experiencing chronic pain. More than 25% of adults in the United States suffer from a diagnosable mental disorder in a given year. Almost half of those with any mental disorder meet criteria for two or more disorders. Major depressive disorder affects 6.7% of the adult US population annually and is the leading cause of disability for Americans aged 15 to 44 years. Generalized anxiety disorder is diagnosed in 3.1% of the US population aged 18 years or older in any given year. There are many other anxiety disorders which increase this percentage rate overall. Substance abuse disorders affect 7.3% of the population. Currently, opioids are the most widely prescribed drug in the United States, the second most abused drug in the United States, and a survey found 94% of physicians failed to identify drug abuse.

2. What is the prevalence of psychological comorbidities in patients with chronic pain?

   The prevalence of psychiatric comorbidities in the population of patients with chronic pain is approximately twice that of the general US population. It has been noted that just more than 50% of patients entering a chronic pain program met criteria for both an Axis I and Axis II Diagnostic and Statistical Manual of Mental Disorders (DSM) diagnosis. In studies that have evaluated the degree to which chronic pain patients have experienced the following childhood issues: physical, sexual, or psychological abuse, abandonment, and/or having chemically dependent parents, 48% to 58% of chronic pain patients reported experiencing three or more of these events and 77% to 84% reported experiencing two or more of these events.

3. What are the recommendations for psychological assessment of patients with chronic pain?

   The need to routinely include a proper behavioral assessment as part of a pain treatment plan has been supported by evidence-based clinical practice guidelines, such as those promulgated for the treatment of low back pain. The first recommendation in this document states that a focused history should be taken, which should include an assessment of psychosocial risk factors that predict risk for chronic disabling back pain.

4. What are the barriers to psychological assessment?

   Many patients arrive anxious, confused, and even embarrassed about receiving a psychological evaluation. Chronic pain sufferers often view pain as a purely medical phenomenon, and many have never met with a psychologist. Unless the referring clinician has explained the rationale for the referral to a psychologist, the patient may have a myriad of negative thoughts and emotions related to the evaluation. Such barriers are assessed and remediated early in the process of a psychological evaluation to the degree possible. However, for a subset of patients, a sense of discomfort leads to a lack of openness, which can result in incomplete and at times inaccurate information provided to the psychologist during the clinical interview. Assessments are used to detect invalid approaches to the evaluation.

5. What are the components of a proper behavior assessment?

   A thorough psychological evaluation of the patient with chronic pain often consists of two main components—a structured interview with behavioral observation and an extensive psychometric assessment. Together these evaluations provide a picture of the patient's current psychological state and the factors contributing to this. From here, a management plan may be constructed.

6. **What are the elements of a proper clinical interview?**

The clinical interview begins with observations of the person's appearance, mannerisms, and postures. Pain behaviors may be observed as the patient enters the room, sits down, or transitions between positions. This phase also includes an assessment of the patient's mood and affect. During the interview itself, evaluation of the person's fund of knowledge and attention span are also completed.

The interview includes a detailed history of the presenting pain problem, including prior treatments (pharmacologic, surgical, and physical) and the person's response to those. The patient's current pain treatment plan should also be recorded. Any prior experience with mental health treatment should also be included. It is often helpful to ask the person about a typical day to better understand the impact of both the physical and emotional components of the disorder on their daily activities.

7. **What is a somatoform disorder?**

A somatoform disorder is a psychological disorder in which a person experiences physical symptoms without a clear medical reason. Pain is often one of these presenting symptoms. It is important to note that patients are truly experiencing these symptoms. Given the subjective nature of many pain states, it is important not to simply dismiss a patient's pain complaints as representing a somatoform disorder without a thorough medical and psychological evaluation.

8. **What is a factitious disorder?**

A factitious disorder is a condition in which a person presents themselves as having symptoms that do not exist. This is often done by the patient for reasons of secondary gain (attention, compensation, maintaining of the sick role).

9. **What is a personality disorder?**

A personality disorder is a psychological condition characterized by a persistent maladaptive pattern of behaviors that impair a person's ability to relate to people and society. These may be grouped into clusters. Cluster A disorders involve suspicious or peculiar thought patterns, such as paranoia, and inability to detect social cues. Cluster B disorders involve overly emotional or dramatic behaviors, such as antisocial and borderline personality disorders. Cluster C disorders involve anxious or fearful behaviors such as obsessive-compulsive or dependent personality disorders.

10. **What is secondary gain?**

Secondary gain is defined as an advantage that is due to illness (whether real or not). Patients may have several benefits by remaining in the sick role. They may be due financial compensation, either from legal actions or other benefits provided as a result of an illness or injury. Moreover, a person may seek the additional attention and/or love that comes from maintaining the sick role or, conversely, allow them to avoid certain situations (social, work, or other obligations). A person may also be able to maintain access to opioids or other medications through continuing in the sick role.

11. **Why perform psychometric assessment?**

Standardized psychometric assessment accomplishes a number of goals. First, it allows an anxious, embarrassed, and/or defensive patient to endorse on a questionnaire the experience of pain he or she is experiencing, which he or she may feel uncomfortable reporting verbally. Psychometric assessment also allows for one individual's results to be compared with normative data on thousands of others, to better understand the meaning of the results obtained in relation to others experiencing pain. For example, knowing a patient is at the 97th percentile for catastrophizing thoughts related to pain is more valuable and predictive information than simply knowing the individual has some negative thinking patterns based on a clinical interview. Lastly, psychometric assessment allows for sophisticated validity testing. An invalid approach to testing could have many explanations, including defensiveness, severe psychiatric problems, English as a second language, malingering, illiteracy, and secondary gain.

12. **Why it is important to evaluate the validity of the patient's psychological evaluation?**

It is of critical importance to assess the validity of the pain patient's approach to the evaluation. An invalid approach to testing could have many explanations, including defensiveness, severe psychiatric problems, English as a second language, malingering, secondary gain, and illiteracy. Patients have been identified completing whole questionnaire packets with no ability to read, which, if undetected, could result in erroneous conclusions being drawn about functioning and lead to treatment plans that do not relate to the patient's unique symptom pattern. Invalid patient presentations (patients falsely representing themselves) must be identified to determine the utility of the assessment and to develop an effective treatment plan. Furthermore, invalid psychological testing has implications for the medical evaluations provided as well. Pain cannot be directly measured, is subjective, and requires self-report. Providers rely heavily on patient communication to assess pain and related variables. Determining if a particular patient is presenting in an invalid manner is essential to determining a treatment plan.

13. **What is the Minnesota Multiphasic Personality Inventory?**
Although there are dozens of psychometric measures used by pain psychologists in the assessment of chronic pain patients, the Minnesota Multiphasic Personality Inventory (MMPI) is the most commonly used tool. It is often found to be among the best predictors of outcome from pain treatment. It was originally published in 1943 and revised several times. It consists of hundreds of statements requiring the patient to indicate if the statement is true or false. There are 10 clinical scales, generally labeled just as numbers at this time, but initially labeled as: hypochondriasis, depression, hysteria, psychopathic deviate, masculinity-femininity, paranoia, psychasthenia, schizophrenia, mania, and social introversion. There are also several scales to determine the validity of the evaluation. If all the subscales are included, more than 120 MMPI-2 scales exist (clinical, validity, restructured clinical, content, content component, and supplementary).

14. **What MMPI scales are the most predictive of outcomes?**
Certain scale scores of the MMPI, including scales 1 and 3, originally named Hs: Hypochondriasis and Hy: Hysteria, respectively, have been among the most powerful predictors of outcome. These scales were originally designed to assess psychopathology manifesting in physical symptoms. Scale 1 measures preoccupation with the body and fears of illness and disease, which are heightened but not delusional. Scale 3 measures excessive reactions to stress, sometimes "hysterical" reactions, and often identifies those with somatic symptoms that develop or are substantially exacerbated in response to stress. The MMPI has been used in hundreds of studies, and nearly every study examining these two scales has found one or both to be significant predictors of outcome. In many of the studies, elevations on one or both of these scales were the strongest predictors of outcome when compared with all other variables in the study, including dozens of other psychological and medical variables.

15. **What other psychometric scales are frequently used to assess pain?**
The McGill Pain Questionnaire is another commonly administered tool to assess and track pain outcomes. This was developed by Dr. Melzack in the 1970s. It is divided into three sections—pain quality, exacerbating/alleviating factors over time, and pain intensity. The Brief Pain Inventory (BPI) and the BPI-facial includes items regarding pain intensity (visual analog scale [VAS]) and location (shade in drawing), as well as questions about the interference with daily activities caused by the pain. There are more than 50 measures in use to assess various aspects of chronic pain patients, including pain coping strategies, emotional impact, negative thinking styles, perceived disability, functional ability, spousal interactions, quality of life, and opioid risk potential.

16. **What tools are commonly used to track functional outcomes in patients with pain?**
The Short Form Health Survey was developed by the RAND Corporation to track quality of life in patients with pain. This consists of 36 questions assessing the functional, social, and emotional effects that the pain imposes on the person's life. The Oswestry Disability Index consists of 10 questions regarding functional limitations, primarily aimed at patients with low back pain.

17. **Do childhood psychological factors influence surgical outcome?**
Studies have demonstrated decreasing surgical success rate with increasing number of patient childhood psychological factors, such as physical and sexual abuse. In one study, those who reported 0 factors obtained a 95% surgical success rate, those with 1 or 2 of the negative childhood events had a 73% surgical success rate, and those with 3 or more of the events obtained only a 15% surgical success rate.

18. **What items should be explored in relation to a person's employment?**
The person's current work status (working, not working, never worked, on disability) should be discussed, as well as their intentions in regard to this. Preinjury job satisfaction level is a

well-known predictor of return to work. Determining whether a patient has no desire to return to his or her former occupation (whether due to pain, dissatisfaction, secondary gain or other reason) is important in devising an overall diagnostic and treatment plan. If people do desire to return to their former position, it needs to be determined if this is feasible with any pain treatment. Are there social or physical barriers to this? What has the patients' performance been at their job(s) over time? What are the physical requirements of their job? What are the positive or negative financial and social impacts of patients resuming their prior position, taking a different position, or remaining off work?

19. **How does chronic pain affect a person's social interactions?**
Chronic pain reduces a person's ability to engage in productive social interactions, both at home and through employment. Patients may not desire to engage with family and friends due to functional and energy limitations due to pain. Self-esteem may also be negatively impacted by pain. However, it has also been shown that supportive social interactions reduce pain responses. Moreover, an individual's pain tolerance may be positively correlated with their social network size.

20. **What types of gender-specific pain responses are there?**
Certain factors, such as catastrophizing and a history of sexual abuse, are more common in women. Both of these are associated with increased pain duration and pain rating intensity. Women are more likely to suffer from migraines, fibromyalgia, irritable bowel syndrome, and temporomandibular joint pain disorder. Woman have been shown to have lower thresholds for heat pain but not ischemic or pressure pain. Men are generally less willing than women to report pain or seek medical advice for pain. Some studies have shown that women may be more sensitive to the analgesic effects of opioids. Some studies that have looked at gender differences in postoperative pain have shown that women tend to report high pain levels immediately postoperatively but that long-term pain outcomes appear similar between men and women.

21. **What psychosocial factors may be predictive of worse outcome from treatment for pain?**
These factors include depression, anxiety, anger, passive coping strategies, job dissatisfaction, pain sensitivity, higher disability levels, disputed compensation claims, negative thinking styles, somatization, abuse history, substance abuse, psychiatric history, and support system. These factors may be stronger predictors of pain treatment outcomes than either physical examination findings or severity and duration of pain.

22. **Why perform presurgical psychological assessment?**
The presurgical evaluation provides valuable information about risk factors and prognosis that can be used in this decision-making process. The evaluation does not determine if a surgery will occur or not, that is a decision between the medical provider and the patient. Failing to identify known risk factors and proceeding with surgery can lead to failed surgical outcomes and all of the negative consequences that follow. In many instances, the poor surgical outcome may be incorrectly attributed to other factors (poor surgical technique or incorrect preoperative diagnosis) rather than understanding the psychological factors that have contributed to the situation.

23. **Can clinicians best identify those patients with psychological comorbidities?**
Some clinicians believe that they can effectively assess which patients have good or poor outcomes, but studies have shown this not to be the case. It has been shown that clinicians' impressions of a patient's level of psychological distress are often inaccurate and underestimate the true level of psychological dysfunction.

24. **What types of psychological risk factors influence surgical outcome?**
Key psychological risk factors include depression, anxiety, anger, pain catastrophizing, secondary gain, active psychosis, malingering, secondary gain, and somatoform disorders. Childhood trauma, sexual or physical abuse, and substance abuse are also significant risk factors for poor surgical outcome. The accuracy of such systems using factors such as these to predict surgical outcomes (exclusive of medical factors) in 2- to 4-year follow-up studies have ranged from 75% to 82%. Individuals receiving a poor prognosis have been found to obtain far less pain relief and improvement in functional ability, are more likely to have additional spine surgeries, and take more medication.

25. **What is the effect of psychological factors on surgical outcomes?**
Psychological evaluation models have been shown to properly predict those patients at higher risk for poor surgical outcome. A 5-year follow-up of patients found to have a poor prognosis for surgery

demonstrated a 14.6-time higher failure rate than patients with a good prognosis. In contrast to this, having low levels of psychosocial risk results in a significantly higher chance of achieving good surgical outcomes in properly selected patients.

26. **How do psychometric scales predict outcome from surgery for pain conditions?**
Several studies have concluded that psychometric and psychosocial variables can be the most powerful predictors of surgical outcome. Several studies have found that the MMPI Hs scores, nonorganic signs, and abnormal pain drawing scores significantly predicted lumbar surgery outcome, whereas type of surgery, postoperative complications, duration of pain, and diagnosis were not predictive. It has also been found that MMPI scores contributed far more to the surgical outcome prediction than medical factors, neurologic signs, imaging studies, etc.

27. **Do psychometric scales predict return to work after surgery for pain?**
Prospective studies using the MMPI found it to be predictive of the development of chronic pain and the failure to return to work following injury. In these studies, patients in the upper quintile on Scale 3 were twice as likely to develop chronic low back pain as other employees. Of 421 acute pain patients, those with elevated Scale 3 score were less likely to be working at 1-year follow-up.

28. **How does psychological evaluation relate to outcome from neuromodulation for pain?**
Multiple studies have investigated the relationship between psychological comorbidities and outcome from both pain treatment in general and especially from implanted neurostimulation therapy. Logistic regression of MMPI scores showed that patients with lower depression and higher mania (energy) subscale scores were more likely to achieve greater than 50% pain reduction from spinal cord stimulation (SCS). Several factors were found to be significantly associated with good outcome (continued >50% pain reduction) 1 year after implant—lower sleep interference scores, lower depression scores, lower catastrophizing, and better preimplant confidence in performing daily activities.

29. **What is the best way to approach referral for behavioral assessment?**
A pragmatic matter worth discussion at the close of a chapter on behavioral assessment of pain relates directly to the manner in which medical providers make referrals to pain psychologists. It is critical to avoid damaging rapport with chronic pain sufferers, many of whom perceive their pain to be 100% physical. Having a reasonable explanation for the purpose of the referral is beneficial.

Many chronic pain sufferers have never seen a mental health provider for professional purposes, despite the previous data demonstrating the number of pain patients with risks such as depression, anxiety, substance abuse, and/or a past abuse history. Such patients may have a negative reaction to a referral for mental health care because of a perceived negative stigma of requiring mental health treatment. A brief explanation from the provider to the patient about effects of chronic pain on so many aspects of the human experience often resolves, and can even serve to validate, what so many chronic pain sufferers experience.

A message that resonates with nearly all pain patients can be composed, rehearsed, and used to effectively make such a referral. An example of such a message that both normalizes the process and validates the pain experience is, "Every patient I have seen with a chronic medical disorder has had his or her life impacted in many ways. Chronic pain often impacts occupational, social, emotional, and sexual functioning, as well as family relationships, financial security, and general health due to decreased activity, increased weight, lower self-esteem, and can lead to increases in substance abuse, depression, anxiety, etc. It is important to treat you as a whole person, not just as a damaged body part, and there is over 50 years of research clearly demonstrating that a multidimensional problem such as chronic pain is most effectively treated with a multidisciplinary team approach to evaluation and treatment. Please take this handout and contact Dr. _____ to schedule an appointment. At our next appointment, we will discuss how your meeting went with Dr. ____."

It is helpful to have preprinted handouts from a pain psychologist with titles such as "What is a Presurgical Psychological Evaluation," "What is Health Psychology," and "What can a Pain Psychologist Do for Me?" Providing such a handout further normalizes the process as a regular practice, the information on the handout demystifies the purpose and activities the patient can expect, while also reducing office staff time providing additional information on these matters, contact information of the pain psychologist, office locations, etc. The minute spent providing a statement like the previous one can be made up by providing such a handout and can result in a more positively rated experience for the patients under your care.

KEY POINTS

1. Psychological factors have a significant impact on a patient's response to treatment.
2. A formal evaluation by a psychologist skilled in the evaluation of patients with chronic pain is important to the development of an overall plan of care.
3. A complete psychological evaluation involves both a structured clinical interview and use of psychometric assessment tools.
4. Psychological factors may carry more weight than medical factors in determining outcome from surgery in patients suffering from pain.

BIBLIOGRAPHY

1. Kessler RC, Demler O, Frank RG, et al. Prevalence and treatment of mental disorders, 1990 to 2003. *N Engl J Med.* 2005;352(24):2515-2523.
2. Schofferman J, Anderson D, Hines R, Smith G, White A. Childhood psychological trauma correlates with unsuccessful lumbar spine surgery. *Spine.* 1992;17(suppl 6):S138-S144.
3. Main CJ. The modified somatic perception questionnaire (MSPQ). *J Psychosom Res.* 1983;27(6):503-514.
4. Main CJ, Wood PL, Hollis S, Spanswick CC, Waddell G. The Distress and Risk Assessment Method. A simple patient classification to identify distress and evaluate the risk of poor outcome. *Spine.* 1992;17(1):42-52.
5. Dzioba RB, Doxey NC. A prospective investigation into the orthopaedic and psychologic predictors of outcome of first lumbar surgery following industrial injury. *Spine.* 1984;9(6):614-623.
6. Junge A, Frohlich M, Ahrens S, et al. Predictors of bad and good outcome of lumbar spine surgery. A prospective clinical study with 2 years' follow up. *Spine.* 1996;21(9):1056-1064, discussion 1064-1055.
7. Spengler DM, Ouellette EA, Battie M, Zeh J. Elective discectomy for herniation of a lumbar disc. Additional experience with an objective method. *J Bone Joint Surg Am.* 1990;72(2):230-237.
8. Sorenson LV. Preoperative psychological testing with the MMPI at first operation for prolapsed lumbar disc. *Dan Med Bull.* 1992;39:5.
9. Block AR, Ohnmeiss DD, Guyer RD, Rashbaum RF, Hochschuler SH. The use of presurgical psychological screening to predict the outcome of spine surgery. *Spine J.* 2001;1(4):274-282.
10. Bigos SJ, Battie MC, Spengler DM, et al. A longitudinal, prospective study of industrial back injury reporting. *Clin Orthop Relat Res.* 1992;279:21-34.
11. Melzack R. The McGill Pain Questionnaire: major properties and scoring methods. *Pain.* 1975;1(3):277-299.
12. Wiesenfeld-Hallin Z. Sex differences in pain perception. *Gend Med.* 2005;2(3):137-145.
13. Doleys DM. Psychological factors in spinal cord stimulation therapy: brief review and discussion. *Neurosurg Focus.* 2006;21(6):E1.
14. Dolce JJ, Crocker MF, Doleys DM. Prediction of outcome among chronic pain patients. *Behav Res Ther.* 1986;24(3):313-319.

CHAPTER 8

NEUROIMAGING IN THE PATIENT WITH PAIN

Gaetano Pastena

1. **What are the main modalities used to image patients in pain and advantages and disadvantages of each?**

   Radiography (plain x-ray), computed tomography (CT), and magnetic resonance imaging (MRI) are the mainstays of imaging.

   Plain radiographs use ionizing radiation (x-rays) to produce an image. They are quick, cheap, readily available, and also good at imaging high-density structures like hardware or bone. Plain radiographs are limited when evaluating complex or curved structures or discriminating different soft tissue structures from one another.

   A CT scan is created by a rotating x-ray tube. X-rays are projected through the patient and a computer performs a mathematic reconstruction of a cross sectional image. The radiation is higher than a conventional x-ray, but CT is readily available, very fast, and gives excellent resolution of bones and good visualization of soft tissues, as well as a very good look at complex structures in cross section. CT is superior for detailed bone visualization in particular.

   MRI uses very strong magnets and radiofrequencies to affect protons and produce an image without any ionizing radiation. The length of exam is longer, and availability is often less than that of CT. This modality is also excellent at visualizing cross-sectional anatomy and soft tissue contrast (the ability to discriminate one tissue type from another) is superior to other modalities—structures such as nerves, intervertebral discs, and ligaments are well seen and evaluated on MRI.

2. **What are T1 and T2 magnetic resonance imaging sequences?**

   MRI produces images by "flipping" proton spins. Spins are changed from one orientation to another (longitudinal to lateral), and the relaxation is measured. The recovery of the longitudinal magnetization is the T1 time and the decay of lateral magnetization is the T2 time. Since different tissues relax at different rates, this contrast in recovery and decay times is used to produce the images.

   Standard T1 images are very good at detecting fat (and subsequently nerves using that fat as intrinsic contrast), subacute hemorrhage, protein, melanin, and gadolinium contrast. T2 images are very good at detecting edema and fluid, demyelination, gliosis, and some forms of hemorrhage.

3. **Is "open" magnetic resonance imaging as good as regular magnetic resonance imaging?**

   Older "open" type MRI scanners do not produce the same strength magnetic field as closed traditional scanners and therefore cannot produce the same quality images. However, wide-bore scanners and "open" design scanners have now been developed with higher field strengths, which may be helpful to patients with claustrophobia.

   The field strength, which is usually lower in fully "open" scanners, is important because it directly influences the amount of signal produced. Higher field strengths lead to more signal, which can be used for higher resolution, faster imaging times, or better signal to improve image quality.

4. **What are contraindications to magnetic resonance imaging?**

   Ferromagnetic clips, noncompatible cardiac pacemakers, metallic foreign bodies in sensitive anatomic regions, and certain medical devices can all be contraindications to an MRI. The dangers lie in both movement of an object or device from the magnetic current as well as in effects of the rapidly changing gradients, which can produce heating and/or induce electric currents. Many devices and clips today are certified as safe for MRI under set conditions; check with the manufacturer of the device or clip or with your local radiology department before ordering an MRI for those patients which you may be unsure of.

5. How are radiography, magnetic resonance imaging, and computed tomography complementary for the evaluation of the patient with back pain?

Radiography is very useful for a quick look at the structure of the spine, while MRI and CT provide a more detailed cross sectional evaluation. CT is most useful for evaluation of the vertebrae themselves and can detect even subtle fracture lines and bone lesions. Plain CT, however, is not very useful for visualizing the spinal cord or nerve roots, and for this MRI is best.

MRI is excellent at resolving subtle edema in the bone marrow or soft tissue structures such as the spinal cord, as well as seeing the intervertebral discs in great detail and their relation to neural structures.

6. When is computed tomography of the spine useful versus magnetic resonance imaging?

The advantage of CT lies in its speed, availability, and superior bone visualization, which make it ideal for use in the acute and/or traumatic evaluation of the spine. CT is also very useful to assess pathologic processes that may produce mineralization, such as ankylosing spondylitis or ossification of the posterior longitudinal ligament.

In most other situations, MRI is superior for visualization of the vertebrae (including marrow edema), discs and ligaments, the paraspinal soft tissues, and the spinal cord and nerves. MRI does not visualize metal hardware well due to artifacts produced during interaction with the magnetic field, even by nonferrogenic material; CT or radiography are thus better for assessing metallic hardware.

7. How do I know which test to order?

The nature of the pain and the distribution into which it falls are very important in selecting the proper imaging test. Diffuse pain without localization can be very challenging and may necessitate imaging centrally to peripherally to eliminate causes. When the symptoms are more localized, imaging can be performed along the neural pathway related to the pain complaint in question, selecting the area most likely to be the source first and the most appropriate imaging modality, given the advantages noted previously.

When uncertain about a situation, a great resource is your local radiologist, who can help direct referring physicians to the proper exam and also help structure complex protocols for unique cases.

As another resource, the American College of Radiology also publishes guidelines on ordering imaging tests for various indications and subindications—the ACR Appropriateness Criteria. The criteria are periodically updated and available for a range of indications, among which is back pain, indicating which imaging tests are the highest yield for each indication and subindication.*

8. What indications require contrast?

This is one of the most frequently asked questions. Intravenous contrast is used to create a signal difference between two structures that would otherwise not be as apparent. For example, a tumor that avidly takes up contrast becomes readily visible relative to the surrounding tissue.

Each type of contrast creates this differential signal in different ways. For CT, iodine containing contrasts stop more x-rays than would normally be attenuated by a structure making it appear more dense. On MRI, gadolinium containing contrasts shorten the T1 time and therefore increase T1 signal in structures that take it up relative to the surrounding tissue.

A good rule of thumb is that when tumors, infection, or active inflammation (such as demyelination) is being considered, contrast is useful to help discriminate these entities from surrounding tissue.

9. What signs help differentiate a benign and pathologic compression fracture?

Preservation of vertebral body fat, lack of lytic foci (on CT), retropulsion of bone fragments, a wedge deformity, and a fluid cleft have been more closely associated with benign osteoporotic compression fractures.

A convex posterior border (suggesting a lesion protruding), pedicle involvement, paraspinal/extraosseous soft tissue or inflammation, the presence of metastatic lesions at other vertebral levels, lytic destruction of cortical bone, complete replacement of normal high T1 signal fatty marrow, and restriction on diffusion imaging are more associated with pathologic fractures (i.e., neoplasm or infection).

---

*ACR Appropriateness Criteria are available at http://www.acr.org/quality-safety/appropriateness-criteria.

10. **What types of imaging are best for suspected cranial nerve vascular compression syndromes as a cause of pain?**
Imaging of blood vessels can be accomplished both with and without contrast media.

CT angiography (CTA) uses iodine containing contrast to enhance vessels. Visualization of the vasculature is excellent, but the resolution of surrounding structures, such as cranial nerves and other tissue, is better on MRI.

On an MRI, vessels can be visualized with magnetic resonance angiography (MRA), high-resolution contrast-enhanced sequences such as a 3D spoiled gradient (SPGR) after gadolinium contrast administration, or with a high-resolution sequence called a balanced steady-state gradient echo. Of these, a high-resolution balanced steady-state sequence offers the best visualization of the blood vessels in relation to fine structures such as nearby cranial nerves. Different vendors have different names for this sequence (Fast Imaging Employing Steady-State Acquisition [FIESTA] and Balance Fast Field Echo [BFFE] are examples), but the concept is the same and the images produced are very high resolution without a need for extrinsic contrast. Visualization of cranial nerves relative to blood vessels is excellent.

MRA and contrast-enhanced SPGR serve a complementary role to the steady-state sequences for vascular compression evaluation.

11. **In the patient with back pain, what are considered "red flags" for more rapid progression to advanced imaging techniques such as magnetic resonance imaging versus conservative therapy?**
Uncomplicated back pain less than 6 weeks in duration without concerning secondary signs (red flags) has been shown to derive little value from imaging, overall.[1,2]

Findings raising concern for neoplasm, infection, trauma/fracture, and/or severe neurologic impairment would be red flags, necessitating further workup of back pain with advanced imaging early on in the evaluation process.[3]

12. **Case: A 25-year-old male presents with severe pain after a motor vehicle accident, with point tenderness over the lower thoracic region at about T10 to T12 and leg weakness. What is the most appropriate modality for initial evaluation in the emergency department?**
CT is the most appropriate due to availability, speed of exam, and superiority for visualization of complex osseous structures.

The major concern here would be an osseous injury and spinal canal/cord compromise due to trauma.

Radiography is fast, but visualization of complex fractures and subtle findings is limited, and this patient is manifesting focal pain and neurologic symptoms. MRI is excellent for assessment of the cord itself and vertebrae for edema, but the exam time is longer, and it may not be readily available. In this setting, most times MRI serves a supportive role in those patients needing further evaluation of the ligamentous structures around the spine and better visualization of the spinal cord itself.

13. **Case: A 40-year-old female with a known history of IV drug abuse presents with fever, back pain, and urinary incontinence. What is the best modality for workup? Should contrast be used?**
MRI is the most appropriate modality in this situation, and contrast is indicated.

The concern in this case would be for infection, specifically an epidural abscess with neural compression. Contrast is indicated in the setting of infection when possible, though MRI as a modality can also be useful to assess for other causes such as disc herniation.

CT can evaluate for secondary signs of infection such as bone erosion, but MRI is superior for assessment of the soft tissues and discs and visualization of the spinal canal. Radiography is not adequate for assessing for subtle infection or intraspinal fluid collections.

14. **What is functional magnetic resonance imaging and how does it work?**
Functional MRI uses a sequence called BOLD (blood oxygenation level dependent), which is very sensitive to changes in oxygen levels, as the name implies, to analyze subtle increases in blood flow in areas of the brain utilized for specific tasks.

Task-dependent or stimulus-induced functional MRI is performed in blocks of activity or stimulation alternating with rest blocks over a period of a few minutes. Analysis of the data is then performed to look for areas that fit the expected pattern of alternating activity and rest. Pixels that meet statistical threshold values of significance, as defined by the user, are then shown on the image as colors producing a statistical map of function.

Many researchers are using this technology to map and assess the areas of the brain involved in processing pain as well as developing and assessing therapies and responses.

KEY POINTS

1. Contrast is useful to help discriminate tumors, infection, or active inflammation (such as demyelination) from surrounding tissue.
2. In evaluation of vascular compression, MRA and contrast-enhanced SPGR serve a complementary role to steady-state sequences.
3. Further workup of back pain with advanced imaging early on in the evaluation process is often indicated by findings indicating concern for neoplasm, infection, trauma/fracture, and/or severe neurologic impairment.

REFERENCES

1. Modic MT, Obuchowski NA, Ross JS, et al. Acute low back pain and radiculopathy: MR imaging findings and their prognostic role and effect on outcome. *Radiology.* 2005;237(2):597-604.
2. Chou R, Qaseem A, Owens DK, Shekelle P. Diagnostic imaging for low back pain: advice for high-value health care from the American College of Physicians. *Ann Intern Med.* 2011;154(3):181-189.
3. ACR Appropriateness Criteria: Low Back Pain. https://acsearch.acr.org/docs/69483/Narrative/.

CHAPTER 9

CHRONIC PELVIC PAIN

Andrew Dubin

What is chronic pelvic pain (CPP)? By definition, it is pain that is located in the lower abdominal or groin region. It is noncyclical in nature. It has been present for more than 3 to 6 months and is not exclusively associated with intercourse or menstruation. Twenty-five percent of adult community living women have issues of chronic pelvic pain, and in the majority of women the etiology is never fully elucidated.

The limitations of this definition are obvious. It does not address the male population. Men also have issues of chronic pelvic pain; however, they are less likely to seek out medical evaluation.

Establishing the diagnosis presents a challenge. Many times the interplay between the urological, gynecological, as well as gastrointestinal systems can complicate the presentation. Additionally, neurological, endocrinologic, and psychological issues can all add confounding layers to the presentation and pain. Lastly, the musculoskeletal system can have dramatic impact on pelvic pain or can be the primary source generator for pelvic pain.

Unfortunately the musculoskeletal system is not typically thought of as a source of pelvic pain until several providers have been seen, multiple tests have been performed, and in many instances many procedures have been done. In essence it becomes the default organ system.

COMMON PRESENTING COMPLAINTS AND SYMPTOMS

CPP patients commonly present with complaints of pan with Valsalva type activities, such as straining to have a bowel movement. They may note pain with ambulation, prolonged sitting, lumbar flexion, and or extension. A quick look at the following complaints leads one to realize the lack of specificity of these complaints. They can be seen in lumbar degenerative disc disease, disc herniation, as well as in posterior element dysfunction, such as facet joint arthritis. Pain with extension and ambulation can be seen in spinal stenosis. Groin pain with ambulation may be secondary to degenerative joint disease of the hip. Patients may additionally complain of urinary urgency, frequency, as well as sensory dysesthesias in the perineum. Males can complain of erectile dysfunction. The complaints of urinary urgency and frequency not only can be seen in primary urological issues such as benign prostatic hypertrophy but also are frequently noted in patients with cervical or thoracic level myelopathy. Sensory dysesthesias can be seen in myelopathies as well as cauda equine level dysfunction. Erectile dysfunction can be seen in both upper motor neuron as well as lower motor neuron dysfunction. Realizing that pelvic pain can arise from multiple pathologies, the criticality of the history and physical cannot be overemphasized.

This section will focus primarily on the musculoskeletal system as the source generator for pelvic pain as it is the most frequently overlooked system.

The physical exam starts with observation. Note how the patient ambulates. Do they walk with a compensated Trendelenburg gait pattern? Primary hip pathology, as well as a possible profound L 5 radiculopathy, needs to be explored. In the setting of an L 5 radiculopathy that is severe enough to cause a compensated Trendelenburg, an associated foot drop should also be noted. If one is not present, the diagnosis of L 5 radiculopathy is highly unlikely, as nerve function recovers proximal to distal. However, isolated superior gluteal nerve neuropathy, gluteus medius muscle tear, or primary hip pathology all remain in the differential. Observe sitting posture. Patients that are comfortable sitting or sitting forward flexed may have facet joint arthritis, or spinal stenosis. Patients that prefer to stand or sit with lumbar support may have issues of discogenic pain.

A complete pelvic pain workup must include a thorough examination of the musculoskeletal system. It should include an assessment of lumbosacral spine motion, gait evaluation. Additionally manual muscle testing should be performed on both lower extremities to compare side to side and should include assessment of strength of the hip flexors, knee extensors, as well as ankle/toe dorsiflexors and plantar flexors. Given the strength of the ankle plantar flexors, having the patient perform multiple calf raises will sometimes elucidate subtle weakness of S 1 innervated musculature not appreciated on manual muscle testing. Additionally heel walking may bring out slight weakness of ankle dorsiflexors not appreciated on the physical exam.

Evaluation of reflexes is critical—notation of hyperreflexia, ankle clonus, crossed adductors. Positive Babinski raises the specter of a CNS level dysfunction. Abnormal findings in the upper extremities manifesting with overflow reflex activity and hyperreflexia, Hoffmann's sign, with associated sensory symptoms in the hands, and concomitant cervical radicular distribution of weakness raise the specter of cervical level dysfunction. Brain level dysfunction needs to be considered in the setting of diffuse upper and lower extremity hyperreflexia, with long tract signs without a clear-cut cervical radicular pattern of weakness that localizes a cervical root level issue in concert with cervical cord compression. A clear radicular level of weakness in the upper extremities on manual muscle testing with hyperreflexia below is classic for a radiculomyelopathy and warrants MRI imaging of the cervical spine. Diffuse hyperreflexia, with associated weakness in a more diffuse or patchy nonradicular distribution, especially in young women with appropriate historical data (including changing neurological symptoms over time in addition to issues of vision loss, transient foot drop, or wrist drop), should raise an index of suspicion for multiple sclerosis. At that point MRI of the brain and spinal cord both with and without contrast would be very reasonable. Diffuse lower extremity hyporeflexia can be seen in peripheral neuropathies, or polyradiculopathies. Unilateral sensory dysesthesias involving the perineum should raise the question of a symptomatic Tarlov cyst. It is important to remember that not all Tarlov cysts are asymptomatic or incidental findings, and their symptomatic presentation is commonly limited to the perineum, with sensory complaints noted. Additionally, males may note erectile dysfunction, and women may note changes in clitoral sensitivity. In this scenario, detailed physical exam to assess sensation in the perineum as well as reflex testing of the bulbocavernosus reflex in men and the clitoral-anal reflex in women, is critical. Workup for a suspected Tarlov cyst should include sacral MRI as well as needle EMG of the right and left anal sphincter musculature looking for denervation, as well as changes in typical motor unit morphology. Needle EMG of the anal sphincter should only be done by people with significant experience in evaluating this muscle, as the normal anal-sphincter motor units look abnormal in comparison to typical motor units seen in appendicular skeletal muscles. Work by Podnar revealed that in males, abnormal penile sensation in concert with an abnormal or absent bulbocavernosus reflex on physical exam was highly correlative to abnormal electrodiagnostic testing. Unfortunately in women the clitoral-anal reflex can be difficult to obtain on physical exam, and as such in this group, electrophysiologic testing including reflex testing and anal sphincter EMG may have great utility. Normal reflexes in the upper extremities with loss of reflexes in the lower extremities can be seen in patients with peripheral neuropathy. The history will be critical at that point to determine whether or not this is potentially a hereditary neuropathy that has now progressed to the point it is becoming symptomatic versus an acquired neuropathy. Causes of acquired neuropathies can range from cryptogenic, to toxic metabolic, to autoimmune and inflammatory mediated, and require detailed workup to avoid missing treatable causes. Other causes of lower motor neuron findings isolated to the lower extremities can include cauda equina, but this will typically manifest with marked lower extremity weakness in a polyradicular pattern weakness, as well as marked sensory dysfunction in the perineum. While myopathies are not a common cause of pelvic pain, patients who note that their symptoms worsen throughout the day and note cramping pelvic pain, especially after straining during a bowel movement, may be exhibiting findings of muscle fatigue of proximal musculature with prolonged activity. Physical examination and detailed manual muscle testing may reveal a proximal to distal gradient of motor weakness or possibly patterns of weakness such as scapula humeral peroneal or facial scapula humeral peroneal. In these instances, preexercise and postexercise creatine phosphokinase (CPK) levels may be very illustrative, as the patient may have a normal to minimally elevated CPK at rest, only to have it rise markedly 24 to 36 hours post regular and routine exercise. This group of patients may note on direct questioning that they are always sore in their muscles after they exercise, but assume it is normal because they have always felt this way. In most instances the complaint of pelvic level pain in patients with myopathy is secondary to altered gait mechanics, with subsequent overload of the SI joint of lumbar facet joints in patients who stand and walk with excessive lumbar lordosis as a result of manifest proximal weakness. Typically in adults this would be seen in limb girdle dystrophies or adult onset myopathies.

Hip joint pathology can be a common source of pelvic region pain. True intraarticular hip joint pathology will classically cause groin pain. Patients will complain of pain with weight bearing and walking. Pain will improve when they are sedentary. Additionally use of a cane in the contralateral hand will ease their pain. Startup pain is a common phenomenon, but unfortunately is not unique to hip joint pathology. Physical exam findings will classically include replication of groin pain with internal rotation of the affected hip. Proxy referral patterns of pain include radiating anterior thigh pain or referral to the knee with internal rotation of the hip. Intraarticular hip joint pathology can present many challenges when it becomes part of the differential diagnosis for the workup for pelvic pain. It is not an uncommon finding in an aging population and as such can also be associated with degenerative changes in the lumbar spine. The physical exam may help delineate the driver of the patient's pain, but if doubt persists as to the role the hip is playing in the patient's pain complaints, a diagnostic and potentially therapeutic intraarticular hip joint injection, done either under fluoroscopic guidance or ultrasound, can easily be done. A markedly positive response to the injection will quickly confirm the clinical suspicion and a negative response efficiently removes the joint from the equation and allows the physician to turn his or her attention to other potential source generators.

Anterior groin pain and associated pelvic level pain in younger patients may be due to labral pathology. Patients may note that their pain worsens with standing and walking. Unlike hip pain from degenerative joint disease (DJD), patients with femoral acetabular impingement (FAI) with labral pathology may also complain of pain while seated. Additionally, FAI may also have replication of groin pain with external rotation of the hip as well as hip abduction. Complaints of sudden sharp pain with clicking and a sensation of give way weakness can also be seen with FAI. The differential diagnosis is rather extensive when FAI is entertained and includes such entities as iliopsoas impingement, subspine impingement, and ischiofemoral impingement. Iliopsoas impingement, more common in women than men, may be secondary to repetitive traction injury to the tendon with subsequent scarring and adherence of the tendon to the capsule-labrum complex of the hip. This can be seen in younger patients involved in sports and activities that place the patient in positions of extreme hip extension or rapid eccentric loading of the hip flexors. Subspine impingement, more common in men than women, is thought to be the result of a prominent anterior superior iliac spine (ASIS) abnormally contacting the distal femoral neck. Symptoms in this case are typically seen with attempts at deep hip flexion (catchers in softball and baseball). The etiology of the prominent ASIS may be secondary to repetitive avulsion type injury to the ASIS during repetitive knee flexion with hip extension type activities (soccer players). Ischiofemoral impingement is typically more commonly seen in women than in men. It results from a tight space between the ischial tuberosity and the lesser trochanter, causing repetitive impingement and trapping of the quadratus femoris muscle. This is typically a congenital issue, but can develop after hip fracture, or in association with early superior and medial migration of the femoral head in early hip DJD. While imaging studies clearly have a role and place in the workup of anterior groin and pelvic level pain, all findings need to be placed into context. The context grows from the physical exam. Previous work by Silvis et al. revealed a high prevalence of abnormal findings on MRI of pelvis, hip, and groin regions on a cohort of asymptomatic college and professional hockey players. These abnormalities included common adductor and rectus abdominus tendonitis, with associated bone edema in the symphysis pubis. Additionally partial tears as well as complete tears of the above muscles off the pubis were noted. Finally, hip abnormalities including labral tears, as well as osteochondral lesions of the femoral head, were noted. To further cloud the picture, similar findings have been noted on lumbar MRIs in asymptomatic patients.

As one can see, hip joint pathology and its associated groin level pain can present unique challenges as part of the workup for pelvic pain. The physical exam is critical in helping delineate the driver of the patient's pain. Sometimes even after a detailed physical exam, it may still be difficult to determine if intraarticular or extraarticular sources are the primary source generator for the patients' groin- and pelvic-level pain. In these scenarios where doubt persists as to the role intraarticular joint pathology is playing in the patient's pain complaints, a diagnostic and potentially therapeutic intraarticular hip joint injection, either under fluoroscopic guidance or ultrasound, can easily be done. A markedly positive response to the injection will quickly confirm the clinical suspicion, and a negative response efficiently removes the joint from the equation and allows the physician to turn his or her attention to other potential source generators.

In summary, pelvic pain presents many unique challenges for the treating physician. Many of these patients have seen multiple providers and have had multiple procedures performed. These patients not uncommonly present with a high level of frustration as well as a degree of mistrust for the medical community, as they have been shuffled from provider to provider. Obtaining a detailed history and performing a thorough physical can go a long way in elucidating the problem. Sometimes just getting patients to understand why they have their pain goes a long way in helping them manage pain. It all starts with the history and physical, and the trust that develops over time as the patient grows to realize that you as the treating physician are taking a measured, thoughtful approach to their pain.

KEY POINTS

1. Chronic pelvic pain may result from a variety of etiologies, including intrapelvic sources and pain that is referred from nonpelvic sources.
2. Numerous medications may contribute to chronic lower abdominal pain; thus, this needs to be considered when evaluating a patient with chronic pelvic pain.
3. Chronic pelvic pain does not only occur in women.
4. EDX specifically needle EMG of the anal sphincter is highly sensitive for evaluation of S2-S4 nerve function.
5. Physical examination of the pelvic pain patient must include assessment of lower extremity strength and reflexes.

BIBLIOGRAPHY

1. Mui J, Allaire C, Williams C, Yong PJ. Abdominal Wall Pain in Women with Chronic Pelvic Pain. *J Obstet Gynaecol Can.* 2016;38(2):154-159.
2. Ploteau S, Cardaillac C, Perrouin-Verbe MA, Riant T, Labat JJ. Pudendal neuralgia due to pudendal nerve entrapment: warning signs observed in two cases and review of the literature. *Pain Physician.* 2016;19(3):E449-E454.
3. Speer LM, Mushkbar S, Erbele T. Chronic pelvic pain in women. *Am Fam Physician.* 2016;93(5):380-387.
4. Podnar S. Utility of sphincter electromyography and sacral reflex studies in women with cauda equina lesions. *Neurourol Urodyn.* 2014;33(4):426-430.
5. Podnar S. Cauda equina lesions as a complication of spinal surgery. *Eur Spine J.* 2010;19(3):451-457.

URGENT ISSUES IN PAIN

Steven Lange, Youngwon Youn, Sara Gannon, Julia Prusik and Julie G. Pilitsis

CHAPTER 10

1. **What is acute pain?**
   Acute pain is characterized as pain lasting less than 6 months. This pain is provoked by a specific disease or injury, and is usually amenable to immediate intervention; at other times, however, it is a harbinger for more serious disease processes.

2. **What is radiculopathy?**
   Radiculopathy is categorized as sensory or motor dysfunction marked by nerve compression that may cause pain, numbness, tingling, or weakness along the course of a nerve. The pain can also radiate along the limb of the dermatome corresponding to the affected nerve root. Lumbosacral radiculopathy is three times as likely as its cervical counterpart. The pathology of the disease takes place on the nerve fibers, from their spinal cord departure to their entrance in the intervertebral foramen and intervertebral canal, where sensory and motor neurons join in the spinal nerve.

3. **When does radiculopathy require urgent care?**
   Disc herniation and foraminal stenosis are the most common sources of nerve compression, though tumors, trauma, and synovial cysts are also other etiologies. When the cauda equina is involved, immediate attention is required, as symptoms may become irreversible. Patients may develop saddle anesthesia, urinary/bowel incontinence/retention, and motor deficits.

4. **How can pain be medically managed?**
   Medical management of acute radiculopathy includes oral steroids, antiinflammatory medications (nonsteroidal antiinflammatory drugs), muscle relaxants, and narcotics. However, patients can become refractory to pharmacotherapy, and other options must be considered. Epidural steroid injections and physical therapy (PT) are other options.

5. **How can physical therapy be a curative treatment of radiculopathy?**
   In addition to pharmacotherapy, PT is often used in multimodal regimens to restore range of motion and strengthen musculature. Stretching exercises can be combined with electrical stimulation to alleviate pain, and isometric contraction and resistance training may further help the patient.

6. **How effective are epidural injections in previously irresponsive patients?**
   Image-guided epidural steroid injections are approved in cases irresponsive to other treatments. Level IV data indicate that transforaminal epidural injections may provide relief for 60% of patients, with short-term relief negating the need for surgery in 25% of patients who are cleared to undergo intervention.

7. **When is it appropriate to use selective diagnostic nerve root block in addition to magnetic resonance imaging and electromyography?**
   Selective diagnostic nerve root block (SNRB) is often employed when magnetic resonance imaging (MRI) and electromyography show multilevel pathology. In a recent study, correlation between SNRB results and the level with most severe degree of MRI degeneration was 60%, and correlation between SNRB results and levels decided by neurological deficits/dermatome radicular pain distribution was 28%. SNRB may help in the preoperative investigation of patients in accordance with MRI pathology, neurological examination, and pain distribution.

8. **What is cauda equina syndrome?**
   Cauda equina syndrome is a medical emergency that consists of damage to the bundle of spinal nerves called the cauda equina, usually via lumbar disc herniation. Cauda equina syndrome can result in a combination of saddle anesthesia, abnormal lower extremity reflexes, and bilateral leg

weakness. Involvement of the S2, S3, and S4 nerve roots can produce a distended atonic bladder with urinary retention or overflow incontinence, constipation, decreased rectal tone, fecal continence, or loss of erection. It is essential to detect and treat cauda equina syndrome promptly to avoid irreversible deficits. Urgent surgery is required.

9. **What is herpes zoster or shingles?**
Shingles is a viral condition resulting from reactivation of latent varicella-zoster virus. The most debilitating complication of herpes zoster is pain associated with acute neuritis and postherpetic neuralgia. This pain is usually the first presenting symptom and exhibits characteristic stimulus-independent burning and throbbing pain that is often described as electrical. Pain is soon accompanied by a red maculopapular rash that evolves into a dermatomal vesicular rash, usually in the T3 to L3 levels. Shingles is most severe in immunocompromised individuals and bone marrow transplant recipients.

10. **What are the initial symptoms of herpes zoster?**
Diagnosis and treatment occur in the acute phase upon presentation of a unilateral dermatomal rash, usually on the trunk. Pain is commonly precipitated by movement (mechanical allodynia) or thermal change (warm or cold allodynia), and may extend beyond the margins of the original eruption. Acute herpes zoster can be associated with severe psychosocial dysfunction, including impaired sleep, decreased appetite, and diminished libido that affects a patient's quality of life, normal daily function, and social activity.

11. **How easily is herpes zoster treated?**
Patients with herpes zoster benefit from oral antiviral therapy with acyclovir, valacyclovir, or famciclovir. These may reduce the duration of viral shedding, hasten rash healing, reduce the severity and duration of acute pain, and reduce the risk of progression to postherpetic neuralgia. Additionally, acute pain from herpes zoster can be effectively controlled through the application of nerve blocks.

12. **Why does postherpetic neuralgia occur?**
Postherpetic neuralgia may be due to hypersensitivity of the primary afferent neuron that initially responded to the tissue damage during the acute zoster. Central and peripheral nervous system damage and dorsal horn atrophy may be observed in postherpetic neuralgia.

13. **How are acute neuritis and postherpetic neuralgia treated?**
Antiinflammatories and tramadol are often used as first-line medications. Gabapentin, pregabalin, amitriptyline, hydrochloride, and fluphenazine hydrochloride have been reported as beneficial pharmaceutics for pain relief as well. The lidocaine patch is efficacious in treatment of patients with allodynia, has excellent safety and tolerability, and may be left on the skin for 12 to 18 hours. Stronger opioids and tricyclic antidepressants are considered as second-line agents, while topical capsaicin and valproate are third-line therapies.

14. **When does care for complex regional pain syndrome become urgent?**
Complex regional pain syndrome (CRPS) is a chronic pain condition, often affecting at least one of the limbs, and is considered to be a neuroinflammatory disorder. Although a chronic condition, patients benefit drastically from early diagnosis and treatment, specifically within 6 months. Early and aggressive treatment has been shown to effectively stop the natural progression of the disease. Treatments include PT, neuropathic medication, stellate ganglion blocks, and spinal cord stimulation.

15. **What are status migraines?**
Migraines that last longer than 72 hours are referred to as status migraines. These are due to lack of treatment or incorrect treatment, such as overmedication. They can lead to fatigue, sleep loss, confusion, and sometimes auras.

16. **What are the treatment options for status migraines and refractory migraines?**
Steroids and sumatriptan are often used to mitigate status migrainosus. Muscle relaxants have also been used for refractory migraines. In addition, management of chronic pain with implanted devices is common for pain that does not respond to other methods of treatment. The analgesic effects of spinal cord stimulators are provided by mild electrical stimulation to the epidural space. Similarly, intrathecal pumps are surgically implanted devices with a pump unit placed in the abdomen and a catheter connecting the unit to the intrathecal space of the spinal cord. Intrathecal pumps are favorable for various reasons, including their acute drug application capabilities, avoidance of broad opioid use, and tempering of the side effects that exist when administered in other forms.

KEY POINTS

1. Radiculopathy requires urgent care when resulting in unrelenting pain or motor deficits such as food drop as it can indicate cauda equine of the spinal cord.
2. Herpes zoster should be treated to avoid complication like post herpetic neuralgia characterized by burning pain.
3. CRPS patients should be diagnosed and treated within 6 months as they are highly responsive to treatments such as PT, neuropathic medication, stellate ganglion blocks, as well as spinal cord stimulation.
4. Patients with status migrainosus or with migraines unresponsive to traditional treatments may benefit from muscle relaxants, intrathecal pumps, and spinal cord stimulation.

BIBLIOGRAPHY

1. Ahn UM, Ahn NU, Buchowski JM, et al. Cauda equina syndrome secondary to lumbar disc herniation: a meta-analysis of surgical outcomes. *Spine.* 2000;25(12):1515-1522.
2. Braunwald E, Fauci A, Kasper D, et al. *Harrison's Principles of Internal Medicine.* 15th edition. New York: McGraw-Hill; 2001.
3. Bruggeman AJ, Decker RC. Surgical treatment and outcomes of lumbar radiculopathy. *Phys Med Rehabil Clin N Am.* 2011;22(1):161-177.
4. Harden RN, Oaklander AL, Burton AW, et al. Complex regional pain syndrome: practical diagnostic and treatment guidelines, 4th edition. *Pain Med.* 2013;14:180-229.
5. Kost RG, Straus SE. Postherpetic neuralgia—pathogenesis, treatment, and prevention. *N Engl J Med.* 1996;335(1):32-42.
6. Freitag FG, Schloemer F. Medical management of adult headache. *Otolaryngol Clin North Am.* 2014;47(2):221-237. doi:10.1016/j.otc.2013.11.002.
7. Sampathkumar P, Drage LA, Martin DP. Herpes zoster (shingles) and postherpetic neuralgia. *Mayo Clin Proc.* 2009;84(3):274-280.

CHAPTER 11

MIGRAINE

Grace Forde

1. **Is migraine an important public health problem?**
   Migraine is a major public health problem by almost any standard. It is a highly prevalent disorder that affects approximately 14.9% of the US population and produces enormous suffering for individuals and their families. Recent estimates indicate that 47 million Americans suffer from migraine headaches; many experience severe pain and significant levels of headache-related disability. The overall age-adjusted 3-month prevalence of migraine in females was 19.1% and in males 9.0%, but this varied substantially depending on age. The prevalence of migraine was highest in females ages 18 to 44, where the 3-month prevalence of migraine or severe headache was 23.5%.

   In one study the economic cost to employers ranged from 5.6 to 17.2 billion dollars annually, due to decreased productivity and missed work days. These indirect costs resulting from missed work and disability greatly exceed direct medical expenditures on migraine treatment. In addition, headaches are the seventh leading reason for outpatient visits in the United States and account for 2% to 4% of all emergency room visits.

2. **What are the phases of the migraine attack?**
   It is useful to divide the migraine attack into four phases: premonitory, aura, headache, and resolution. The premonitory phase typically occurs hours or days before the headache. The aura usually occurs within 1 hour of headache onset but may begin during the headache. The headache phase is characterized by pain and associated symptoms. In the resolution phase, spontaneous pain subsides, but other symptoms are present. It is important to recognize that no phase is obligatory for migraine and that most patients do not experience all four phases.

3. **Describe the premonitory phase.**
   Premonitory features include changes in mood or behavior that precede the headache by hours or days. This phase is sometimes referred to as the *postdrome*. Patients may feel depressed, euphoric, irritable, or restless, and occasionally report fatigue or hyperactivity. Constitutional symptoms may include changes in appetite, fluid balance, and bowel function. Some patients report food cravings; others describe a poorly characterized feeling that an attack is coming. Premonitory features vary from person to person and from attack to attack.

4. **Describe the aura.**
   The aura consists of focal neurologic symptoms that usually precede, but that may accompany, the attack. Only 20% to 30% of migraine sufferers ever experience auras, and most people who have attacks with aura also have attacks without aura. Aura symptoms typically develop slowly, over 5 to 20 minutes, and usually last 60 minutes. Auras most commonly involve changes in vision, although changes in motor and sensory function may also occur. The classic visual aura of the migraine is characterized by both positive symptom features, such as flashes of light (scintillations) or zigzag lines (fortification spectra), and negative symptom features, such as visual loss (scotoma). The visual aura may begin in a small portion of the visual field and gradually expand to encompass an entire visual hemifield. Some individuals also describe tunnel vision due to a loss of peripheral vision, as if looking down the barrel of a gun.

   Sensory auras are also characterized by a mix of positive (tingling) and negative features (numbness), sometimes beginning on one side of the face or hand and slowly expanding to encompass an entire side of the body. Hemiparesis may occur, and if the dominant hemisphere is involved, dysphasia or aphasia may develop.

5. **How do you differentiate migraine aura from other kinds of focal episodes of neurologic dysfunction?**
   Transient neurologic deficits may have several causes. These include migraine aura, epileptic seizure, cerebrovascular disorder, metabolic derangements, and psychiatric disease. Seizure is most typically characterized by positive phenomena such as tonic or tonic/clonic movements. A

cerebrovascular event is most often characterized by negative phenomena, such as weakness. Both seizures and stroke tend to come on relatively suddenly. The gradual evolution of symptom features and the mix of positive and negative features, as well as the temporal association with headache, help identify migraine aura. The patient's age and risk-factor profile may also point the clinician in one diagnostic direction or another. It may not always be possible to differentiate migraine aura from other causes of focal neurologic dysfunction on the basis of history and physical examination alone; therefore, additional diagnostic testing (e.g., neuroimaging, electroencephalogram [EEG], bloodwork) should be considered as appropriate.

6. What are the characteristics of the headache phase?
The headache phase of migraine is characterized by a combination of pain and associated symptoms. Migraine pain has four characteristic features, and most migraine sufferers experience at least two of these. Migraine pain is typically:
- Unilateral (may be bilateral at onset or may begin on one side and then become generalized)
- Pulsatile (85% of patients, but this description is not specific for migraine)
- Moderate to severe in intensity
- Aggravated by routine physical activities (e.g., climbing stairs, head movement)
    By definition, the pain of migraine must be accompanied by other features. Nausea occurs in about 75% of patients and vomiting in up to one-third. Many patients experience sensory sensitivity in the form of photophobia, phonophobia, and osmophobia. Other accompanying features include anorexia or food cravings, blurry vision, nasal stuffiness, abdominal cramps, polyuria, and pallor. Although impaired concentration is common, measurable memory impairment has rarely been documented.

7. What is the resolution phase?
The resolution phase of the migraine attack begins as the pain wanes. Following the headache, the patient may feel irritable, listless, tired, or washed-out. Many patients report residual scalp tenderness in the distribution of the remitted spontaneous pain. Some patients feel unusually refreshed or euphoric after a migraine attack.

8. What feature or features are absolutely required to diagnose migraine?
It is important to recognize that no single headache feature or no single associated symptom is pathognomonic for migraine. For example, 20% to 30% of migraineurs have auras; the physician who relies exclusively on aura will usually miss the diagnosis. If nausea occurs in 75% of patients, the clinician who relies exclusively on nausea will miss 25% of cases.
    In 1988 the International Headache Society provided a classification system for headache disorders. That system defined seven different types of migraine. The two most important types are migraine without aura and migraine with aura (Boxes 11.1 and 11.2).

Box 11.1. Diagnostic Criteria for Migraine Without Aura

- At least five attacks fulfilling B–D.
- Headache attacks lasting 4–72 hours (untreated or unsuccessfully treated).
- Headache has at least two of the following characteristics:
  a. Unilateral location
  b. Pulsating quality
  c. Moderate or severe intensity (inhibits or prohibits daily activities)
  d. Aggravation by walking stairs or similar routine physical activity
- During headache at least one of the following: (1) nausea and/or vomiting, (2) photophobia and phonophobia.
- At least one of the following:
  a. History, physical, and neurologic examinations do not suggest secondary headache.
  b. History and/or physical and/or neurologic examinations do suggest such disorder, but it is ruled out by appropriate investigations.
  c. Such disorder is present, but migraine attacks do not occur for the first time in close temporal relation to the disorder.

Box 11.2. Diagnostic Criteria for Migraine With Aura

- At least two attacks fulfilling B.
- At least three of the following four characteristics:
  a. One or more fully reversible aura symptoms indicating focal cerebral cortical and/or brain stem dysfunction.
  b. At least one aura symptom develops gradually over more than 4 minutes, or two or more symptoms occur in succession.
  c. No aura symptom lasts more than 60 min. If more than one aura symptom is present, accepted duration is proportionally increased.
  d. Headache follows aura with a free interval of less than 60 min. (It may also begin before or simultaneously with the aura.)
- At least one of the following:
  a. History, physical, and neurologic examinations do not suggest secondary headache.
  b. History and/or physical and/or neurologic examinations do suggest such disorder, but it is ruled out by appropriate investigations.
  c. Such disorder is present, but migraine attacks do not occur for the first time in close temporal relation to the disorder.

---

9. **Describe considerations for diagnostic testing.**

   Diagnostic testing in migraine serves primarily to exclude secondary causes of headache. The first step is to identify red flags that suggest the possibility of secondary headache (see Chapter 13). If the patient has no history of red flags, the general medical and neurologic exams sometimes raise the possibility of secondary headache. If there is a possibility of secondary headache, an appropriate diagnostic workup is required.

   In the absence of alarms, the second step is to try to diagnose a specific primary headache disorder. If the patient has typical migraine or tension-type headache (TTH), it is appropriate to proceed with treatment. If there are atypical headache features, even in the absence of red flags, consider diagnostic testing to exclude secondary causes. If treatment is initiated and the expected response to therapy is not obtained, revisit the issue of secondary headache. However, because migraine and TTH are so common, it is neither appropriate nor cost-effective to obtain neuroimaging for every patient.

10. **What diagnostic tests are required to establish the diagnosis of migraine?**

    There are no diagnostic tests required to diagnose migraine.

11. **Why is migraine considered a neurologic disease?**

    Migraine is viewed as a disease of the brain. Changes in the brain give rise to inflammatory changes in cranial and meningeal blood vessels, which in turn produce pain. The premonitory phase, with its characteristic changes in mood, behavior, and autonomic function, is best understood on the basis of central nervous system dysfunction. Neuroimaging procedures, including positron emission tomography (PET), EEG, and magnetoencephalography, demonstrate abnormalities of the brain during or between attacks in patients with migraine. Finally, the drugs used to treat migraine often act on the brain, cranial nerves, or the cranial blood vessels. These include the triptans and others, for example.

12. **Describe the mechanism of the aura.**

    The phenomenon of "spreading cortical depression" may underlie the aura of migraine. Spreading depression was originally described as a wave of excitation (depolarization) followed by a wave of inhibition that spreads over the cortical surface of experimental animals after mechanical or chemical stimulation. Neuronal activity decreases during a wave of inhibition, producing decreased cerebral blood flow through the mechanism of cerebral autoregulation. As a consequence, inhibition is accompanied by a wave of spreading oligemia (decreased blood flow).

    In migraine with aura, cerebral blood flow studies demonstrate a wave of oligemia that accompanies the aura, as predicted by the model of spreading depression. This wave of oligemia progresses at a rate of 2 to 3 mm/minute, the same rate reported for spreading depression in experimental animals. In addition, the rate of spreading oligemia and spreading depression corresponds with the evolution of the scintillating scotoma that marches across the visual field of the typical migraine aura. Spreading oligemia has been demonstrated using xenon inhalation and magnetic resonance imaging.

13. What is the substrate of migraine pain?

The work of Michael Moskowitz and colleagues suggests that the trigeminovascular system may be a final common pathway for migraine pain. The trigeminovascular system includes the trigeminal nerve and the cranial blood vessels that it innervates. The trigeminal nerve endings contain a wide range of neurotransmitters, including substance P, calcitonin gene-related peptide, and neurokinin A. Release of these transmitters causes a sterile inflammatory response within the cranial blood vessels accompanied by extravasation of plasma proteins. The fibers of the trigeminal nerve provide an interface between the blood circulation and the brain. The pain associated with migraine may result from the activation of trigeminal sensory afferents and the development of a neurogenically mediated inflammatory response.

14. What is the role of serotonin in migraine?

Serotonin plays a prominent role in pathophysiologic models of migraine. Blood levels of serotonin decrease during a migraine attack. Urinary concentrations of serotonin's metabolites increase during a migraine attack. A serotonin-releasing factor is present in the plasma of migraine patients during attacks but not at other times. In addition, activation of the serotonergic dorsal raphe nucleus causes migraine-like headaches. Finally, evidence from PET demonstrates increased metabolism in the brainstem in the region of the serotonergic dorsal raphe nucleus during migraine attacks.

15. What role might serotonin receptors play in migraine?

The neuropharmacology of serotonin has become increasingly complex in recent years. There are many classes of serotonin receptors in the brain and blood vessels, and many subclasses as well.

The 5-HT1 receptors might play a role in acute migraine therapy on at least two levels. One subtype of the 5-HT1 receptor is found on cranial blood vessels (5-HT1b), and another is found on trigeminal nerve endings (5HT1d). Activation of 5-HT1b receptors produces a vasoconstrictor response that may also play a role in relieving the pain of migraine. Activation of the 5-HT1d receptors on the trigeminal nerve terminal blocks the release of the mediators of neurogenic inflammation. Many of the acute treatments for migraine, including ergotamine, dihydroergotamine, and the triptans, are 5-HT1 agonists. The triptans are selective agonists for the 5HT1b/1d receptors. Receptors of this class are also found within the brain. The relative importance of these receptors on blood vessels, on trigeminal nerve endings, and within the brain remains uncertain.

Many of the medications used as preventive treatments for migraine act on 5-HT2 receptors. Tricyclic antidepressants may act by downregulating the 5-HT2 receptor.

16. What is the role of genetics in the pathophysiology of migraine?

We have long known that migraine is a familial disorder. Twin studies demonstrate that identical twins are more likely to be concordant for migraine than fraternal twins. More recently, specific genetic linkages have been identified for the rare subtype of migraine known as familial hemiplegic migraine (FHM). FHM is characterized by hemiplegic migraine aura and is an autosomal dominant disorder. A locus on chromosome 19 for FHM has been identified; it codes for a pq type calcium channel, which has also been implicated in cerebellar ataxia. The genetic studies suggest that migraine may be caused by abnormalities in ion channels, a "calcium channelopathy." The chromosome 19 locus plays a role in some, but not all, families with FHM. Given that FHM is genetically heterogeneous, it seems virtually certain that there are multiple genetic forms for the other types of migraine, and it is also quite likely that there are nongenetic forms of the syndrome.

17. List the steps in managing migraine.

The US Headache Consortium Guidelines illuminate an approach to managing migraine:
1. Make a specific diagnosis.
2. Assess the impact of illness and comorbidities.
3. Develop a specific treatment plan.
4. Identify factors that trigger the patient's headache, and counsel avoidance.
5. Introduce other behavioral interventions.
6. Provide medications to treat acute attacks.
7. If indicated, provide preventive medications.
8. Follow the patient, and modify treatment as necessary.

Obtaining a thorough headache history and understanding the impact of migraine on the patient's life are critical preludes to treatment. Educate patients and their relatives about the nature of migraine and the approach to therapy.

18. **How do you help patients identify their headache triggers?**
The first step toward helping patients identify their headache triggers is to take a history, and the next step is to encourage them to keep a detailed headache history. The headache diary should include how quickly the headache peaks, the duration and severity of the attack, as well as any potential triggers. The onset and duration of the menstrual cycle should also be captured in the diary. Medications taken to treat the attack and the length of time it takes to work and whether the headache is completely relieved or only subsides is very important to capture. Many dietary triggers contain biologically active chemicals that act on blood vessels or the brain to initiate an attack. Often, patients are aware that alcohol, chocolate, or certain medications trigger their headaches. Despite the long list of putative triggers (Table 11.1), it is important to recognize that triggers vary widely from one person to another. Trigger factors may be difficult to identify because they cause a headache one day but not the next. For example, a small glass of wine may not lead to a headache, but a half bottle of wine will initiate an attack. Chocolate may cause headaches during menses or at a time of stress, but not at other times of the month. Patients should understand that triggers do not necessarily initiate an attack with every exposure. In addition, vulnerability to triggers varies widely from person to person.

19. **What other nonpharmacologic options for migraine treatment are available?**
In discussing nonpharmacologic treatment with patients, it is important to distinguish exacerbating factors from the fundamental cause of migraine. Stress worsens most illnesses, including asthma, heart disease, and ulcers. Just as stress can precipitate headaches, relaxation methods, including biofeedback, can diminish their severity or frequency. Behavioral interventions are often effective treatments and help give the patient a feeling of control.
Nonpharmacologic prevention strategies include changing the diet, learning relaxation methods, using biofeedback, and applying cognitive-behavioral therapy. Biofeedback is a relaxation method that gives patients information about a measured physiologic parameter such as muscle activity (electromyography) or skin temperature. Biofeedback training can help decrease the frequency of attacks by reducing reactivity to stress. It can also be used to treat acute attacks in patients who have learned the methods well.

20. **Is migraine associated with psychiatric disease?**
Yes. Migraine is associated with depression, anxiety disorders, and manic-depressive illness. This comorbidity does not imply that migraine has psychogenic mechanisms. Perhaps perturbations in particular brain systems, such as the serotonin system, predispose patients both to migraine and to certain forms of psychiatric illness. When comorbid psychiatric disease is present, it is important to address it in treatment.

Table 11.1. Selected Migraine Trigger Factors

Alcohol	Hunger
Aspartame	Light (bright or flashing)
Barometric pressure changes	Medication overuse
Cheese	Menstruation
Cigarette smoke	Monosodium glutamate
Dehydration	Odors (perfume, gasoline, solvents)
Estrogens	Oral contraceptives
Excessive or insufficient sleep	Stress and worry
Head trauma	

21. Differentiate acute and preventive pharmacotherapy for migraine.

The drugs used to treat migraine are generally classified as acute agents and preventive agents. Acute therapy is administered at the time of the attack to relieve pain and the associated symptoms of migraine, and to restore the ability to function. Preventive therapy is taken on a daily basis, whether or not headache is present, to reduce the frequency and severity of attacks. An exception to this approach to preventive therapy would be the use of onabotulinum toxin A (Botox) for chronic migraine, which is administered every 12 weeks via injection. Additional preventive injection therapies are under investigation. Almost everyone with migraine needs acute treatments. A minority of migraine sufferers require preventive treatments.

22. What is an appropriate strategy for migraine pharmacotherapy?

There are a number of acute treatment options for migraine. When migraine is mild or moderate, simple analgesics such as aspirin, acetaminophen, or nonsteroidal antiinflammatory drugs (NSAIDs) may be sufficient. Caffeine enhances the effectiveness of simple analgesics (e.g., Excedrin, Anacin) and may have special benefits in migraine if used infrequently, less than 4 times a month. The addition of a barbiturate increases treatment effects in some patients (e.g., Fiorinal, Fioricent, Esgic); however, these compounds may be associated with an increased risk of sedation, rebound headache, tolerance, physical dependence and addiction, so use them cautiously. Isometheptene is a simple, safe, vasoactive compound that can be used in combination with analgesics to relieve headache. When nausea or vomiting is present, adding an antiemetic/prokinetic agent, such as metoclopramide, may enhance the effectiveness of the simple analgesics.

In addition, there is a category of migraine-specific acute treatments. These include ergotamine, dihydroergotamine, and the triptans.

23. How do the migraine-specific acute treatments work?

Migraine-specific acute treatments are believed to act on presynaptic 5-HT1 receptors on trigeminal nerve endings, on the blood vessels, and within the brain itself. Activation of the 5-HT1 receptor blocks the release of substance P, calcitonin gene–related peptide, and neurokinin A, and ameliorates the development of neurogenic inflammation. Ergotamine and dihydroergotamine activate a broad range of receptors, whereas the triptans are highly selective for the 5-HT1 class of receptors. Other 5-HT1 agonist drugs are currently in development for the acute treatment of migraine.

24. What triptans are available?

As of this writing there are eight triptans marketed in the United States: sumatriptan (Imitrex), zolmitriptan (Zomig), rizatriptan (Maxalt), naratriptan (Amerge), almotriptan (Axert), frovatriptan (Frova), eletriptan (Relpax), and sumatriptan/naproxen sodium (Treximet).

25. How do the available triptans compare?

The marketed triptans are highly effective acute treatments for migraine. They are all agonists at 5HT1b/d receptors. They differ in pharmacokinetic profiles, modes of metabolism, available routes of administration, and to some degree, efficacy and tolerability. Sumatriptan was the first available agent in this class and is the most extensively studied and widely used of these agents. It is marketed in three oral doses (25, 50, and 100 mg), as 5- and 20-mg nasal spray, and as 4- and 6-mg subcutaneous injection. Zolmitriptan is available as 2.5- and 5-mg tablets, 2.5- and 5-mg nasal spray, and 2.5- and 5-mg rapidly dissolvable oral wafers. Rixatriptan is available as 5- and 10-mg tablets and 5- and 10-mg wafers; it has efficacy advantages but similar tolerability to sumatriptan. Naratriptan is available as 1- and 2.5-mg tablets; it is less effective than sumatriptan but has superior tolerability and a lower rate of headache recurrence. Almotriptan is available as 6.25- and 12.5-mg tablet and has similar efficacy but superior tolerability to sumatriptan. Frovatriptan is available as 2.5-mg oral tablets, eletriptan is available as 20- and 40-mg oral tablets, and treximet is available as an 80/500-mg tablet.

26. How do you choose from among the acute treatment options?

Acute treatments should be matched to the overall severity of the patient's illness, the severity of the patient's attack, the profile of associated symptoms, and the patient's treatment preferences. This strategy of individualizing treatment from the first is termed *stratified care* and is recommended by the US Headache Consortium. It is supported by a randomized trial.

Simple analgesics and combination analgesics may be adequate for mild to moderate migraine attacks. More severe attacks often require specific migraine therapy. In addition, when nausea or vomiting is prominent, the associated gastric paresis may limit the effectiveness of oral agents. In this context, nonoral agents such as injections, suppositories, and nasal sprays offer advantages. Patients often have strong treatment preferences for one route versus another. Some patients consider suppositories anathema, and others would prefer to avoid injections. Many patients favor nasal sprays as the nonoral route of choice.

Treatment requirements also vary with the context of an attack. If an attack begins before a major business meeting, a rapid parenteral treatment may be needed. If the attack begins on a Saturday morning, the patient may prefer to use a slower oral treatment. Optimal therapy often requires that patients receive more than one treatment. The following are some examples of how treatment is tailored to match patient needs:

- For the patient who awakens with severe, full-blown attacks with prominent nausea and vomiting, non-oral therapy may be the only effective option.
- For patients who have attacks that begin gradually or who are unsure if the attack will be mild or severe, it is best to begin with oral agents and escalate therapy if the attack increases in severity.
- For a patient with both moderate and severe attacks, treatment may begin with an NSAID (plus metoclopramide), and a triptan can be used either as an "escape medication" or for the more severe attacks.

27. **What is the role of triptans in acute migraine therapy?**
The triptans are the most effective and most specific of the available acute treatments for migraine. Response rates to the 6-mg subcutaneous injection of sumatriptan are about 70% to 90%, depending on the study. Response to 50-mg sumatriptan tablets develops more slowly, with overall response rates of about 60% at 2 hours. The choice between oral and injectable triptans should be based on the need for rapid relief and the effectiveness of the alternative routes of administration. If the headaches begin slowly and gradually progress in severity, oral triptans are appropriate and preferred by most patients. For patients who awaken with disabling headache, who require very rapid relief, or who have prominent gastrointestinal disturbances, parenteral treatment offers important advantages.

Note that subcutaneous sumatriptan should not be given during the aura. It is best to wait until pain develops before treating.

28. **When should acute medications be given during the migraine attack?**
Acute medications work most effectively when given while pain is still mild; this has been shown in post hoc analyses for aspirin plus metoclopramide, ergotamine, and sumatriptan, and in specifically designed clinical trials for sumatriptan. The benefits of early treatment need to be balanced against the risks of rebound headache caused by medication overuse. For patients who can identify headaches likely to become disabling, outcomes may improve with early treatment. Though all treatments work best if given while pain is mild, these effects appear most pronounced for triptans.

29. **What are the contraindications for the triptans?**
All of the 5-HT1 agonists are contraindicated in patients with a history of myocardial infarction, ischemic heart disease, migraine with prolonged or complicated aura, and other forms of vascular compromise. Carefully evaluate patients with risk factors for heart disease before prescribing a triptan. Serious side effects are extremely rare, but mild side effects are common. These side effects include pain at the injection site, tingling, flushing, burning, warmth, and hot sensations. In addition, noncardiac chest pressure occurs in approximately 4% of migraine sufferers; be sure to advise patients of these adverse events. Treximet is also contraindicated for anyone in whom an NSAID is contraindicated.

30. **How do you treat the nausea and vomiting of migraine?**
The associated symptoms of migraine, including nausea and vomiting, may be as disabling as the head pain in some patients. Gastric stasis and delayed gastric emptying can decrease the effectiveness of all medications. Most acute medications relieve the nausea and the pain together. Triptans effectively relieve both pain and nausea. Antiemetics such as metoclopramide, promethazine, or prochlorperazine may be used to treat both the nausea and the pain of migraine.

31. **What is the role of opiates in the treatment of migraine?**
Oral opioids, usually in the form of aspirin or acetaminophen and codeine (with or without caffeine and butalbital), are widely prescribed. If these agents relieve pain and restore the ability to function, they provide an appropriate therapeutic option. However, because of the risk of tolerance, physical

dependence, addiction, and rebound headache, they are best reserved for compliant patients with relatively infrequent attacks.

Injectable opioids and antiemetics are still widely used in urgent care settings. In double-blind studies, these drugs have proved to be moderately effective at relieving pain. Pain relief may be accompanied by sedation, limiting the ability of these agents to restore normal function.

32. What is the role of transnasal butorphanol (Stadol)?

Transnasal butorphanol (TB) is a mixed opiate agonist-antagonist available as a nasal spray and sold under the brand name Stadol. The convenient route of administration leads to rapid absorption and pain relief, even in patients with prominent nausea and vomiting. This therapeutic option is especially useful in patients with nocturnal headaches or prominent gastrointestinal symptoms, as well as those with contraindications, side effects, or lack of response to the migraine-specific agents.

TB produces sedation or orthostatic hypotension in about half of patients. Use should be limited to 2 headache days per week. Patients should be instructed to lie down after administration of the drug to minimize side effects.

33. Who should get preventive therapy?

Acute treatment is necessary for virtually everyone with migraine, but preventive medication should be used only under special circumstances, including the following:

- When patients have two or more attacks per month that produce disability lasting 3 or more days per month
- If symptomatic medication is contraindicated or ineffective (Even patients with less frequent pain and disability may be good candidates for preventive treatment in this case.)
- When abortive medication is required more than twice a week
- When headache attacks produce profound, prolonged disruption

34. What are the preventive treatment choices?

The major groups of medication used for migraine prophylaxis include the beta-blockers, antidepressants, serotonin antagonists, anticonvulsants, and calcium-channel blockers. Many of these agents work either by blocking 5-HT2 receptor sites or by downregulating them. Onabotulinum toxin type A is FDA approved for chronic migraine. Chronic migraine is defined as headaches occurring at least 15 days a month, 8 of which are migraine type, for more than 3 months with a minimum duration of 4 hours without treatment.

35. How do you choose from among the preventive treatment options?

If preventive medication is indicated, treatments are selected primarily based on side-effect profiles (Table 11.2) and comorbid conditions. For example, in a patient with migraine and hypertension, beta-blockers or calcium-channel blockers can be used to treat both conditions simultaneously. Similarly, in a patient with migraine and depression, antidepressants may be especially useful. In the patient with migraine and epilepsy, divalproex sodium or topiramate may be appropriate for both. For a patient with migraine and manic-depressive illness, divalproex sodium provides an opportunity to treat two conditions with a single drug.

Comorbid illnesses may also impose therapeutic restrictions. For example, in the patient with migraine and low blood pressure, beta-blockers and calcium-channel blockers are difficult to use. Similarly, in the patient with migraine and epilepsy, caution is advisable because tricyclic antidepressants may lower seizure threshold. The patient with migraine and asthma or Raynaud's syndrome probably should not be treated with beta-blockers. Finally, in patients concerned about sedation or increased appetite, tricyclic antidepressants are not an appropriate choice.

36. What are the principles of using preventive drugs?

In general, drugs should be started at a relatively low dose to avoid side effects. The dose should then be gradually increased until therapeutic effects develop, side effects develop, or the ceiling dose for the agent in question is reached. Because of the need to gradually increase the dose of most of these drugs, a therapeutic trial may take several months. Patients should be advised that treatment effects develop slowly, so that therapy is not discontinued prematurely. An adequate therapeutic trial is at least 8 weeks on a particular medication titrated up to a therapeutic dose, unless intolerable side effects occur. If one agent fails after an adequate therapeutic trial, it is best to choose an agent from a different therapeutic category. However, in the presence of strong relative indications or contraindications, it may be appropriate to choose a second agent within the same category.

Table 11.2. Preventive Agents for Migraine

CATEGORY	DRUG NAME	TOTAL DAILY DOSE	DAILY FREQUENCY	SIDE EFFECTS
Beta-blocker	Propranolol	80–320 mg	2–4 times	Fatigue, depression, light-headedness, impotence. Should not be used or should be used with caution if patient suffers from asthma, emphysema, heart failure, or diabetes.
	Nadolol	40–160 mg	Once	
	Atenolol**	50–100 mg	Once	
	Timolol**	10–60 mg	1–3 times	
Calcium-channel blockers	Verapamil	240–480 mg	1–4 times*	Light-headedness, constipation.
Tricyclic antidepressants	Amitriptyline	50–150 mg	Divided or at bedtime	Drowsiness, dry mouth, weight gain, blurred vision, constipation, difficulty urinating. Should not be used if patient suffers from glaucoma, prostate disorders, or arrhythmias.
	Nortriptyline	50–150 mg		
	Doxepin	50–150 mg		
Cyproheptadine		12–32 mg	3–4 times	Drowsiness, increased appetite, weight gain.
Antiepileptic Divalproex**		500–2000 mg daily	2–4 times	Tremor, sedation, weight gain, hair loss, hepatic dysfunction.
Topamax**		100–400 mg	Divided 2–3 times a day	Cognitive dysfunction, paresthesias, weight loss, eye pain.
Zonisamide		100–400 mg	Divided 2–3 times a day	Side effects same as Topamax but less frequent and less severe.
Lamotrigine		100–200 mg	Divided 2 times a day	Rash and possible Stevens Johnson syndrome.
Levaracitam		500–2000 mg	Divided 2 times a day	Sedation, fatigue
Muscle relaxer	Tizanadine	4–24 mg	Divided 2–4 times a day	Sedation, dry mouth
Onabotulinum***	Toxin A	200 units	Every 12 weeks	

*Ordinary verapamil must be administered in divided doses. There is a sustained release preparation that can be used once daily.
**FDA approved for treatment of migraines.
***FDA approved for chronic daily headaches.

37. **What is chronic or transformed migraine?**

   Chronic or transformed migraine is the single most common condition seen in headache specialty centers in the United States. The patient with chronic migraine typically begins with ordinary attacks of episodic migraine. Over time, attacks increase in frequency but may decrease in average severity. The patient is left with a condition characterized by daily or near-daily attacks that resemble TTH, often with superimposed interval headaches with most or all of the features of full-blown migraine. Chronic migraine must be defined based on a longitudinal history of headache, not simply the headache features at the time of consultation. Chronic migraine is defined as experiencing 15 or more headaches monthly, of which 8 are migraines, for more than 3 months, lasting more than 4 hours/day.

38. **Why is chronic migraine a formidable therapeutic challenge?**

   Eighty percent of patients with transformed migraine overuse analgesics, combination tablets, or ergot alkaloids. These medications sustain the cycle of ongoing daily headache through the mechanism of medication withdrawal. The key to treatment is eliminating the overused medications. Preventive therapies generally do not become fully effective until the pattern of medication overuse is broken.

39. **How is chronic migraine treated?**

   The best approach to treating transformed migraine is prevention. Rebound headaches can be prevented by restricting the use of all acute medications to 2 or at most 3 days/week. Particular caution is needed with analgesics containing caffeine, narcotics, or barbiturates and ergotamine. NSAIDs can be used more frequently with minimal risk of rebound headache. Triptans have been reported to cause rebound headaches. In the outpatient setting, the treatment of rebound headache generally involves substituting an NSAID for the overused medication. Particular caution is needed to avoid barbiturate and opiate withdrawal. At times, rebound headaches may require inpatient therapy.

   Onabotulinum toxin type A (Botox) is derived from the anaerobic bacteria *Clostridium botulinum*. It has been FDA approved for the treatment of CM since October 2010. CM are defined as greater than 15 headache days a month for more than 3 months and at least 8 of these days have migraine features. These headaches should last at least 4 hours. The injections are done every 12 weeks.

40. **Who needs inpatient treatment, and why?**

   The overwhelming majority of migraine sufferers do not require inpatient treatment. Inpatient treatment is indicated when patients experience frequent disabling attacks that do not respond to optimal outpatient therapy. Patients with significant medical or psychiatric comorbidities, patients who are emotionally exhausted by ongoing pain, and patients who are fearful of headache pain sometimes require inpatient therapy. For these patients, early inpatient treatment may be optimally cost-effective.

   The key to inpatient treatment of transformed migraine is the use of parenteral drugs such as intravenous dihydroergotamine in combination with metoclopramide. These agents are often given every 8 hours over a period of several days to taper the pattern of medication overuse. At the same time, an effective program of migraine prevention is initiated, and various behavioral modalities of pain control are introduced.

41. **What are the emerging treatments for migraines?**

   Early phase II studies showed positive results for calcitonin gene related peptide (CGRP) inhibitors in episodic and chronic migraine. This class of drug is now in phase III trials. All available data point to CGRP antibodies as a step forward in migraine prevention, with potential advantages in tolerability and treatment adherence; however, the ideal dose and long-term neurological and systemic safety must be refined.

KEY POINTS

1. Migraine is a highly prevalent health problem that affects approximately 11% of the US population.
2. There are no specific tests that are required to diagnose migraine; rather, diagnostic testing is used when the clinical suspicion is high that a secondary headache disorder is present.
3. Acute migraine treatment will be necessary for virtually everyone with migraine.
4. Preventive medication should be used for patients who have two or more attacks per month that produce disability lasting 3 or more days per month, when acute migraine therapies are contraindicated or ineffective, when abortive medication is required more than twice a week, and/or when headache attacks produce profound, prolonged disruption.

BIBLIOGRAPHY

1. Goadsby PJ, Lipton RB, Ferrari MD. Migraine: current understanding and management. *N Engl J Med.* 2001;346:257-270.
2. Headache Classification Subcommittee of the International Headache Society. The international classification of headache disorders. *Cephalgia.* 2013;32(9):629-808.
3. Lipton RB, Goadsby PJ, Sawyer J, et al. Migraine: diagnosis and assessment of disability, 3rd ed. *Rev Contemp Pharmacother.* 2000;11:63-73.
4. Silberstein SD, Holland S, Freitag F. Evidence-based guideline update: Pharmacologic treatment for episodic migraine prevention in adults: report of the Quality Standards Subcommittee of the American Academy of Neurology and the American Headache Society. *Neurology.* 2012;78(17):1337-1345.
5. Silberstein SD, Saper JR, Freitag FG. Migraine: diagnosis and treatment. In: Silberstein SD, Lipton RB, Dalessio DJ, eds. *Wolff's Headache and Other Head Pain.* 7th ed. New York: Oxford University Press; 2001:121-238.
6. Burch RC, Loder S, Loder E, Smitherman TA. The prevalence and burden of migraine and severe headache in the United States: updated statistics from government health surveillance studies. *Headache.* 2015;55(1):22-34.

CLUSTER HEADACHE

Grace Forde

CHAPTER 12

1. **What is a cluster headache?**

   Like migraine, cluster is a primary headache disorder but with significantly different clinical features. Cluster headaches are characterized by attacks of excruciatingly severe, unilateral head pain. Attacks last 15 to 180 minutes and recur from once every other day up to 8 times daily. These painful episodes are associated with autonomic features, including ptosis, miosis, conjunctival injection, lacrimation, and rhinorrhea, on the side of the pain.

   In episodic cluster, attacks occur in "clusters" lasting weeks to months, separated by periods of pain-free "remission" lasting months to years. Times of frequent headache are called "cluster periods."

   The second edition of the International Classification of Headache Disorders (ICHD II) defines five clinical criteria for cluster headache (Box 12.1).

2. **Are cluster headaches common? Who is affected?**

   Fortunately, cluster headache is relatively rare, affecting approximately 0.05% to 0.1% of the US population. Cluster headache is one of only two headache disorders that occur more often in men. Men are affected 3.5 to 7 times more often than women. In contrast, migraine occurs in women 3 times more often than in men. Most patients begin experiencing cluster headache between the ages of 20 and 50 (mean age is 30), though the age of onset ranges from early childhood through age 80.

   Women with cluster have a later average age of onset than men. Unlike migraine, there is no link between menses and cluster headaches; like migraine, clusters may disappear during pregnancy and may be triggered by the use of oral contraceptives.

3. **What are the characteristics of cluster headaches?**

   The pain of cluster begins abruptly, usually without warning, and reaches maximum intensity within 1 to 15 minutes. The pain is excruciating, deep, and boring, and is often described as a "red-hot poker" in or behind the affected eye. The pain is usually most severe in the orbital and retroorbital regions and may radiate into the ipsilateral temple, upper teeth and gums, and neck. Unlike migraine pain, which may alternate sides, the pain of cluster is generally unilateral; only 10% to 15% of sufferers report side-shift in subsequent bouts. Rarely, patients with typical cluster report that an aura—identical to that described in migraine—precedes an attack.

4. **When do bouts occur?**

   The majority of cluster sufferers note a phenomenon called periodicity—attacks recur around the same time each day during the entire cluster cycle. Approximately 75% of attacks occur between 9 p.m. and 10 a.m. About half of all cluster sufferers report nocturnal attacks that awaken them from sleep. Attacks typically occur within 2 hours of falling asleep and are often associated with rapid eye movement sleep.

   Manzoni et al. studied attack characteristics in 180 cluster sufferers and noted a higher incidence of individual attacks occurring between 1 a.m. and 2 a.m., 1 p.m. and 3 p.m., and at 9 p.m. Thus cluster patients cycle in and out of cluster periods, but during cluster periods the individual headaches occur with regular patterns. For these reasons, cluster is considered a chronobiologic disorder.

5. **What is the explanation for periodicity of cluster headache?**

   Recent evidence points to a dysfunctional hypothalamic pacemaker. The suprachiasmatic nucleus of the hypothalamus controls circadian rhythms such as the sleep-wake cycle and regulates the secretion of melatonin by the pineal gland. Dysfunction of the suprachiasmatic nucleus could explain the periodicity of cluster headache. Positron emission tomography scans during acute bouts of cluster headache have revealed increased activation in the region of the hypothalamic gray matter.

> **Box 12.1.** International Classification of Headache Disorders Diagnostic Criteria for Cluster Headache
>
> 1. At least five attacks fulfilling B–D
> 2. Severe or very unilateral orbital, supraorbital, and/or temporal pain lasting 15 to 180 min if untreated[1]
> 3. Headache is accompanied by at least one of the following signs, which have to be present on the pain side:
>   a. Ipsilateral conjunctival injection and/or lacrimation
>   b. Ipsilateral nasal congestion and or rhinorrhea
>   c. Ipsilateral eyelid edema
>   d. Ipsilateral forehead and facial sweating
>   e. Ipsilateral miosis and/or ptosis
>   f. A sense of restlessness or agitation
> 4. Attacks have a frequency from one every other day to 8 per day[2]
> 5. Not attributed to another disorder[3]
>
> [1]During part (but less than half) of the time-course of cluster headache, attacks may be less severe and/or of shorter or longer duration.
> [2]During part (but less than half) of the time-course of cluster headache, attacks may be less frequent.
> [3]History and physical and neurologic examinations do not suggest any of the disorders listed in groups 5 to 12, or history and/or physical and/or neurologic examinations do suggest such disorder, but it is ruled out by appropriate investigations, or such disorder is present, but attacks do not occur for the first time in close temporal relation to the disorder.

6. **What is known about the pathophysiology of cluster headaches?**
   Although the exact pathophysiologic mechanism is not fully understood, recent work has given us insight into the pathways and structures that are most likely involved. The pain of cluster is carried into the central nervous system through the nociceptive branches of the first division of the trigeminal nerve. This branch (V_1), innervates the pain-sensitive intracranial structures such as the dura and its blood vessels, and activation of the trigeminovascular pathway causes the release of substance P and calcitonin gene-related peptide (CGRP). CGRP release produces vasodilation of the dural blood vessels and induces neurogenic inflammation. Activation of this system in cluster is evidenced by the findings of increased blood levels of CGRP in the external jugular vein during an acute attack of cluster.
   The autonomic features that accompany the pain suggest that there is activation of the cranial parasympathetic pathway. Fibers within this pathway originate from neurons arising within the superior salivatory nucleus. These first-order neurons travel with the seventh cranial nerve, synapsing in the pterygopalatine ganglia. The postganglionic fibers supply vasomotor and secretory innervation to the cerebral vessels, lacrimal glands, and nasal mucosal glands, which produces the clinical features seen with cluster. A marker for cranial parasympathetic activation, vasoactive intestinal peptide (VIP), is also elevated in the external jugular blood during cluster attacks. These pathways have been termed the "trigeminal autonomic reflex."
   The Horner syndrome that accompanies cluster is postganglionic and likely located within the cavernous sinus, because it is here that the sympathetic, parasympathetic, and trigeminal fibers meet. It is possible, therefore, that activation of both the trigeminovascular and cranial parasympathetic systems occurs in the setting of a disordered hypothalamic pacemaker that may be dysfunctional during the cluster period.

7. **Are cluster headaches triggered by the same things as migraine?**
   A very small minority of cluster sufferers report that typical migraine triggers induce their headaches. These include stress, relaxation after stress, exposure to heat or cold, and certain foods such as chocolate, dairy, or eggs. Alcohol is a common precipitant of cluster headache, affecting more than half of all sufferers. Alcohol tends to trigger attacks 5 to 45 minutes after ingestion. Interestingly, this trigger is present only during the active "cluster" phase of the disorder; imbibing alcohol-containing beverages during the "remission" phase does not trigger an attack. Sublingual nitroglycerine can also induce attacks.

8. **Are there different types of cluster?**
   Yes. Typical cluster may be divided into two forms: episodic and chronic. About 90% of cluster sufferers experience the episodic form, in which discrete attacks recur in cycles, usually lasting 1 to

3 months, separated by pain-free remissions lasting from 1 month to several years. Many patients with episodic cluster headaches experience one or two bouts yearly (typically in the spring or fall).

In chronic cluster, attacks recur on a daily or near-daily basis for more than 1 year without remission or with remissions lasting less than 1 month. Chronic cluster has two temporal profiles: (1) in some patients the chronic form begins from onset (previously classified as primary chronic), and (2) others begin with an initially episodic form that evolves into the chronic form (previously called "secondary chronic"). The evolving subtype affects approximately 10% of cluster sufferers, and may occur more frequently in patients who experience a later onset of the episodic form.

The ICHD II also considers the paroxysmal hemicranias as a form of cluster headache (see Chapter 14).

9. **How are cluster headaches diagnosed?**
   The diagnosis of cluster headache rests primarily on the history. Despite the distinctive features of the headache, cluster sufferers consult an average of five physicians prior to receiving the correct diagnosis. Their severe headaches are often misdiagnosed as migraine. Or, if pain radiates into the upper teeth and gums, it is mistakenly related to dental pathology. Frontal pain, nasal congestion, and/or rhinorrhea may be attributed to sinus disease. Refer to Box 11.1.

10. **How is cluster headache differentiated from the paroxysmal hemicranias?**
    Features of cluster that distinguish it from the paroxysmal hemicranias include the following: an overwhelming male predominance, a lack of mechanical trigger mechanisms, a lesser number of daily attacks, a longer duration of each attack, and specific patterns of treatment response (Table 12.1).

11. **How do you determine whether a headache is cluster or migraine?**
    Cluster is differentiated from migraine by a number of important features. Migraine tends to be more prevalent in females, begins at an earlier age, demonstrates side-shift from attack to attack, and is associated with nausea, vomiting, photophobia, phonophobia, and osmophobia. In migraine, attacks

Table 12.1. Differential Diagnosis of Cluster Headaches

	CLUSTER	HEMICRANIA CONTINUA	MIGRAINE	PAROXYSMAL HEMICRANIAS
Sex F:M	1:6	1.8:1	3:1	2.13:1
Age of onset	20–40	11–58	Teens-20s	6–81
Pain quality	Stabbing, boring	Baseline dull ache, superimposed throbbing/stabbing	Throbbing, pulsatile	Stabbing, pulsatile, throbbing
Site of maximal pain	Orbit/temple	Orbit/temple	Temple/forehead	Orbit/temple
Attacks per day	0–8	Varies	0–1	1–40
Duration of untreated attacks	15–180 min (average 20–45)	2–45 mins	4–72 h	2–120 min (average 2–25)
Autonomic features	+	+ (but less pronounced than cluster)	−	+
Aura	−	−	+ in 15–20%	−
Patient's behavior during attack	Pacing/rocking	Pacing or rest	Rest/sleep	Pacing/rocking
Oxygen may abort acute attacks	+ in 80%	−	+ in 20%	−

last longer, do not occur multiple times daily, and are usually not associated with autonomic features ipsilateral to the pain. Additionally, only rarely is there an aura in cluster (see Question 3). During cluster, patients pace, sit upright in a chair, or bang their heads against a wall, whereas migraine patients lie quietly in a dark room and attempt to sleep. Of note, recumbency actually increases the pain of cluster.

There are headaches with features of both migraine and cluster that cannot be adequately categorized in either group. These patients often have an intermediate disorder referred to as "cluster-migraine variant."

12. **How is cluster headache differentiated from hemicrania continua?**
Hemicrania continua is an underrecognized, benign disorder characterized by continuous, baseline, low-level discomfort. Sufferers report exacerbations of more severe pain, lasting from 5 minutes to a few days, superimposed on the baseline pain. These exacerbations are often associated with the ipsilateral autonomic features of cluster, although if present, they tend to be less pronounced than in cluster. The disorder is mistaken for cluster if the clinician or patient focuses on the exacerbations and misses the continuous, less severe pain. Hemicrania continua is uniquely responsive to treatment with indomethacin and fails to remit with standard anticluster therapy.

13. **Is it possible to prevent cluster attacks?**
Yes. Nearly all patients with cluster headache require preventive treatment. The short duration, high frequency, and remarkable severity of attacks make acute treatment unsatisfactory. A variety of anticluster agents can be used (Table 12.2).

Most headache specialists begin treatment with verapamil and a prednisone taper. Prednisone usually induces a rapid remission, but it has too many side effects for long-term use. Verapamil is generally safe and well tolerated, but its benefits develop over 1 to 2 weeks. Accordingly, prednisone is started at 60 to 80 mg daily for 1 week. In the second week, prednisone is tapered by 10 mg per day. Verapamil is started at a dose of 240 mg daily and often increased to 480 mg per day if tolerated. Sometimes, additional dose escalations are required. Prednisone is intended to induce a rapid remission; verapamil is intended to prevent attacks until the cluster cycle is over.

If verapamil fails, lithium carbonate may also be tried. Lithium tends to be more efficacious in the chronic form. Valproic acid has been proven useful in both forms.

14. **How long should prophylactic therapy be continued?**
Patients should be maintained on preventive medications for slightly longer than their typical cycles; for example, if the cluster period usually lasts 6 weeks, keep patients on their anticluster regimen for 8 weeks and then gradually taper the preventive medications. Recurrences are treated by adjusting the dosage upward, and then retapering at a later date.

Table 12.2. Treatment of Cluster Headaches

DRUG	DOSE (mg/day)	COMMENTS
Medications Used Preventively		
Verapamil	240–960	Useful in all forms; sometimes doses above the 480-mg maximum on the label are required
Valproic acid	500–3000	Useful in all forms
Lithium carbonate	300–1500	Best for chronic cluster
Medications Used Abortively		
Oxygen	8–10 mg L/min via face mask for 10–15 min	—
Sumatriptan	6 mg SQ	Maximum of two injections daily
DHE	0.5–1 mg SQ/IM	Maximum 2 mg/day and 6 mg/week

DHE, Dihydroergotamine; *IM*, intramuscular; *SQ*, subcutaneous.

15. **How are acute attacks treated?**
    The two acute treatment alternatives for cluster are oxygen and sumatriptan. Oxygen is usually administered via a face mask or nasal cannula for 10 to 15 minutes. Subcutaneous sumatriptan 6 mg rapidly aborts attacks of cluster in 5 to 10 minutes in most patients. Unfortunately, the drug cannot be given more than twice daily, and sufferers may have more than two attacks daily. Dihydroergotamine (DHE) 0.5–1.0 mg administered intramuscularly or subcutaneously is also effective. Ergot suppositories at bedtime may prevent nighttime headaches in patients with nocturnal attacks.
    DHE is not specifically indicated for cluster headache. Sumatriptan has received FDA approval for treatment of cluster headaches.

16. **If these medications fail to break the attacks, what else can be done?**
    Medically refractory patients can be treated in a number of ways. Hospitalization and treatment with repetitive DHE and metoclopramide every 8 hours has been proven to break cluster cycles. Alternatively, ipsilateral occipital nerve blocks occasionally help. For patients refractory to these treatments, percutaneous glycerol injections into the trigeminal cistern, percutaneous radiofrequency trigeminal rhizotomy, or decompression of the nervus intermedius can be tried. Recently, success has been reported in a small series of patients with intractable cluster headaches treated with hypothalamic deep brain stimulation.
    Alternative and complementary therapies should be tried because cluster headaches can be so debilitating. Melatonin has shown modest effectiveness in treating nighttime attacks. There is also some evidence that capsaicin, used intranasally, might reduce the frequency and severity of the cluster headache attack.

17. **Name a few potentially dangerous syndromes that can present with symptoms similar to cluster headache.**
    The differential diagnosis has to include any syndromes that can present with retroorbital pain and ptosis. One of the more serious syndromes is carotid artery dissection. Pain is sometimes felt behind the eye, and because the sympathetic fibers ascend with the carotid artery, Horner syndrome may be present. Similarly, disease in the cavernous sinus can produce periorbital pain and ptosis. However, in these patients the pupil is usually large, rather than small, because the ptosis is due to a third-nerve palsy, rather than sympathetic dysfunction.

KEY POINTS

1. Cluster headaches are characterized by attacks of excruciatingly severe, unilateral head pain; 75% of the attacks occur between 9 p.m. and 10 a.m.
2. The pain of cluster begins abruptly, usually without warning, and reaches maximum intensity within 1 to 15 minutes. The pain is excruciating, deep, and boring, and is often described as a "red-hot poker" in or behind the affected eye.
3. In contrast to migraine, men are affected more commonly than women.
4. Both acute and chronic forms of cluster headache exist.
5. The practitioner should be aware of the specific acute and prophylactic therapies that are effective for cluster headache.

BIBLIOGRAPHY

1. Bahra A, May A, Goadsby PJ. Cluster headache: a prospective clinical study with diagnostic implications. *Neurology.* 2002;58(3):354-361.
2. Ekbom K, Hardebo JE. Cluster headache: etiology, diagnosis and management. *Drugs.* 2002;62(1):61-69.
3. Headache Classification Subcommittee of the International Headache Society. The international classification of headache disorders. *Cephalalgia.* 2013;32(9):629-808.
4. Leone M, Bussone G. A review of hormonal findings in cluster headache: evidence for hypothalamic involvement. *Cephalalgia.* 1993;13:309-317.
5. Leone M, Franzini A, Broggi G, Bussone G. Hypothalamic deep brain stimulation for intractable cluster headache: a 3 year follow-up. *Neurol Sci.* 2003;24(suppl 2):143-145.
6. Manzoni GC, Terzano MG, Bono G, et al. Cluster headache—clinical features in 180 patients. *Cephalalgia.* 1983;3:21-30.

7. May A, Bahra A, Büchel C, Frackowiak RS, Goadsby PJ. Hypothalamic activation in cluster headache attacks. *Lancet.* 1998;351:275-278.
8. May A, Bahra A, Büchel C, Frackowiak RS, Goadsby PJ. PET and MRA findings in cluster headache and MRA in experimental pain. *Neurology.* 2000;55(9):1328-1335.
9. Newman LC, Goadsby P, Lipton RB. Cluster and related headaches. *Med Clin North Am.* 2001;85:997-1016.
10. Newman LC, Lipton RB, Solomon S. Hemicrania continua: ten new cases and a review of the literature. *Neurology.* 1994;44:2111-2114.
11. Swanson JW, Yanagihara T, Stang PE, et al. Incidence of cluster headaches: a population-based study in Olmstead County, Minnesota. *Neurology.* 1994;44:433-437.
12. Taha JM, Tew JM Jr. Long-term results of radio frequency rhizotomy in the treatment of cluster headache. *Headache.* 1995;35:193-196.

CHAPTER 13

TENSION-TYPE HEADACHE

Grace Forde

1. **Is there a medical term for the headaches of everyday life?**
   Yes. The most common form of primary headache is tension-type headache (TTH). Almost everyone experiences a TTH at one time or another, and about 40% of the population has had one within the past year. Although occurrence is slightly higher in females, the gender ratio is very close to 1:1. TTH affects individuals of all ages but is most common in middle life. It is seven times more common than migraine but is much less disabling. Nonetheless, because it is so common, TTH causes a societal impact equivalent to or greater than that of migraine.

2. **What is meant by "primary" and "secondary" headache?**
   In primary headaches, the headache is the problem. In secondary headaches, the headache is symptomatic of an underlying condition such as a brain tumor.

3. **What is the approach to diagnosing tension-type headache?**
   The steps in the diagnosis of TTH resemble the steps in the diagnosis of migraine. Secondary headache disorders are excluded based on a directed history and a careful general medical and neurologic examination. If red flags are present, a workup is required to diagnose or exclude secondary causes of headache. If no such red flags are noted by history or exam, the next step is to diagnose a specific primary headache disorder. If the patient fits neatly into a standard diagnostic category, a diagnosis is assigned and treatment is initiated. If the headache is atypical and does not meet criteria for a primary headache disorder, revisit the possibility of a secondary headache.

4. **How is tension-type headache defined?**
   TTH are characterized by recurrent attacks of head pain without specific associated features. To diagnose TTH, the International Headache Society requires a history of at least 10 lifetime attacks. Early in the course of TTH, however, patients will not yet have experienced that number of attacks. To make the diagnosis, two of the following four pain features should be present:
   - Pain on both sides of the head (bilateral pain)
   - Pain that is a steady ache or a pressure pain
   - Pain that is mild or moderate in severity
   - Pain that is not exacerbated by routine physical activity

   The pain of TTH is often bifrontal, bioccipital, or nuchal. It may be described as a squeezing sensation akin to wearing a hat that is too tight, as a headband of pain, or as a pressure sensation at the vertex of the head. On occasion, the pain is associated with palpation tenderness of the pericranial muscles. Headaches typically last from 30 minutes to several days, but a duration of several hours is most common.

5. **What is the frequency of tension-type headache?**
   TTH is the most common type of headache experienced, with a lifetime prevalence of 88% in women and 69% in men. They can occur daily especially during periods of stress and anxiety.

6. **Are there different types of tension-type headache?**
   It is traditional to divide TTH into two broad groups: episodic and chronic. By definition, episodic attacks occur less than 15 days/month (or 180 days/year), and chronic headache occurs 15 or more days per month for at least 6 months (or 180 days/year). Otherwise, the clinical features of the attacks are quite similar. Chronic TTH affects about 3% of the population.

7. **Discuss chronic tension-type headache in relation to chronic migraine**
   The differential diagnosis of chronic TTH includes chronic (or transformed) migraine. Although both chronic TTH and transformed migraine are characterized by frequent attacks of mild to moderate headache, these disorders are different. As the name implies, chronic migraine evolves out of

episodic migraine, as headaches increase in frequency and decrease in severity, and the specific migraine features remit. Chronic TTH may arise de novo or in individuals with episodic TTH. Those with chronic migraine may have occasional episodes of full-blown migraine.

8. **What is the differential diagnosis of tension-type headache?**
TTH must be distinguished from other primary and secondary headache disorders. Its bilateral location, mild to moderate pain intensity, and absence of autonomic features make differentiating it from cluster headache relatively easy (see Chapter 12). Its distinction from migraine is discussed in Question 9. Underlying structural or metabolic causes must be considered in patients who have headaches resembling TTH.

Early in their course, brain tumors and other intracranial mass lesions tend to produce bilateral, dull headaches, which may be difficult to distinguish from TTH. Headaches resulting from brain tumors tend to progress in frequency and severity, and they are often associated with focal neurologic symptoms and signs or evidence of increased intracranial pressure. When headaches of similar profile have been present for months or years and the neurologic exam is normal, secondary headaches are unlikely.

9. **How are tension-type headache and migraine differentiated?**
The diagnostic features of TTH and migraine contrast rather sharply.

Migraine Pain	TTH Pain
Unilateral	Bilateral
Throbbing or pulsatile	Steady ache or squeezing/pressure sensation
Moderate to severe	Mild or moderate
Aggravated by routine physical activity (e.g., climbing stairs)	Not aggravated

In addition, TTH is characterized by an absence of the migraine-defining associated symptoms. Specifically, episodic TTH is generally not accompanied by aura or nausea and only rarely by photophobia or phonophobia (not both).

10. **How are tension-type headache and sinus headache differentiated?**
TTH and sinus headache are often confused. This is especially likely when the headache is frontal in distribution; the location over the frontal and/or the maxillary sinuses creates diagnostic confusion. Sinus headaches are associated with sinus tenderness, fever, postnasal drip, and purulent nasal discharge. Sinus headaches rarely cause brief, recurrent headaches.

11. **What is the pathophysiology of tension-type headache?**
The mechanism of pain in TTH remains uncertain. This disorder was once called "muscle contraction headache," based on the assumption that excessive contraction of skeletal muscles of the neck and shoulder girdle produced pain. The term "tension headache" was sometimes used to suggest that stress or psychological tension was the fundamental cause of the disorder. The term "TTH" is intended to imply that we do not know what, if anything, is "tense." Although there are excess levels of muscle contraction in TTH, these levels do not exceed those found in patients with migraine. Although stress is a trigger for some people with TTH, the disorder can occur in the absence of stress, and high levels of stress can occur without TTH.

Some believe that TTH is a form of mild migraine, but response to the drug sumatriptan suggests that this is true only in some patients. According to the spectrum study, sumatriptan effectively treats TTH in individuals who also have migraine. In individuals without migraine, sumatriptan is ineffective (see Chapter 11). Factors that exacerbate TTH include oromandibular dysfunction, psychosocial stress, psychiatric disorders, and drug overuse.

12. **Is tension-type headache a genetic disorder?**
There is no clear evidence that episodic TTH runs in families. Recent studies do suggest that chronic TTH, like migraine, aggregates within families.

13. **What are the approaches to treating tension-type headache?**
The treatment of TTH, like the treatment of migraine, can be divided into two major categories: nonpharmacologic and pharmacologic therapies. The pharmacologic therapies are divided into acute (abortive) and preventive (prophylactic). Note that patients with mild and infrequent TTHs may simply

be looking for a diagnosis and reassurance that the headaches do not have a serious cause. These patients may not need prescription drugs.

14. **What are trigger factors?**
Trigger factors precipitate headache in a biologically vulnerable individual, but they are not the fundamental cause of headache. When devising a treatment plan, it is important to begin by identifying factors that exacerbate or trigger headaches and to distinguish trigger factors from causes. Psychological stress, perhaps related to a job or to a family situation, may be an important trigger factor. The traditional triggers of migraine, including dietary factors, missed meals, disrupted sleep, changes in the weather, and hormonal factors, occasionally contribute to TTH.

15. **True or false: Caffeine can trigger a headache.**
This is partially true: caffeine withdrawal can trigger a headache. If a patient drinks several cups of caffeinated beverages or takes caffeine-containing medications on a daily basis, the absence of caffeine can trigger headache. Some patients awaken on weekend mornings with a headache because they slept through their regular cup of coffee. Caffeine withdrawal headaches are quite common even in moderate caffeine users.

16. **What are the nonpharmacologic treatment options for episodic tension-type headache?**
Resolving stressful situations sometimes improves headache control. Stress management methods, including relaxation techniques or biofeedback, often are helpful. Cognitive-behavioral therapy also can be useful. Some patients find that postural factors (such as working long hours with an awkward head position) contribute to headache. For these patients, ergonomic changes in the workplace or simply getting up to stretch may be helpful. Regular meals, consistent sleep patterns, and exercise can help eliminate headache.
When TTH is associated with spasm or tenderness of the pericranial or cervical musculature, physical modalities, such as local application of heat or ice packs and the use of a cervical pillow, are sometimes helpful. Diathermy, physical therapy, massage, and trigger point injections are also employed. Transcutaneous electrical nerve stimulation has been reported to alleviate TTH.

17. **What are the acute treatment options for episodic tension-type headache?**
TTH can be treated with simple over-the-counter (OTC) analgesics such as aspirin, acetaminophen (Tylenol), ibuprofen (Advil, Nuprin), naproxen sodium (Aleve), and ketoprofen (Actron, Orudis KT). When OTC medications do not provide adequate relief, prescription drugs can be tried. Nonsteroidal antiinflammatory agents (NSAIDs) such as naproxen sodium (Anaprox), 550 mg, or diflunisal (Dolobid), 500 mg, may succeed when OTC NSAIDs could not. Transnasal opioids (Stadol NS) can be useful for severe TTHs refractory to other treatments; however, one must be very concerned with the potential for overuse of these types of agents. In general, acute medications should not be used more than 2 or at most 3 days/week to avoid rebound headaches.

18. **What is rebound headache?**
The medications that are used to relieve headache can become a cause of headache if overused. Virtually any medication can cause rebound headache, and therefore it is important to limit the dose of all acute medications. The medications that are most likely to cause rebound headaches are the combination analgesics such as the caffeine and butalbital-containing products. These include but are not limited to Fioricet, Fiorinal, Esgic, Excedrin, and Excedrin migraine. On average, episodic TTHs occur twice per month. In chronic TTH, with 15 or more headache days per month, the risk of rebound headache is substantial.

19. **Why is caffeine found in so many headache remedies?**
When caffeine is taken at the time of a headache, it increases the efficacy of analgesics. For this reason, patients often learn to drink a cup of coffee when they take a painkiller or use combination drugs that contain caffeine. The best advice is to limit caffeine intake on nonheadache days (to one cup of coffee or tea a day) and to save caffeine for its medicinal effects on headache days. Note that caffeine free and decaf are not the same thing—decaf still has caffeine, just less.

20. **Do preventive medications have a role in the treatment of tension-type headache?**
Preventive treatment is used for only a small minority of patients who suffer from TTH. Preventive medication should be considered in patients who have disability because of headaches 3 or more

days each month. In addition, preventive medication may play a role in treatment of patients at risk for rebound headache because of a frequent need for analgesics. If acute medication is ineffective or contraindicated, preventive therapy is a treatment option. Finally, if the patient has a comorbid condition (such as depression) that requires treatment, it is appropriate to treat both the headache disorder and the comorbid condition with a single drug, when possible.

21. **What are the preventive treatments of choice for tension-type headache?**
The most widely used drugs are the antidepressants. The tricyclic antidepressants are a standard choice. I prefer nortriptyline (Pamelor) and doxepin (Sinequan) because they have fewer anticholinergic side effects than amitriptyline (Elavil). The usual regimen starts with a low bedtime dose (10 or 25 mg), and the dose is gradually increased as needed and as tolerated. The selective serotonin-reuptake inhibitors (SSRIs) are sometimes used for prevention of TTH. Fluoxetine (Prozac) has been shown to be effective in a small controlled study of chronic daily headache. The other SSRIs have not been studied but are widely used.

If antidepressants are unsuccessful or contraindicated, many of the drugs used for the prevention of migraine may also be used for TTH. Calcium-channel blockers and divalproex sodium are generally more successful than beta-blockers. Daily administration of long-acting NSAIDs such as naproxen sodium is also sometimes used for prevention. The muscle relaxer tizanidine (Zanaflex) has also shown benefit in patients, especially in patients with chronic TTH.

22. **Are the management approaches for chronic tension-type headache and episodic tension-type headache the same or different?**
Behavioral interventions to reduce the frequency of attack are especially important for chronic TTH. Although the acute treatment options are similar, because of the frequency of attacks, patients with chronic TTH are at increased risk for rebound headache. Use of acute treatments that cause rebound headache should be avoided or severely limited. It is usually desirable to treat these patients with preventive medications.

KEY POINTS

1. TTH is the most common type of headache experienced.
2. The mechanism of TTH is uncertain.
3. Both symptomatic and prophylactic therapies are available for the treatment of TTH. Prophylactic agents should be considered for those patients with TTH who are experiencing more than 3 days of headache-related disability each month.

BIBLIOGRAPHY

1. Couch JR. Medical management of recurrent tension-type headache. In: Tollison CD, Kunkel RS, eds. *Headache Diagnosis and Treatment.* Baltimore: Williams and Wilkins; 1993:151-162.
2. Headache Classification Subcommittee of the International Headache Society. The international classification of headache disorders, 2nd ed. *Cephalgia.* 2004;24(suppl 1):9-160.
3. Jensen R, Bendtsen L, Olesen J. Muscular factors are of importance in tension-type headache. *Headache.* 1998;38:10-17.
4. Lipton RB, Bigal ME, Steiner TJ, Silberstein SD, Olesen J. Classification of primary headaches. *Neurology.* 2004;63(3):427-435.
5. Rasmussen BK, Jensen R, Schroll M, Olesen J. Epidemiology of headache in a general population: a prevalence study. *J Clin Epidemiol.* 1991;44:1147-1157.
6. Schwarts BS, Stewart WF, Simon D, Lipton RB. Epidemiology of tension-type headache. *JAMA.* 1998;279:381-383.
7. Selby G, Lance JW. Observation in 500 cases of migraine and allied vascular headaches. *J Neurol Neurosurg Psychiatry.* 1960;23:23-32.
8. Solomon S, Newman LC. Episodic tension-type headache. In: Silberstein SD, Lipton RB, Dalessio DJ, eds. *Wolff's Headache and Other Head Pain.* 7th ed. New York: Oxford University Press; 2001:238-246.
9. Warner JS. The outcome of treating patients with suspected rebound headache. *Headache.* 2001;41(7):685-692.
10. Martin MT. The diagnostic evaluation of secondary headache disorders. *Headache.* 2011;51(2):347.
11. Yancey J, Sheridan R, Koren K. Chronic daily headache:diagnosis and management. *Am Fam Physician.* 2014;89(8):642-648.

CHAPTER 14

THE PAROXYSMAL HEMICRANIAS

Grace Forde

1. **What are the paroxysmal hemicranias?**
   The paroxysmal hemicranias (PHs) are a group of rare, benign headache disorders that resemble cluster headache in most ways but are less responsive to medications typically effective for cluster headache. The PHs are characterized by severe, excruciating, throbbing, boring, or pulsatile pain affecting the orbital, supraorbital, and temporal regions. These pains are associated with at least one of the following signs or symptoms ipsilateral to the painful side:
   - Conjunctival injection
   - Lacrimation
   - Nasal congestion
   - Rhinorrhea
   - Ptosis
   - Eyelid edema

   Attacks occur from 1 to 40 times daily, usually exceeding eight attacks in a 24-hour period. Duration is typically 2 to 30 minutes, but on rare occasions attacks last as long as 2 hours. Headaches may occur any time during the day or night, and there is often a predisposition to nocturnal attacks, in which the patient is awakened from a sound sleep by an incapacitating headache.

2. **Are there different clinical variations of the paroxysmal hemicranias?**
   Yes. Although there has been controversy regarding the nomenclature of the PH, there appear to be three related forms:
   - Chronic paroxysmal hemicrania (CPH), in which multiple headaches occur daily for years on end without remission or with remission periods of less than 1 month
   - Episodic paroxysmal hemicrania (EPH), in which there are discrete phases characterized by frequent daily attacks separated by long-term, pain-free remissions
   - Pre-CPH, in which an initially episodic form of these headaches ultimately evolves into the chronic unremitting form

   Some authors prefer alternative nomenclature. At present, only CPH and EPH are recognized in the International Headache Society's diagnostic system, as outlined in the third edition of the International Classification of Headache Disorders (ICHD III beta).

3. **What distinguishes the paroxysmal hemicranias from cluster headache?**
   The major distinguishing features of the PH and cluster headache lie in the frequency of the attack, the duration of the attack, and the response to treatment. In addition, the PHs do not show the striking preponderance among males that characterizes cluster headache. In cluster headache, attacks are less frequent but of longer duration—one or two a day with a typical duration of 30 minutes to 2 hours. Attacks in the PH exceed five a day and last 2 to 25 minutes each.

4. **Do the paroxysmal hemicranias differ pathophysiologically from cluster headache?**
   The PHs, like cluster headache, belong to a group of headache disorders known as the trigeminal autonomic cephalgias (TACs). The TACs are characterized by cyclical episodes of severe headaches that are associated with cranial autonomic activation. These disorders share a common pathophysiologic mechanism, the trigeminal autonomic reflex (see Chapter 12).

   Like cluster headaches, the PH can be triggered by alcohol. Approximately 10% of patients with CPH report that attacks are precipitated either by bending or by rotating the head. Headache attacks may also be triggered by exerting external pressure against the transverse process of the C4

to C5, the C2 root, or the greater occipital nerve. Headaches may be precipitated within a few seconds of the trigger (range 5 to 60 seconds), sometimes in rapid succession without any refractory period.

5. **Does it matter whether we call these headaches clusters or paroxysmal hemicranias?**

   Yes. The differential diagnosis is exceptionally important, as the PHs are often resistant to the medications that typically prevent cluster headaches. The PHs are uniquely responsive to treatment with indomethacin. In fact, the International Headache Society has deemed response to indomethacin therapy a sine qua non for establishing the diagnosis. Some headache specialists believe that there are patients with paroxysmal hemicrania refractory to indomethacin.

6. **Once the diagnosis of episodic or chronic paroxysmal hemicrania is established, are any further workups necessary?**

   Although the PHs are benign by definition, there have been patients with clear medical or structural etiologies of this clinical disorder. For example, to date, there have been a number of published cases of patients with CPH-like headaches associated with collagen vascular diseases, malignant brain tumors, arteriovenous malformations, and ischemic stroke. Neuroimaging is therefore recommended in all cases with the presumptive diagnosis of either CPH or EPH in those patients presenting for the first time or in those presenting with a change in their typical pattern, to exclude other causes of these rare headaches. Several of these patients have also responded to indomethacin.

7. **Once the diagnosis is established and neuroimaging is normal, how are these headaches treated?**

   The hallmark of PHs is the absolute cessation of the headache with indomethacin. Initial therapy consists of 25 mg indomethacin 3 times daily. If there is no response or if there is a partial response after 1 week, increase the dose to 50 mg 3 times a day, and on rare occasion up to 75 mg 3 times a day. Complete resolution of the headache is prompt, usually occurring within 1 or 2 days of initiating the effective dose. Occasionally, suppositories are better tolerated than oral indomethacin. Very rarely, some patients require indomethacin doses as high as 300 mg/day. Recent reports suggest that a need for high indomethacin doses may be an ominous sign pointing to an underlying specific medical or structural etiology. Advise patients of the risk of gastritis and ulcer disease, as well as the other side effects of indomethacin. In patients with CPH who are on indomethacin, consider concurrent treatment with misoprostol or histamine (H-2) receptor antagonists or a proton pump inhibitor.

8. **True or false: Breakthrough headaches do not occur with indomethacin therapy.**

   False. Some patients experience breakthrough headaches at the end of dosing intervals. These headaches are usually eliminated by increasing the dose or shortening the dosing interval. For patients with breakthrough headaches in the early morning hours, slow-release indomethacin at night may be helpful.

9. **If indomethacin fails to treat the headaches, what then?**

   If indomethacin fails to successfully treat the headaches, reconsider the diagnosis and make sure there is no underlying cause. If upon further review the diagnosis of CPH or EPH is still likely, a range of drugs may show partial to complete relief in certain groups of patients. These include verapamil, acetylsalicylic acid, ibuprofen, naproxen, or paracetamol. These agents are not nearly as effective as indomethacin and should not be used as first-line therapy.

   Neuromodulatory procedures, such as greater occipital nerve blockade, blockade of sphenopalatine ganglion, and neurostimulation of the posterior hypothalamus, are reserved for patients with refractory PH.

10. **What is SUNCT and SUNA syndrome?**

    SUNCT is an acronym for short-lasting, unilateral, neuralgiform headache attacks with conjunctival injection and tearing. SUNA is an acronym for short-lasting unilateral neuralgiform headache attacks with autonomic symptoms. They are rare and often disabling primary headache disorders. They belong to the group of disorders known as the TACs (see Question 4). SUNCT and SUNA should be considered clinical phenotypes of the same syndrome. They are characterized by very frequent attacks of extremely short-lasting, unilateral headaches. The headaches of the SUNCT and SUNA syndromes recur from 3 to 200 times per day; each attack lasts 5 to 240 seconds each. As the name suggests, individual attacks are associated with ipsilateral conjunctival injection and lacrimation. Brain MRI should always be performed with a dedicated view to exclude neurovascular compression. The high percentage of remission after microvascular decompression (MVD) supports the pathogenetic role of neurovascular compression.

11. **How are SUNCT and SUNA treated?**
SUNCT and SUNA are very refractory to treatment. Treatment with medications used for cluster and the TACs are ineffective for SUNCT and SUNA. Lamotrigine, as an oral preventative treatment, and lidocaine, as an intravenous transitional treatment, seem to be the most effective therapies. For medically intractable chronic forms of SUNCT and SUNA, several surgical approaches have been tried. These include ablative procedures involving the trigeminal nerve or the Gasserian ganglion, MVD of the trigeminal nerve, and neurostimulation techniques.

KEY POINTS

1. The PHs are a group of rare, benign headache disorders that resemble cluster headache in most ways but differ from cluster headache because they do not respond to anticluster medications and are generally more frequent and of shorter duration than cluster headache.
2. The PHs are uniquely responsive to indomethacin.
3. There are secondary causes of the PHs, including collagen vascular disorders and brain tumor; therefore, for all patients who are suspected of having the diagnosis of one of the PHs, neuroimaging is recommended.

BIBLIOGRAPHY

1. Antonaci F, Sjaastad O. Chronic paroxysmal hemicranias (CPH): a review of the clinical manifestations. *Headache.* 1989;29:648-656.
2. Goadsby PJ. Trigeminal autonomic cephalgias (TACs). *Acta Neurol Belg.* 2001;101(1):10-19.
3. Goadsby PJ, Lipton RB. A review of paroxysmal hemicranias, SUNCT syndrome and other short-lasting headaches with autonomic features, including new cases. *Brain.* 1997;120:193-209.
4. Haggag KJ, Russell D. Chronic paroxysmal hemicrania. In: Olesen J, Tfelt-Hansen P, Welch KMA, eds. *The Headaches.* New York: Raven Press; 1993:601-608.
5. Kudrow L, Esperanza P, Vijayan N. Episodic paroxysmal hemicrania. *Cephalalgia.* 1987;7:197-201.
6. Medina JL. Organic headaches mimicking chronic paroxysmal hemicrania. *Headache.* 1992;32:73-74.
7. Newman LC. Effective management of ice pick pains, SUNCT, and episodic and chronic paroxysmal hemicrania. *Curr Pain Headache Rep.* 2001;5(3):292-299.
8. Newman LC, Goadsby P, Lipton RB. Cluster and related headaches. *Med Clin North Am.* 2001;85:997-1016.
9. Newman LC, Gordon ML, Lipton RB, Kanner R, Solomon S. Episodic paroxysmal hemicrania: two new cases and a literature review. *Neurology.* 1992;42:964-966.
10. Newman LC, Lipton RB. Paroxysmal hemicranias. In: Goadsby PJ, Silberstein SD, eds. *Headache.* Blue Books of Practical Neurology. Vol. 17. Boston: Butterworth-Heinemann; 1997:243-250.
11. Sjaastad O, Dale I. Evidence for a new (?), treatable headache entity. *Headache.* 1974;14:105-108.
12. Sjaastad O, Stovner LJ, Stolt-Nielson A, Antonaci F, Fredriksen TA. CPH and hemicrania continua: requirements of high indomethacin dosages—an ominous sign. *Headache.* 1995;35:363-367.
13. Prakash S, Patell R. Paroxysmal hemicrania: an update. *Curr Pain Headache Rep.* 2014;18(4):407.
14. Lambru G, Matharu MS. SUNCT, SUNA and trigeminal neuralgia: different disorders or variants of the same disorder? *Curr Opin Neurol.* 2014;27(3):325-331.
15. Lambru G, Matharu MS. SUNCT and SUNA: medical and surgical treatments. *Neurol Sci.* 2013;34(suppl 1):S75-S81.

IV. UNCOMMON HEADACHE SYNDROMES

SUBARACHNOID HEMORRHAGE

Alexandra R. Paul and Alan S. Boulos

CHAPTER 15

1. **How is the headache of subarachnoid hemorrhage often described?**
   Headache following subarachnoid hemorrhage is often described by patients as "the worst headache of my life" or as a "thunderclap headache." A thunderclap headache has been described as an acute, severe, and explosive headache that immediately reaches maximal intensity. The term "thunderclap headache" originates from 1986 from Day and Raskin, because of the similarities to being struck by a thunderbolt.

2. **What is a sentinel headache?**
   Many patients who do present with subarachnoid hemorrhage often describe a preceding "sentinel headache," which has been found to occur in 10% to 40% of patients. The sentinel headache has been attributed to a possible small leak in the aneurysm or sudden enlargement of the aneurysm.

3. **What is the most common cause of spontaneous subarachnoid hemorrhage?**
   Saccular aneurysm rupture is the cause in 85% of spontaneous cases. Other causes of subarachnoid hemorrhage include arteriovenous malformation (AVM) rupture, vasculitis, trauma, or dissection. In approximately 10% of cases of spontaneous subarachnoid hemorrhage, no aneurysm or AVM is found and the diagnosis of perimesencephalic subarachnoid hemorrhage is made. The cause of perimesencephalic subarachnoid hemorrhage is generally a diagnosis of exclusion and thought to be secondary to a venous bleed.

4. **What is the prevalence of saccular aneurysms?**
   In the general asymptomatic population, saccular aneurysms have been found in 3.2% of patients in autopsy series.

5. **What are possible physical examination findings in a patient with subarachnoid hemorrhage?**
   Patients presenting with subarachnoid hemorrhage typically do not demonstrate any localizing signs. They may be lethargic or have meningismus. The exception is in cases of ruptured posterior communicating artery aneurysms. The posterior communicating artery is in close proximity to the third cranial nerve, and ruptured posterior communicating artery aneurysms can cause a third nerve palsy. In these cases the patient typically presents with a painless mydriasis and lateral eye deviation in combination with headache.

6. **How is the diagnosis of subarachnoid hemorrhage made?**
   If the patient presents within 6 hours of headache onset, the sensitivity of a noncontrast computed tomography (CT) is 100% (Fig. 15.1). The sensitivity decreases to 93% within 24 hours of onset and 80% at 3 days. A lumbar puncture may be required to demonstrate the presence of blood, particularly if the headache was remote in time. Xanthochromia in the fourth tube of cerebrospinal fluid is most accurate. Magnetic resonance imaging (MRI) sequences are also very sensitive for detecting acute subarachnoid hemorrhage.

7. **What are the criteria from the International Headache Society for subarachnoid hemorrhage?**
   1. Severe headache of sudden onset fulfilling criteria C and D
   2. Neuroimaging (CT or MRI T2 or flair sequences) or cerebrospinal fluid evidence of nontraumatic subarachnoid hemorrhage with or without other clinical signs
   3. Headache develops simultaneously with hemorrhage
   4. Headache resolves within 1 month

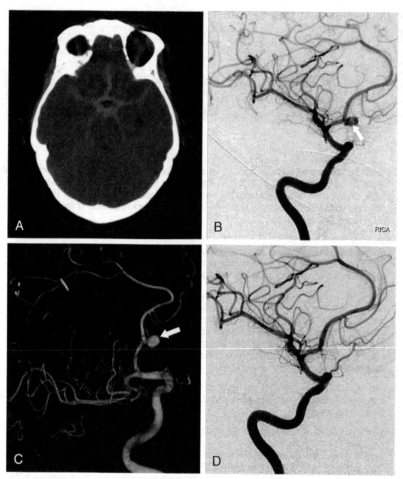

Figure 15.1. (A) Classic appearance of subarachnoid hemorrhage on a noncontrast computed tomography scan. Acute blood is visualized filling the basal cisterns. (B) The 6 mm ruptured anterior communicating artery aneurysm *(red arrow)* visualized on angiography. (C) A 3D reconstruction of the aneurysm. (D) Postcoiling angiogram demonstrating near complete occlusion of the aneurysm.

8. What is the pathophysiologic cause of a headache from subarachnoid hemorrhage?

The pain caused by aneurysmal rupture may be related to stretching of the blood vessel wall. Another theory is that there is a temporary rise in intracranial pressure to equal the mean arterial pressure in order to abate the bleeding from the aneurysm. Other potential etiologies are likely to exist, however, as patients with nonaneurysmal rupture also have severe headaches. Possible causes include increased local inflammation and irritation of the surrounding blood vessel, vasospasm, and mechanical stimulation of trigeminovascular afferents or meningeal irritation and inflammation. It is possible that all of the above are causes of the headache following subarachnoid hemorrhage, but at different points along the course of the disease.

9. What are potential causes for a delayed headache in a patient with subarachnoid hemorrhage?

The most important causes to rule out for a patient with a delayed headache following subarachnoid hemorrhage are hydrocephalus and aneurysm re-rupture. If these causes have been excluded, the later phases of headache are more likely due to vasospasm and aseptic meningitis.

10. How should the headache from subarachnoid hemorrhage be treated?

The 2013 European Stroke Organization Guidelines for the Management of Intracranial Aneurysms and Subarachnoid Hemorrhage recommend acetaminophen, and in cases of severe pain, opiates, to treat subarachnoid hemorrhage associated headaches. Unfortunately opiates are often associated with nausea, vomiting, ileus, urinary retention, depressed respiratory drive, hallucinations, hypotension, and possible acute withdrawal. The treatment of headaches from subarachnoid hemorrhage is often complicated by concerns for altered mental status and the need for frequent neurologic exams. New studies are evaluating the use of gabapentin in reducing the acute and chronic pain associated with subarachnoid hemorrhage. Decadron may be beneficial during the two inflammatory peaks at day 13 and day 18.

KEY POINTS

1. The complaint of "the worst headache of my life" or "thunderclap headache" should prompt evaluation for subarachnoid hemorrhage.
2. CT scan is positive for subarachnoid hemorrhage in the majority of cases. In rare cases, a lumbar puncture or MRI is required to make the diagnosis.
3. Treatment of subarachnoid hemorrhage headaches is complicated by the need for frequent neurologic assessments. Low dose opiate analgesics, acetaminophen, and gabapentin have all been used successfully.

BIBLIOGRAPHY

1. Chen SP, Ayata C. Spreading depression in primary and secondary headache. *Curr Pain Headache Rep.* 2016;20:44.
2. Day JW, Raskin NH. Thunderclap headache: symptom of unruptured cerebral aneurysm. *Lancet.* 1986;2:1247-1248.
3. Dhakal LP, Harriott AM, Capobianco DJ, Freeman WD. Headache and its approach in today's neurointensive care unit. *Neurocrit Care.* 2016;25(2):320-334.
4. Dhakal LP, Hodge DO, Nagel J, et al. Safety and tolerability of gabapentin for aneurysmal subarachnoid hemorrhage(sah) headache and meningismus. *Neurocrit Care.* 2015;22:414-421.
5. Dreier JP, Major S, Manning A, et al. Cortical spreading ischaemia is a novel process involved in ischaemic damage in patients with aneurysmal subarachnoid haemorrhage. *Brain.* 2009;132(Pt 7):1866-1881.
6. Ju YE, Schwedt TJ. Abrupt onset severe headaches. *Semin Neurol.* 2010;30:192-200.
7. Linn FH, Wijdicks EF, van der Graaf Y, et al. Prospective study of sentineal headache in aneurysmal subarachnoid haemorrhage. *Lancet.* 1994;344:590-593.
8. Mortimer AM, Bradley MD, Stoodley NG, Renowden SA. Thunderclap headache: diagnostic considerations and neuroimaging features. *Clin Radiol.* 2013;68:e101-e113.
9. Polmear A. Sentineal headaches in aneurysmal subarachnoid haemorrhage: what is the true incidence? A systematic review. *Cephalalgia.* 2003;23:935-941.
10. Steiner T, Juvela S, Unterberg A, et al. European Stroke Organization guidelines for the management of intracranial aneurysms and subarachnoid haemorrhage. *Cerebrovasc Dis.* 2013;35:93-112.
11. Suarez JI, Tarr RW, Selman WR. Aneurysmal subarachnoid hemorrhage. *N Engl J Med.* 2006;354(4):387-396.
12. Vlak MH, Algra A, Brandenburg R, Rinkel GJ. Prevalence of unruptured intracranial aneurysms, with emphasis on sex, age, comorbidity, country, and time period: a systematic review and meta-analysis. *Lancet Neurol.* 2011;10:626.
13. Woitzik J, Dreier JP, Hecht N, et al. Delayed cerebral ischemia and spreading depolarization in absence of angiographic vasospasm after subarachnoid hemorrhage. *J Cereb Blood Flow Metab.* 2012;32(2):203-212.

CHAPTER 16

PAIN ASSOCIATED WITH BRAIN TUMOR

Adedamola Adepoju, Benjamin Yim, Nataly Raviv and Tyler J. Kenning

1. **What is the classic description of brain tumor headache?**

   The classical brain tumor headache is commonly described as a severe early morning headache, associated with nausea and vomiting. The headache starts initially as episodic, and nocturnal, which usually awakens patients from sleep. As the tumor progresses, the headache becomes intermittent, then constant. It is influenced by position, most notably bending down or when recumbent. It is worsened with activities that increase intracranial pressure, such as cough, sneeze, emesis, and Valsalva maneuver. The headache is presumably expected to improve with ambulation. However, studies have demonstrated that few patients actually have the classical presentation of brain tumor headache, and as a result, morning headache that wakes patients up but improves during the day is not diagnostic.

2. **What was the theoretical basis for the pathophysiology of classic brain tumor headache?**

   Brain tumor headache is believed to be caused by two processes: The first is the regional traction and stimulation of pain-sensitive structures including cranial nerves, blood vessel, and dura. The second is the global and generalized traction of the brain structures from high intracranial pressure, which is worsened by recumbency position and physiological states that increase intracranial pressure such as CO_2 retention, cerebral vasodilation, and peritumoral edema. The mild CO_2 retention caused by hypoventilation during sleep is believed to be the inciting factor for the increased pain associated with brain tumors early in the day.

   The progressive nature of brain tumor headache is believed to correspond to the transition from local to global traction of cranial structures as brain tumor size increases. In addition, the positional change in brain tumor headache is due to changes in the intracranial pressure in which venous outflow congestion such as laying down increases intracranial pressure. Conversely, ambulation and upright position increase venous outflow and decrease intracranial pressure, and hence improve brain tumor headache.

3. **How commonly do patients with brain tumors have the "classic history" of a brain tumor headache?**

   Only about 17% of patients with brain tumors present with the "classic" headache syndrome. Instead, brain tumor headaches are mostly diffuse, and nondescriptive or tension-type headaches. Migrainous headaches are found in a small number of patients. However, not all tension-like headaches are associated with a brain tumor. In patients with new headaches without a prior cancer diagnosis, the risk of a brain tumor is low (0.15%). If the headache fits the criteria for a primary headache disorder, that risk is even lower (0.045%).

4. **How often do brain tumor headaches determine the localization and laterality of brain tumors?**

   Studies show that the location of the headache does not correlate well with the location of a brain tumor, especially for supratentorial brain tumors. Instead, these tumors often result in diffuse headaches that are unilateral in less than 50% of patients. When unilateral, however, brain tumor headaches are almost always on the same side as the tumor. Posterior fossa tumors are different, and they have strong association with occipital rather than frontal or temporal headaches.

5. **If brain tumor headaches are most commonly tension like, how do you differentiate between a benign tension-type headache and a brain tumor headache?**

   A tension-like headache is the most common type of brain tumor headache. It is found in 77% of patients, while the migrainous headache is found in 5% to 10%. There are a number of factors that differentiate the more common tension-type headache from headaches due to a brain tumor. The most important is the presence of neurologic symptoms, including focal deficits associated with tumor location and symptoms related to raised intracranial pressure—namely nausea, vomiting, and decreased level of consciousness. An abnormal neurologic exam is not commonly associated with a benign headache, except for Horner syndrome in cluster headache. This abnormality occurs in over 50% of patients with brain tumor headaches.

Time course is another factor that differentiates a tension-like brain tumor headache from a regular tension headache. A new-onset headache that develops over time is more likely to represent a space-occupying lesion than a chronic headache that has been stable over an existing period. Furthermore, development of a new onset headache in a patient with a history of cancer should raise the suspicion for possible cerebral metastasis, and appropriate neuro-imaging should be obtained. New onset progressive headaches in elderly patients with no prior history should also alert the clinician to the possibility of a brain tumor.

6. What "red flags" should prompt evaluation for a brain tumor?
"Red flags" include headaches that have acutely changed in character, especially if there are new, more severe, or progressive symptoms. Other concerning headache symptoms are those on exertion or with onset at night or in the early morning, associated with fever, systemic symptoms, meningismus, or new neurologic signs, precipitated by Valsalva maneuvers. Lastly, if a new headache occurs in an adult (especially the elderly) or young child or in a cancer patient, cranial imaging should be performed to diagnose a potential brain tumor (Table 16.1).

7. Name and describe circumstances under which extracerebral cancer can cause headache and/or facial pain.
Extracranial cancers can cause headache by several mechanisms. Tumors of the neck and mediastinum compressing or invading major venous drainage pathways, such as the jugular veins or superior vena cava, can increase intracranial pressure due to venous outflow compromise. Systemic malignancies can also induce hypercoagulable states and subsequent venous sinus thrombosis, producing increased intracranial pressure and possibly decreased levels of consciousness. Extracranial tumors can also cause referred pain due to compression of adjacent neurovascular structures. For example, sinonasal and facial tumors can stimulate or invade the trigeminal nerve to cause referred head pain. Similarly, upper cervical masses compressing the nerve roots can cause posterior fossa pain and headache.

8. Is the pathology of the brain tumor important in determining the clinical presentation?
The pathology of brain tumor has limited bearing on the clinical presentation. Location is the most important factor and dictates clinical presentation. Supratentorial tumors can be associated with focal motor and sensory deficits, speech and language difficulties, memory difficulty, and personality changes. Infratentorial tumors are associated with noncommunicating hydrocephalus, cranial nerve palsies from brain stem compression, and hemiparesis. Noncommunicating hydrocephalus is due to cerebrospinal fluid (CSF) outflow obstruction, and it produces symptoms such as nausea, vomiting, papilledema, vision abnormalities, and "sunsetting" of eyes.

9. What is Parinaud syndrome?
Parinaud syndrome is caused by masses of the pineal region compressing the midbrain tectum. It is characterized by difficulty with ocular convergence, upgaze palsy, light-near dissociation, eyelid retraction, and convergence nystagmus.

Table 16.1. Headache Red Flags That Require Further Evaluation for a Brain Tumor
Prior headaches that have changed in character
New, severe, progressive headaches
Occur with exertion or onset at night or early morning
Associated with fever, other systemic symptoms, meningismus, or new neurologic signs
Precipitated by Valsalva maneuvers
New symptoms in young child or adult (especially the elderly)
New symptoms in a patient with a prior cancer diagnosis

10. **What is a "ball-valve" headache?**

Some masses may be loosely based on a tissue pedicle, allowing for mobilization with positional changes. For example, this may occur in colloid cysts, which most commonly arise in the third ventricle and may account for the fluctuating symptoms with these masses, as they may swing back and forth with positional changes of the head. As the patient's head moves to a new position, the cyst may shift and block the foramen of Monro and the outflow of CSF from the lateral ventricle, causing an acute increase in intracranial pressure. The on-and-off occlusion of the foramen of Monro causes episodic headache, which is termed the "ball-valve effect."

11. **How commonly is headache the presenting complaint in patients with metastatic brain tumors?**

Headache is a common feature of metastatic brain tumor. The development of a new headache or change in the quality of headache in patients with a systemic malignancy is an ominous sign for intracranial metastasis. About 32% to 54% patients with systemic cancer who present with new or changed headache have an intracranial metastasis which is a common symptom in these patients

12. **In what clinical scenarios does a brain tumor headache require urgent treatment?**

There are few emergencies associated with brain tumor headache. Although it has an indolent presentation, the acute change in the nature of the headache with severe neurologic deficit could be an indication of worsening conditions. The most common cause of acute change in brain tumor headache is due to hemorrhage. Some primary brain and metastatic tumors such as oligodendroglioma, hemangioblastoma, melanoma, renal cell carcinoma, choriocarcinoma, and lung cancer have the propensity to bleed. Melanoma has a high frequency of intraparenchymal hemorrhage, and in some instances, a patient may present to the emergency department with acute neurologic deficits due to the hemorrhage. Hemorrhage in the supratentorial space would present with focal and lateralizing neurologic signs, while posterior fossa hemorrhage with brain stem compression can render patients unresponsive and possibly lead to death if neurosurgical intervention is not provided in a timely fashion.

Brain tumor headache associated with increased intracranial pressure can present with nonfocal neurologic signs such as a decreased loss of consciousness, nausea, and vomiting. CSF flow obstruction with tumors located within the ventricular space, such as central neurocytoma, ependymoma, and colloid cyst, or those compressing the ventricular outlets can cause acute change in headache with signs of increased intracranial pressure.

Brain tumors resulting in significant brain parenchymal irritation or mass effect often cause severe vasogenic edema. This can result in a change in headache character that may be accompanied by focal neurologic symptoms and signs of increased intracranial pressure. Corticosteroids reduce the vasogenic edema and typically provide headache relief associated with the edema. At one point, the "steroid test" was used as a diagnostic tool for brain tumor headaches. A dramatic response to steroid administration strengthened the diagnosis, on the theory that peritumoral edema was resolving. Over the years, however, it has become increasingly clear that steroids can relieve many types of headaches—not just those resulting from brain tumors.

13. **Which systemic tumors commonly metastasize to the brain and why do they cause headache?**

Lung cancer, breast cancer, colorectal cancer, and melanoma are some of the most common cancers that metastasize to the brain for reasons that are not completely understood. There are studies showing that the brain presents a microenvironment niche that favors the growth of these tumors. Cancer cells can seed multiple areas in the brain including structures with nociceptive receptors such as meninges, blood vessels, and cranial nerves, which cause headache. These cells can also inflame these structures, leading to headache.

14. **Under what circumstances is a brain tumor likely to produce severe headaches with little or no neurologic focality?**

Tumors that arise in relatively "clinically silent" areas of the brain may reach very large sizes before producing signs and/or symptoms. Tumors arising in and/or around the frontal lobes, for example, may grow to large sizes without producing focal neurologic deficits. Usually, however, there is some change in personality or cognition. Additionally, these can produce Foster-Kennedy syndrome, where there is papilledema in the contralateral eye, optic atrophy in the ipsilateral eye, and anosmia. This most commonly occurs in tumors of the anterior cranial base, such as meningiomas, that cause compression of the optic and olfactory nerves. These tumors can be very sizeable before detection.

Intraventricular tumors such as central neurocytoma, and ependymoma, can obstruct the flow of CSF within the ventricle and cause hydrocephalus without focal deficit. Hydrocephalus is associated with progressive headache, nausea, emesis, and a decreased level of consciousness.

15. **Do primary brain tumors cause headaches?**
There are two types of primary brain tumor: extra- and intraaxial brain tumors. Extraaxial brain tumors develop around the brain mostly from the meninges and the bone. Intraaxial primary brain tumors develop from the brain parenchyma, in which glioma is the most common type. Both types of primary brain can cause headache either through the local traction of pain-sensitive structures surrounding the tumor or global traction from increased intracranial pressure.

16. **What is the preferred treatment for brain tumor headaches?**
The definite treatment for brain tumor headache is often surgical resection. In the interim, medical management including steroids can minimize the vasogenic edema and increased intracranial pressure associated with many brain tumors. In an acute setting, mannitol and hypertonic saline can also provide relief from headache by also reducing intracranial pressure.

Radiation, an adjuvant therapy for brain tumor, can worsen headache through inflammation and increased swelling secondary to tissue necrosis. In this setting, steroids can minimize the inflammation and edema associated with necrosis.

17. **What percentage of brain tumor patients experience headaches?**
Approximately 50% to 70% of brain tumor patients report headaches. Patients with a history of primary headaches are more likely to experience headaches in the setting of brain tumor—64% versus 38% of headache-naïve patients.

18. **What is pituitary apoplexy, and how do affected patients commonly present?**
Pituitary apoplexy is a syndrome commonly associated with a pituitary tumor that develops following an acute hemorrhage into or infarction of the tumor. Patients may present with sudden onset of severe headache accompanied by visual loss, ophthalmoplegia, facial numbness, altered mental status, cardiovascular collapse, and hormonal dysfunction. Treatment involves medical management with corticosteroid replacement for any pituitary insufficiency and evaluation of electrolytes with appropriate treatment. Surgical decompression of the tumor may also be indicated if there are symptoms of mass effect from the tumor, such as vision loss or ophthalmoplegia.

19. **A 60-year-old woman complains of progressive, unilateral headache and facial pain. On examination, she shows nystagmus, hearing loss, facial weakness, and ataxia. What is the likely diagnosis?**
This constellation of symptoms is suggestive of a mass lesion involving cranial nerves V, VII, and VIII, as well as the cerebellum. This can be due to a tumor located within the cerebellopontine angle. The most common masses to occur in this location are vestibular schwannomas or meningiomas. Less commonly, a metastatic tumor can result in similar symptoms. Of note, patients may also develop headaches secondary to elevated intracranial pressure and hydrocephalus with vestibular schwannomas attributed to increased protein content within the CSF or mass effect upon the fourth ventricular outlet.

20. **A middle-aged man has progressive headaches and is found to have a frontal glioma. His headaches become worse, and he develops diplopia that is most pronounced on distant gaze and not present on near gaze. What is a likely explanation?**
Diplopia on distant gaze is most likely due to sixth nerve palsy, which limits the eyes' movement laterally and is a false localizing sign of chronic high intracranial pressure. Focusing on near objects mostly involves bilateral third nerves to converge the eyes towards the midline. Conversely, focusing on faraway objects involves the sixth nerve, and its disruption results in diplopia on distant gaze. The sixth cranial nerve has the longest course of travel in the brain and increased intracranial pressure is believed to stretch the nerve and cause its dysfunction.

21. A 60-year-old man with glioblastoma has undergone a full course of radiation therapy with some improvement. Six months later, he complains of increasing headache and increasing neurologic deficits referable to the area of the original tumor. What is the differential diagnosis? How would you differentiate between the two main possibilities?

The differential diagnosis in this setting includes recurrent tumor or radiation necrosis. Radiation necrosis typically occurs about 3 to 9 months after radiation, and there are studies that show it can persist for several years. Unfortunately the two diagnoses are similar on routine neuroimaging techniques, and it takes specific imaging tests such as magnetic resonance spectroscopy and perfusion to differentiate between them. However, none of these tests are definitive, but rather just suggestive, of a diagnosis.

Acknowledgment

We would like to acknowledge the work of the chapter's authors from the first edition of this book, Ronald Kanner, MD, FAAN, FACP and Charles E. Argoff, MD.

KEY POINTS

1. Brain tumor headaches are often diffuse, nondescript, and similar to tension headaches. The classically described morning headache is not common with brain tumors and not diagnostic.
2. The incidence of brain tumor in patients with tension headaches is low, and neuro-imaging is not typically indicated unless there are "red flags" present, including failure of medical therapy or a change in the character, quality, or intensity of the symptoms.
3. Headache can be the only symptom of a brain tumor. Brain tumor headaches, however, are often commonly associated with other neurologic signs, including focal neurologic deficit, evidence of increased intracranial pressure, and/or seizures.
4. Acute changes in brain tumor headache that require emergent treatment are typically those associated with hemorrhage and hydrocephalus.

BIBLIOGRAPHY

1. Boiardi A, Salmaggi A, Eoli M, Lamperti E, Silvani A. Headache in brain tumors: a symptom of reappraise critically. *Neurol Sci.* 2004;25:S143-S147.
2. Chidel MA, Suh JH, Barnett GH. Brain metastases: presentation, evaluation, and management. *Cleve Clin J Med.* 2000;67:120-127.
3. Friedman BW, Lipton RB. Headache emergencies: diagnosis and management. *Neurol Clin.* 2012;30:2012.
4. Goffaux P, Fortin D. Brain tumor headaches: from bedside to bench. *Neurosurgery.* 2010;2:459-466.
5. Jamieson DG, Hargreaves R. The role of neuroimaging in headache. *J Neuroimaging.* 2002;12:42-51.
6. Kahn K, Finkel A. It is a tumor—current review of headache and brain tumor. *Curr Pain Headache Rep.* 2014;18:421.
7. Kirby S, Purdy RA. Headaches and brain tumors. *Neurol Clin.* 2014;32:423-432.
8. Larner AJ. Not all morning headaches are due to brain tumors. *Pract Neurol.* 2009;9:80-84.
9. Posner JB. *Intracranial Metastases. Neurological Complications of Cancer.* Philadelphia: FA Davis; 1995:77-110.
10. Purdy RA, Kirby S. Headaches and brain tumors. *Neurol Clin.* 2004;22:39.
11. Siepmann DB, Siegel A, Lewis PJ. Tl-201 SPECT and F-18 FDG PET for assessment of glioma recurrence versus radiation necrosis. *Clin Nucl Med.* 2005;30:199-200.
12. Valentinis L, Tuniz F, Valent F, et al. Headache attributed to intracranial tumours: a prospective cohort study. *Cephalalgia.* 2010;30:389-398.

HEADACHE RELATED TO INCREASED OR DECREASED INTRACRANIAL PRESSURE

Kevin S. Chen, Parag G. Patil and Karin M. Muraszko

CHAPTER 17

1. What is the normal range for intracranial pressure and how is it measured?

Surprisingly, definitions of "normal" intracranial pressure (ICP) vary depending on the source, but studies suggest median opening pressure is about 17 cmH_2O, with the 95% confidence interval ranging from 10 to 25 cmH_2O. Typically, ICP is measured by lumbar puncture (LP) with the patient lying in a lateral position with legs extended. More invasive means of measuring ICP that require burr holes placed in the skull include epidural, subdural, and intraparenchymal ICP monitors, as well as external ventriculostomy catheters.

2. Describe the Monro-Kellie doctrine.

The Monro-Kellie doctrine pertains to the balance of forces that contribute to cerebral perfusion pressure (CPP). The intracranial contents are treated as being contained within a rigid box. Therefore the net CPP is the difference between the pressure of blood entering the intracranial space (as measured by the mean arterial pressure [MAP]) and the resistance from ICP. In other words, CPP = MAP − ICP. Contributors to ICP include brain tissue, interstitial fluid, intracranial blood, cerebrospinal fluid (CSF), and any mass lesions (tumors, hematomas, etc.). These parameters may be manipulated (e.g., CSF drainage, osmotic agents, surgical evacuation, etc.) to optimize CPP. Derived largely from the trauma literature, an optimal CPP is 50 to 70 mmHg.

3. Under what circumstances is the pressure measured by lumbar puncture not a true reflection of intracranial pressure?

When measured at the level of the cauda equina by LP, the opening pressure (OP) is used as a surrogate measure of ICP, which is referenced at the foramen of Monro (Fig. 17.1). The LP is performed low in the thecal sac to avoid injury to the spinal cord. To accurately estimate ICP by the OP, the patient must be positioned laterally such that the foramen of Monro is horizontally level with the LP site. If the head is elevated (or the LP performed in the sitting position), the fluid column between the foramen of Monro and the LP site will increase fluid pressure at the site of access, giving a falsely elevated OP. Conversely, if the LP is performed prone (as is often done in interventional radiology), one must use extension tubing to place the manometer at the level of the foramen of Monro; otherwise the manometer placed on the patient's back will give a falsely low OP. In addition, any structural blockage of CSF flow to the lumbar cistern may result in inaccurate OP measurement.

4. How is cerebrospinal fluid formed and reabsorbed?

CSF is chiefly formed by the vasculature of the choroid plexus, employing active transport of water and solutes across the blood-brain barrier into the cerebral ventricles. CSF exits the ventricular system via the foramina of Magendie and Luschka, flowing into the subarachnoid spaces surrounding the brain and spinal cord. The total subarachnoid space contains about 150 mL of CSF in adults, but the production of CSF is about 400 to 600 mL per day. Therefore, in a single 24-hour period, the entire volume of CSF is exchanged about 3 to 4 times. CSF is chiefly resorbed via the dural venous sinuses. Recently, interstitial glial-lymphatic channels as well as true lymphatics have been described as contributing to CSF egress.

5. Why does increased or decreased intracranial pressure cause headaches?

While the brain parenchyma contains no nociceptive receptors, the overlying dura takes sensory innervation from cranial nerves and upper cervical nerves and can be quite sensitive to pain. The dura detects pressure and stretch caused by abnormally elevated or diminished ICP.

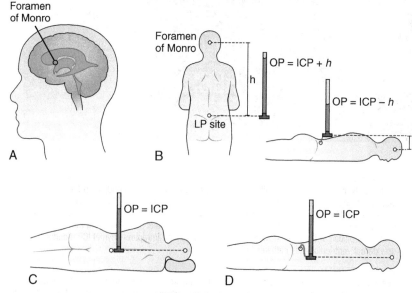

Figure 17.1. A, Intracranial pressure *(ICP)* is made with reference to the foramen of Monro, where the lateral ventricles join the third ventricle in the midline. The opening pressure *(OP)* obtained during lumbar puncture *(LP)* is used to infer ICP at this site. **B,** Erroneous measurements of the OP can be made during LP if the manometer is significantly below the level of the foramen of Monro (e.g., patient sitting upright, OP = ICP + *h*) or above the foramen of Monro (e.g., patient prone, OP = ICP − *h*). **C,** For the OP to accurately reflect true ICP, the manometer must be held at the level of the foramen of Monro, which can be achieved with the patient in the lateral position, or **D,** using extension tubing to adjust the level of the manometer accordingly.

6. **What clinical characteristics suggest headache is due to elevated intracranial pressure?**
   Headaches resulting from elevated ICP are typically described as positional, worsening when the patient lies flat (diminished CSF and venous outflow from the intracranial space), as well as with Valsalva maneuvers (straining, coughing, laughing, etc.). After sleeping recumbent through the night, headaches can be worst upon waking in the morning, or can even wake the patient from sleep. These positional headaches should improve quickly after sitting or standing upright. Along with headache, patients often present with nausea/vomiting, visual disturbances (diplopia or diminished acuity), disorientation, or even altered mental status.

7. **What neurologic signs can be seen with diffuse increases in intracranial pressure?**
   Neurologic signs of global increased ICP are often manifested by diminished level of consciousness, ranging from confusion and drowsiness, to obtundation and coma in severe cases. On funduscopic examination, bilateral papilledema with engorged retinal veins can be seen, although this may take hours to develop. Severely elevated ICP may also produce unilateral or bilateral abducens nerve palsies. In cases of chronic elevated ICP, as described later, persistent pressure on the optic nerves and visual disturbances are a chief concern.

8. **Describe the risks of performing lumbar puncture in patients with increased intracranial pressure.**
   Normally the subarachnoid spaces freely communicate and redistribute CSF to normalize pressures throughout the CSF. However, if a compartment is abnormally isolated (e.g., large posterior fossa tumor blocking CSF flow across foramen magnum) or pressure gradients are set up (e.g., expanding hematoma or cerebral edema surrounding a tumor), the act of exposing the lumbar cistern to normal air pressure via LP may acutely exacerbate pressure gradients in the central nervous system. This can cause an abnormal shift in brain structures and even herniation.

9. **Name the elements that define "Cushing's triad."**
   The classic Cushing's triad of hypertension, bradycardia, and respiratory irregularity may be seen with sudden and acutely elevated ICP.

10. **What is idiopathic intracranial hypertension?**
    Idiopathic intracranial hypertension (IIH), also known as pseudotumor cerebri, is a chronic elevation of ICP that is not secondary to another etiology (tumors, hydrocephalus, etc.). The distribution of IIH favors women over men, particularly women in their childbearing years, as well as in the pediatric population. It is also strongly associated with obesity, although to a lesser extent in prepubertal cases.

11. **What are the diagnostic criteria for idiopathic intracranial hypertension?**
    The formal criteria for IIH have been described in the International Classification of Headache Disorders. To summarize, daily, diffuse/constant headaches or those that are aggravated by Valsalva maneuvers are typical for IIH. Patients may also present with transient visual obscurations and/or pulsatile tinnitus. Neurologic examination is normal except for signs concerning for elevated ICP, including papilledema, enlarged blind spot, visual field deficits, and/or abducens palsy. Uncommonly, patients may present with visual obscurations without headache.

12. **Describe the proper workup of a patient with suspected idiopathic intracranial hypertension.**
    A magnetic resonance imaging (MRI) of the brain to rule out a structural lesion causing elevated ICP is required. This can also rule out hydrocephalus (by contrast, in IIH, patients can exhibit a paradoxical "slit ventricle" syndrome). This evaluation should also include MR venography to rule out venous sinus thrombosis or stenosis. The diagnosis of IIH can be confirmed by LP to measure ICP. Demonstration of elevated ICP by LP is diagnostic (>20 cmH$_2$O in normal weight and >25 cmH$_2$O in obese individuals); relief of symptoms with drainage of CSF can also lend credence to the diagnosis. The CSF fluid analysis must also be normal.

13. **What are the main complications of untreated idiopathic intracranial hypertension?**
    The most concerning complication from untreated IIH is compromise of visual function. Prolonged elevated pressure in the subarachnoid space restricts blood flow to the optic nerve and retina. Therefore patients with IIH may present with visual obscurations or loss of visual fields. Papilledema can be seen on funduscopic examination. Patients with a workup suggestive of IIH should be urgently evaluated by an ophthalmologist, as loss of visual function is the main indication for intervention.

14. **Describe the treatments for idiopathic intracranial hypertension.**
    Given the association of IIH with obesity, weight reduction can be an effective treatment for IIH and reverse visual deficits. Bariatric surgery can also be considered. Pharmacologic treatment includes acetazolamide, which acts to decrease CSF production. With failure of maximal medical therapy, surgical options include CSF diversion (e.g., ventriculoperitoneal or lumboperitoneal shunts). Optic nerve sheath fenestration, a procedure that relieves pressure on the optic nerve, may be appropriate for patients with predominantly visual symptoms and papilledema, but long-term efficacy is debated. In cases associated with venous sinus stenosis, endovascular venous sinus stenting has also shown promise.

15. **What are some mimics of idiopathic intracranial hypertension?**
    Secondary intracranial hypertension results from an identifiable process causing elevated ICP. These should be investigated prior to settling on a diagnosis of IIH. Potential causes for secondary intracranial hypertension include infectious/inflammatory processes, endocrine/metabolic disorders (related to steroid withdrawal, hypothalamic-pituitary-adrenal imbalances, thyroid/parathyroid disorder, or sex hormone imbalance), and drug side effects (e.g., tetracycline antibiotics, nitrofurantoin, vitamin A imbalance, lithium, and certain chemotherapeutics).

16. **How do brain tumors cause increased intracranial pressure?**
    Brain tumors can affect all components of the Monro-Kellie doctrine that contribute to ICP in addition to their own inherent mass effect. Dural-based lesions can compress venous sinuses, hampering outflow of blood from the intracranial space. Tumors can also incite a strong inflammatory reaction, with surrounding vasogenic edema swelling and expanding the brain tissue. All of these can contribute to elevated ICP headaches in brain tumor patients.

17. **What are low-pressure headaches, and what are the clinical characteristics?**
As might be suspected, intracranial hypotension results when ICP is abnormally low. Intracranial hypotension is usually caused by insufficiency of CSF, leading to inadequate buoyancy and positional brain shift. Headaches are typically described as worse when sitting or standing upright but improved when lying flat. Irritation of the dura and meninges can cause neck pain, nausea, and vomiting. Abnormal loss of CSF can also present with hearing loss, thought to result from alterations in cochlear perilymph that communicates with the subarachnoid space. Severe cases can even result in subdural hygromas or subdural hematomas.

18. **Name some common causes of intracranial hypotension.**
The most common cause of intracranial hypotension is from iatrogenic causes, resulting from persistent CSF loss after LP, or when an opening in the dura is made by epidural/spinal anesthesia or spinal operations. Persistent CSF leaks can also be associated with trauma—particularly skull base or sinus fractures associated with dural tears. Rarely CSF leaks can occur spontaneously, sometimes associated with connective tissue diseases but are often idiopathic.

19. **How can low-pressure headache be diagnosed?**
As outlined in the International Classification of Headache Disorders, low-pressure headache symptoms must accompany evidence of CSF leakage on imaging or low ICP (<6 cmH$_2$O) by LP. Often a history of iatrogenic or traumatic cause of CSF leak can be elicited. For cases of spontaneous intracranial hypotension, MRI often reveals leptomeningeal enhancement due to diffuse meningeal irritation. In this case, intrathecal injection of contrast or radionuclide followed by MRI, computed tomography, or positron emission tomography myelography may be able to localize the site of CSF leak.

20. **Describe the treatment options for low-pressure headaches.**
Little prospective data exists for treatment of low-pressure headaches. For small iatrogenic or traumatic CSF leaks, conservative management consists of bed rest with the head positioned to minimize fluid pressure on the leak (i.e., head of bed flat for lumbar leaks, head of bed raised at 30 degrees for skull base leaks). Adequate hydration and/or abdominal binders may also provide some relief, with these CSF leaks often resolving after a short period of conservative management. Pharmacologic treatments for associated headache include caffeine, steroids, or theophylline. For spontaneous intracranial hypotension, an epidural "blood patch" may seal the leak if identified on imaging (usually requiring a myelogram). Surgical interventions are reserved for persistent CSF leaks where a significant dural defect can be identified.

Acknowledgments

Special thanks to Dr. Ronald Kanner, MD, who authored the original chapter that was used to inform the current edition. Special thanks to Holly Wagner for editorial review.

KEY POINTS: HEADACHE RELATED TO INCREASED INTRACRANIAL PRESSURE

1. High-pressure headaches are positional: worse when lying flat, improved when upright.
2. Evaluate the patient first with MRI/MR venography to rule out structural lesions, and then followed by LP to prove elevated ICP.
3. Treatment of IIH is chiefly directed at preserving visual function.

KEY POINTS: HEADACHE RELATED TO DECREASED INTRACRANIAL PRESSURE

1. Low-pressure headaches are positional: worse when upright, improved by lying flat.
2. Often a history of trauma or iatrogenic dural violation can be obtained. If this is not the case, imaging studies such as MRI or myelography can detect signs of low ICP, and may even identify the site of a CSF leak.
3. Conservative measures such as bed rest and hydration are often sufficient for intracranial hypotension to resolve spontaneously. Epidural blood patch may also be effective.

TOP SECRETS

1. Headaches resulting from abnormally high or low ICP are characterized as positional (changing when the patient is lying down versus upright).
2. In an obese woman of childbearing age presenting with positional headaches and visual changes, consider a workup for IIH.
3. In a patient presenting with headache that improves when lying down but worsens when upright, seek a history that may be consistent with persistent CSF leak.

BIBLIOGRAPHY

1. Lee SC, Lueck CJ. Cerebrospinal fluid pressure in adults. *J Neuroophthalmol*. 2014;34:278-283.
2. Oreskovic D, Klarica M. The formation of cerebrospinal fluid: nearly a hundred years of interpretations and misinterpretations. *Brain Res Rev*. 2010;64:241-262.
3. Hoffmann J, Goadsby PJ. Update on intracranial hypertension and hypotension. *Curr Opin Neurol*. 2013;26:240-247.
4. Graff-Radford SB, Schievink WI. High-pressure headaches, low-pressure syndromes, and CSF leaks: diagnosis and management. *Headache*. 2014;54:394-401.
5. Galgano MA, Deshaies EM. An update on the management of pseudotumor cerebri. *Clin Neurol Neurosurg*. 2013;115:252-259.
6. Headache Classification Committee of the International Headache Society. The International Classification of Headache Disorders, 3rd edition (beta version). *Cephalalgia*. 2013;33:629-808.

CHAPTER 18

HEADACHE AND PAIN SYNDROMES ASSOCIATED WITH EMERGENT AND CHRONIC SYSTEMIC DISEASE

Robert A. Duarte and Noah Rosen

1. **How often are headaches a manifestation of systemic disease?**
   Although headache is one of the most common pain complaints for which patients seek medical help, it is uncommonly associated with a serious systemic illness. The vast majority of headaches seen by practitioners are migraine. A smaller number are cluster, tension type, and even fewer are paroxysmal hemicranias. In an emergency room setting, up to 95% of headaches are primary (migraine) and not secondary to a systemic illness.

2. **What do patients believe is the most common systemic cause for episodic headaches?**
   Following "sinuses" as a cause for their headaches, most patients often believe that their headaches could be due to a brain tumor. These suspicions can be quickly dispelled by an imaging study or by obtaining a good history, which should include (1) duration of the headache symptoms, (2) morning awakening with headache, (3) the progressive nature of the headache, and (4) systemic complaints—for example, weight loss. Chronic headaches greater than 5 years' duration are rarely secondary to neoplastic disease. A patient presenting with an episodic headache described as "the worst headache in my life" should be ruled out for subarachnoid hemorrhage and meningitis. Often patients are concerned that their blood pressure could be causing their headaches. In general, controlled hypertension does not lead to episodic or chronic headache. However, labile blood pressure contributes to episodic headaches. And if associated with tachycardia and diaphoresis, a tumor known as *pheochromocytoma* should be part of your differential diagnosis. When a patient presents with headache, altered mental status, and marked elevation in blood pressure, hypertensive encephalopathy must be ruled out.

3. **What is the most common systemic cause of headache?**
   Febrile illnesses are probably the most common cause of headache. Even the common cold is usually associated with a headache. However, when meningitis is superimposed, these headaches become much more severe, may be bursting in character, and rapidly increase over a period of minutes to hours. The most common cause of a sudden, severe headache in children is meningitis. In severe cases, there is stiff neck, nausea, vomiting, and photophobia. These headaches result from a direct irritation of meningeal nociceptors caused by inflammation or infection. With bacterial meningitis, signs are usually fulminant. However, with an aseptic or viral meningitis, signs may be subtle and progressive over hours to days, and the cerebrospinal fluid (CSF) commonly shows just a few cells (mainly lymphocytes) and increased protein.

4. **Describe the headache characteristics associated with Lyme disease.**
   Headache is the most common symptom of neurologic Lyme disease, but rarely is headache the presenting symptom. The headache is located bifrontally and/or in the occipital region and is intermittent. When it does occur, the headache tends to resemble migraine or tension-type headache, but is often associated with cognitive impairment or focal neurologic dysfunction. Headaches associated with Lyme disease are usually seen as part of a meningitic process associated with early-stage dissemination, and they typically are responsive to antibiotic therapy. The CSF is usually abnormal, with pleocytosis.

Investigate for Lyme disease when a patient has new-onset headache, focal neurologic deficits, and residence in a Lyme-endemic region. In general, routine screening for Lyme disease is not recommended in patients with headache.

5. What exogenous substances can precipitate pain or headache?

The most common exogenous agents causing extremity pain are the statins. Reports show that up to 75% of patients on statins report symptoms of muscle pain. The most commonly recognized exogenous substances causing headache are the vasodilators. Amyl nitrite, a substance often used to heighten the sexual experience, is a potent vasodilator and may cause a severe, pounding headache, even in patients who do not have a headache diathesis. Similar reactions may occur in patients taking nitrates for cardiac disease. Alcoholic beverages can also cause headaches, both in the acute and the well-known hangover phase. The exact mechanism is unclear. For the acute headache, it appears to be vasodilatation. The hangover may be due to some vasoactive substances that are in the congeners in the alcoholic beverage.

Caffeine most often causes a headache as a withdrawal symptom. Cocaine, usually a vasorestrictive substance, can also cause headaches. Both of these headaches may be due to transient, severe rises in blood pressure or to a cerebral vasculitis. Monosodium glutamate (MSG) is a clear precipitant in patients who are sensitive to the substance. A generalized, throbbing headache develops within 20 to 25 minutes of eating food containing MSG.

In episodic migraine patients, certain analgesics—even those commonly used to treat headaches—can precipitate a chronic, daily headache syndrome if taken frequently. The headache is often described as a less severe, holocephalic head pain, often associated with generalized malaise and sleep disturbances. These agents include acetaminophen, aspirin, barbiturate-containing agents, ergots, and opioids. Estrogens and oral contraceptives are commonly associated with headaches.

6. What is the typical presentation for colloid cyst headache?

Brief, short-lasting, positional headache is the most common complaint related to colloid cyst, occasionally associated with nausea and vomiting. Rarely, a patient may experience a sudden loss of consciousness at the peak of headache. The location of the headache is bifrontal, frontoparietal, or frontooccipital, and is described as an intense, throbbing sensation, often aggravated by exertion and relieved when lying supine. The underlying mechanism for the headache secondary to a colloid cyst is thought to be due to an intermittent obstruction of the CSF flow through the foramen of Monro by a ball-valve phenomenon causing a transient and sudden increase in intracranial pressure. The physical examination is typically normal. In view of the elevated intracranial pressure, there can be signs of papilledema, nystagmus, sixth-nerve palsies, and extensor plantar responses.

7. Describe the painful neuropathy associated with diabetes.

Diabetic peripheral neuropathy is most commonly described as a distal symmetrical sensorimotor polyneuropathy followed by the autonomic neuropathies. The associated neuropathic pain presenting as an odd, dysesthetic sensation is estimated in up to 50% of people with diabetes. Diabetic amyotrophy can cause a severe, intractable bilateral but asymmetric proximal pain followed by weakness. This pain syndrome may be the initial presenting symptoms of diabetes. Unilateral eye pain can be seen in diabetics with a third nerve palsy.

8. In what degenerative diseases of the nervous system is headache or pain a common complaint?

About one-third of patients with Parkinson's disease report headaches. Between 40% and 60% of patients with Parkinson's disease have chronic pain most described as musculoskeletal pain. Although headaches do not necessarily correlate with the severity of the disease, chronic pain does appear to correlate with age of patient as well as the duration and severity of Parkinson's disease.

About 10% of patients with multiple sclerosis complain of significant headaches, either secondary to the disease process or secondary to specific disease-modifying interventions. Degenerative diseases of the cervical spine often produce a headache that radiates up from the back of the head to the vertex, consistent with an occipital neuralgiform pain. This headache is usually more intense in the morning, after the patient has slept on an elevated pillow, and relieved as the day goes on. Chronic pain has been described in up to 75% of patients in multiple sclerosis including extremity pain, trigeminal neuralgia, Lhermitte's sign, and back pain. Interestingly, there was no association between chronic pain and sites of demyelination.

9. Which central nervous system vasculitides present with headache early in the course of the disease?

Giant cell arteritis and primary angiitis of the central nervous system (CNS). Giant cell arteritis also known as temporal arteritis is the most common form of CNS vasculitis, usually presenting after the age of 50 with new-onset headache and potentially leading to permanent vision loss. Although headache is also a common symptom in primary angiitis of the CNS, it is rarely acute more often following a subacute, chronic course.

10. Describe the pain patterns that are seen in systemic lupus erythematosus.

The prevalence of headache is as high as 70% in patients with systemic lupus erythematosus (SLE). There are three major types of headache in SLE: migraine, tension-type, or associated with lupus cerebritis. Migraine-type headaches seem most common at the onset of SLE. Later in the disease, tension-type headaches are more likely to develop. The headache of lupus cerebritis is accompanied by a clear-cut picture of cerebritis, with confusion and obtundation. Active migraines have been associated with higher disease activity, antiphospholipid antibodies, and Raynaud's phenomena. Approximately 50% of patients with lupus present with diffuse joint and muscular pain.

11. How frequently is headache/pain associated with ischemic cerebrovascular disease?

Approximately 25% of patients with carotid-middle cerebral ischemia and almost 50% of those with vertebrobasilar insufficiency describe new, recurrent, nondescript headaches. Headaches can be the presenting symptom of ischemia, can occur during the actual infarction, or can follow the event, especially if there is hemorrhagic conversion. Strokes have been known to cause a central pain syndrome in up to about 15% of patients. Also known as Dejerine-Roussy syndrome, patients will present with often a patchy distribution of pain described as a severe, burning, dysesthetic sensation recalcitrant to pharmacological pain therapies.

KEY POINTS

1. Although acute and chronic headache syndromes together represent one of the most common pain disorders experienced by patients, headaches, in fact, are uncommonly associated with a serious systemic illness.
2. Chronic pain and headache conditions have become more commonly recognized in degenerative disorders.
3. Ingestion of multiple exogenous substances, including prescription and nonprescription medications, may cause chronic musculoskeletal pain headaches.

BIBLIOGRAPHY

1. Borsook D. Review article—neurological diseases and pain. *Brain.* 2012;135:320-344.
2. Diener HC, Dahlof CGH. Headache associated with chronic use of substances. In: Olesen J, Tfelt-Hansen P, Welch KMA, eds. *The Headaches.* Philadelphia: Lippincott Williams and Wilkins; 2000:871-877.
3. John S, Hajj-Ali R. Headache in autoimmune diseases. *Headache.* 2014;54(3):572-582.
4. Giannini C, Salvarani C, Hunder G, Brown RD. Primary central nervous system vasculitis: pathology and mechanisms. *Acta Neurolpathol.* 2012;123:759-772.

CHAPTER 19

TRIGEMINAL NEURALGIA

Steven Lange, Abigail Bemis, Julia Prusik and Julie G. Pilitsis

1. What is trigeminal neuralgia?

   Trigeminal neuralgia (TN) is a chronic condition characterized by nonpainful stimuli to the face, leading to intense pain. It is most common in women older than 50, although men and younger adults can also be affected. Patients report intermittent, shooting pain to the face that lasts seconds to minutes. The pain usually follows one distribution of the trigeminal nerve: V1, V2, or V3. These are the ophthalmic, maxillary, and mandibular dermatomes, respectively, carrying sensory information from the defined areas of coverage.

   TN can be classified into several subtypes. Type 1 is characterized by predominantly episodic pain, and type 2 is characterized by constant pain. To be defined as trigeminal neuropathic pain, it must result from injury to the nerve due to trauma or surgery. Another classification is trigeminal deafferentation pain, which results from damage due to peripheral nerve ablation, gangliolysis, or rhizotomy attempted to treat facial pain. Postherpetic neuralgia can also occur in the trigeminal distribution. Lastly, atypical facial pain produces facial pain due to a somatoform pain disorder and requires psychological examination for an accurate diagnosis.

2. What are common causes of trigeminal neuralgia?

   In most cases, TN is caused by vascular compression of the nerve, most commonly the superior cerebellar artery (SCA), followed by the anteroinferior cerebellar artery and the basilar artery. Nerve compression may also be due to tumors, dural arteriovenous fistulas, and an ectactic basilar artery. Additionally, the pathophysiology of TN in multiple sclerosis (MS) is different. In MS it is common for demyelination to be present at the root entry zone of the trigeminal nerve in the pons, whereas compression may take place anywhere along the whole course of the nerve for TN in other pathologies.

3. How is trigeminal neuralgia diagnosed?

   A medical history and neurological examination in combination with magnetic resonance imaging is used to determine whether the patient has TN and if there is vascular compression of the nerve. The branch of the trigeminal nerve involved is determined by inspection based on dermatomes V1, V2, and V3 and presence of reflexes in these distributions.

4. How is trigeminal neuralgia treated?

   Treatment of TN begins with medication, most commonly carbamazepine or other anticonvulsants, including gabapentin. Patients prescribed carbamazepine must undergo weekly blood testing during the initial 2 months to monitor levels of carbamazepine therapy. Once an adequate dose has been reached, testing is less frequent but regular to ensure the drug is within acceptable levels in the blood.

   These medications are generally effective in alleviating nerve pain with side effects, including fatigue, headaches, and nausea. Doses vary based on the drug of choice, with the dose for pain mediation commonly being less than the recommended for epileptic patients prescribed the same pharmacologic agent. There have also been multiple reports of the efficacy of antidepressants, muscle relaxants, and steroids in treating TN.

5. How effective are medications as treatments for trigeminal neuralgia?

   Medications are not ubiquitously helpful, or may diminish in effectiveness after use for a certain period of time. In these cases, other treatment options may be considered in dealing with TN, such as physical therapy, holistic options, or invasive options. Physical therapies involving heat treatment, ultrasound, craniosacral manipulation, and massage have been beneficial to some patients. For others, acupuncture, yoga, and meditation have provided relief. Lastly, invasive options such as botulinum toxin type-A, percutaneous procedures, radiosurgery, and open surgery may be considered.

6. **What is microvascular decompression and when is it an appropriate treatment?**
   In cases in which there is vascular compression, the gold standard of surgical treatment is microvascular decompression. Commonly alleviating pain in 70% to 80% of patients at 10 years after treatment, this procedure involves creating an incision behind the ear and displacing the artery in contact with the nerve. Although uncommon, risks of this procedure include potential facial numbness, partial hearing loss, double vision, and in severe cases, stroke.

7. **What are additional procedures to treat trigeminal neuralgia?**
   Percutaneous procedures include balloon compression, radiofrequency ablation, and glycerol rhizotomy. Each of these methods uses a needle to reach the trigeminal nerve through the face and uses glycerol, an inflated balloon, or an electrical current to damage the nerve. These procedures are beneficial and often reduce pain for years. However, problems associated with this type of procedure include recurrent pain, with the patient sometimes experiencing facial numbness and facial muscle weakness. Radiosurgery is another treatment option offered to many patients, which uses a dose of radiation aimed at the root entry zone of the nerve.

8. **What is different about trigeminal neuralgia in multiple sclerosis?**
   Between 1% and 2% of patients with MS present with symptoms of TN. In patients with a history of MS, TN generally presents bilaterally. TN complaints in MS patients are most common between the ages of 60 and 70 years of age, and in these patients a history of hypertension is correlated with a slightly higher incidence of TN. Unfortunately, TN secondary to MS is extremely difficult to treat, as painful symptoms stem from demyelination rather than vascular compression of the nerve root. Therapies effective in traditional TN are often less effective for this mechanism of action, and treatment should focus on MS prior to TN.

KEY POINTS

1. TN is defined by intense localized pain resulting from nonpainful stimuli to the face. It is most commonly caused by vascular compression of a nerve.
2. Medications, specifically anticonvulsants, are the first line of defense against TN.
3. Microvascular decompression is the gold standard surgical treatment for TN.

BIBLIOGRAPHY

1. Braunwald E, Fauci A, Kasper D, et al. *Harrison's Principles of Internal Medicine*. 15th ed. New York: McGraw-Hill; 2001.
2. Burchiel KJ. A new classification for facial pain. *Neurosurgery*. 2003;53(5):1164-1166.
3. Love S, Coakham HB. Trigeminal neuralgia: pathology and pathogenesis. *Brain*. 2001;124(12):2347-2360.
4. Lutz J, Linn J, Mehrkens JH, et al. Trigeminal neuralgia due to neurovascular compression: high-spatial-resolution diffusion-tensor imaging reveals microstructural neural changes. *Radiology*. 2011;258:524-530.
5. Gronseth G, Cruccu G, Alksne J, et al. Practice parameters: the diagnostic evaluation and treatment of trigeminal neuralgia (an evidence-based review): report of the quality standards subcommittee of the American academy of neurology and the European federation of neurological societies. *Neurology*. 2008;71(15):1183-1190.
6. Wiffen PJ, Derry S, Moore RA, McQuay HJ. Carbamazepine for acute and chronic pain in adults. *Cochrane Database Syst Rev*. 2011;(1):CD005451.
7. Verma G. Role of botulinum toxin type-A (BTX-A) in the management of trigeminal neuralgia. *Pain Res Treat*. 2013;Article ID 831094:6 pages.
8. Bolay H, Reuter U, Dunn AK, et al. Intrinsic brain activity triggers trigeminal meningeal afferents in a migraine model. *Nat Med*. 2002;8(2):136-142.
9. Zakrzewska JM, Lopez BC, Kim SE, Coakham HB. Patient reports of satisfaction after microvascular decompression and partial sensory rhizotomy for trigeminal neuralgia. *Neurosurgery*. 2005;56:1304-1311.
10. Krafft R. Trigeminal neuralgia. *Am Fam Physician*. 2008;77(9):1291-1296.
11. Katusic S, Beard CM, Bergstralh E, Kurland LT. Incidence and clinical features of trigeminal neuralgia, Rochester, Minnesota, 1945–1984. *Ann Neurol*. 1990;27(1):89-95.

CHAPTER 20

GLOSSOPHARYNGEAL AND OTHER FACIAL NEURALGIAS

Fady Girgis and Jonathan Miller

1. What is glossopharyngeal neuralgia?

   Glossopharyngeal neuralgia (GPN) is a unilateral severe pain felt in the distribution of the glossopharyngeal nerve, the auricular (Jacobsen's nerve) and pharyngeal branches of the vagus nerve. Pain occurs in the ear, the posterior third of the tongue, and the tonsillar fossa.

2. How does glossopharyngeal neuralgia present?

   Pain is elicited by stimulating trigger points in the cutaneous distribution of the glossopharyngeal or vagus nerves, often with swallowing, chewing, yawning, or coughing. Note that while most triggers mimic those of trigeminal neuralgia, swallowing is specific to GPN. In "classic" GPN, patients are pain-free in between severe episodes that are brief and lancinating. In "symptomatic" GPN, an aching pain is present between the episodes of stabbing pain. Episodes often occur in clusters, and patients tend to sit leaning forward and drool during attacks. Syncope occurs in 10% of cases, due to hypersensitivity of the dorsal motor nucleus of the vagus nerve.

3. How common is glossopharyngeal neuralgia?

   GPN is a rare disorder, 1/100 as common as trigeminal neuralgia. It occurs most frequently in middle-aged men and women.

4. What is the etiology of glossopharyngeal neuralgia?

   The majority of GPN cases are idiopathic or are related to neurovascular compression of cranial nerves IX and X. Tumors involving the jugular foramen can cause GPN as well. Eagle syndrome is another uncommon but well-described cause, where an elongated styloid process or ossified stylohyoid ligament compresses the glossopharyngeal nerve.

5. How is glossopharyngeal neuralgia diagnosed?

   GPN is a clinical diagnosis. Imaging investigations can include magnetic resonance imaging (MRI) to assess for vascular compression and to rule out neoplastic lesions and demyelinating disease. Computed tomography or plain films are also recommended to assess for Eagle syndrome. The diagnosis can often be confirmed by the cessation of pain with a nerve block at the jugular foramen or with application of topical anesthesia to the pharynx.

6. What is the pharmacologic treatment for glossopharyngeal neuralgia?

   Antiepileptic medications such as carbamazepine and gabapentin are commonly used to treat GPN. If syncope is a prominent feature of the disease, atropine can also be used.

7. What are the surgical options for treatment of glossopharyngeal neuralgia?

   Surgical treatment is reserved for cases of drug inefficacy or intolerance. Microvascular decompression of the cranial nerves IX and X is first line, often producing excellent results. If no vascular compression is present, sectioning of the nerve IX and upper rootlets of nerve X can be performed. Other options include percutaneous radiofrequency rhizotomy and radiosurgery. In the event of Eagle syndrome, the pain can be cured by resection of the styloid process.

8. Describe the presentation and treatment of geniculate neuralgia.

   Geniculate neuralgia, also termed nervus intermedius neuralgia, is an extremely rare disorder that affects young to middle-aged women. It presents as brief intermittent episodes of deep stabbing ear pain, triggered by cutaneous stimulation of the auditory canal. The pain can also be associated with increased salivation, a bitter taste, and/or tinnitus. MRI should be used to carefully assess the cerebellopontine angle, looking for vascular compression of cranial nerves V to X. Medical treatment consists of anti-epileptic drugs and surgical treatment involves microvascular decompression or sectioning of the nervus intermedius.

9. What is Ramsay-Hunt syndrome?

Ramsay-Hunt syndrome is a herpetic infection of the geniculate ganglion of the facial nerve. Symptoms include ear and facial pain, lower motor neuron facial weakness, and vesicular eruption around the external auditory canal. Treatment comprises oral acyclovir and corticosteroids.

10. What is the most common presentation of acute herpes zoster of the face?

Ophthalmic zoster, a herpetic eruption in the V1 distribution of the trigeminal nerve, is the most common. Pain may precede the eruption by several days. This type of facial herpes is the most dangerous, as the viral vesicles may involve the eye, leading to blindness in severe untreated cases. In addition to oral antiviral treatment with acyclovir, the eye must be protected from secondary infection. Like other herpes infections, postherpetic neuralgia is a dreaded sequela, and occurs more commonly in the elderly.

11. Describe the presentation and treatment of occipital neuralgia.

Occipital neuralgia is characterized by a sharp pain originating in the back of the head and radiating into the distribution of the greater and/or lesser occipital nerves, and sometimes into the eye. Symptoms can be triggered or unprovoked, and are often associated with dysesthesia in the same distribution. Most cases are unilateral, but bilateral occipital neuralgia does occur. Compression or trauma to the involved nerve(s) is often a cause, but many cases are idiopathic. Medical management with antiepileptic agents is first-line treatment, and local anesthetic injections can transiently relieve the pain and confirm the diagnosis. Surgical treatments include C2/3 ganglionectomy and occipital nerve stimulation.

12. What is Tolosa-Hunt syndrome?

Tolosa-Hunt syndrome is a painful ophthalmoplegia caused by idiopathic inflammation in the region of the superior orbital fissure. Acute-onset deep retro-orbital pain often precedes the onset of diplopia. MRI is a useful modality to confirm inflammation of the cavernous sinus, although sometimes it presents as normal. While the pain will respond well to corticosteroids within 24 to 72 hours of therapy initiation, the ophthalmoparesis can take up to several months to resolve, and in severe cases may be permanent.

13. What is superior laryngeal neuralgia?

The superior laryngeal nerve, a branch of the vagus nerve, innervates the cricothyroid muscle of the larynx. This muscle stretches, tenses, and adducts the vocal cord. Superior laryngeal neuralgia usually appears as a postsurgical complication. There are paroxysms of unilateral submandibular pain, sometimes radiating to the eye, ear, or shoulder. This pain may be indistinguishable from GPN. It lasts from seconds to minutes and is usually provoked by swallowing, straining the voice, turning the head, coughing, sneezing, yawning, or blowing the nose.

14. Define sphenopalatine neuralgia.

Sphenopalatine neuralgia, also termed lower half headache, greater superficial neuralgia, and Sluder's neuralgia, is an uncommon facial pain disorder. Key clinical features include unilateral pain in the face lasting for days and associated with nasal congestion, otalgia, and tinnitus. Unlike trigeminal and GPN, sphenopalatine neuralgia is not commonly associated with a trigger zone. Some authors believe that this is not a separate syndrome and may simply be a variation of cluster headache. Treatment options are limited, but sphenopalatine ganglion blocks have been tried with minimal success.

Acknowledgments

We wish to acknowledge Dr. Robert Duarte and Dr. Charles Argoff for preparing the original version of this chapter.

KEY POINTS

1. GPN shares similar triggers with that of trigeminal neuralgia, such as talking and chewing, but swallowing is a trigger that is often specific to GPN.
2. If GPN occurs in the setting of objective sensory loss or motor weakness, a structural lesion should be considered and imaging investigations pursued.

3. Medications such as carbamazepine are first-line treatments for GPN, and surgical options such as microvascular decompression and/or sectioning of cranial nerves IX and X should be reserved for cases of drug inefficacy or intolerance.
4. The differential diagnosis of facial pain should include trigeminal neuralgia, geniculate neuralgia, occipital neuralgia, Ramsay-Hunt syndrome, Tolosa-Hunt syndrome, superior laryngeal neuralgia, sphenopalatine neuralgia, dental or periodontal disease, and temporomandibular joint pain.

BIBLIOGRAPHY

1. Blumenfeld A, Nikolskaya G. Glossopharyngeal neuralgia. *Curr Pain Headache Rep.* 2013;17:343.
2. Rey-Dios R, Cohen-Gadol AA. Current neurosurgical management of glossopharyngeal neuralgia and technical nuances for microvascular decompression surgery. *Neurosurg Focus.* 2013;34:E8.
3. Siccoli MM, Bassetti CL, Sandor PS. Facial pain: clinical differential diagnosis. *Lancet Neurol.* 2006;5:257-267.
4. Sweet JA, Mitchell LS, Narouze S, et al. Occipital nerve stimulation for the treatment of patients with medically refractory occipital neuralgia: Congress of Neurological Surgeons Systematic Review and Evidence-Based Guideline. *Neurosurgery.* 2015;77:332-341.
5. Tang IP, Freeman SR, Kontorinis G, et al. Geniculate neuralgia: a systematic review. *J Laryngol Otol.* 2014;128:394-399.

CHAPTER 21

ACUTE AND CHRONIC LOW BACK PAIN

Sarah Narayan and Andrew Dubin

ACUTE PAIN

Acute pain stems from a direct injury to soft tissue or bone. This is pain lasting for 4 weeks or less. Time frames are somewhat arbitrary, since it is anticipated that those with acute back pain will either heal on their own or receive the appropriate treatment to recover from their injury. Eighty-four percent of adults will experience back pain some time in their lives. A majority of those with back pain improve over time. Low back pain is one of the leading causes of missed work and doctors visits. This pain can be either localized (axial) versus radiating pain (radicular). We will discuss the more common presentations of acute pain.

Before discussing the common sources of back pain, we must appreciate the anatomy of the lumbar spine. The lumbar spine is made up of five lumbar vertebrae. There is a network of ligaments that surround these bony parts, like Saran Wrap. The sacrum is made up of five fused vertebrae. All lumbar and sacral spinal nerve roots originate at T10 to L1, where the spinal cord terminates at the conus medullaris. The nerve roots come off the spinal cord and travel down the central canal, behind the vertebrae, before exiting at the neural foramina. The lumbar intervertebral discs cushion each vertebra, serving as a shock absorber for the vertebral bodies. The discs also create additional height between the vertebrae to create space for the lumbar nerve roots to exit from. Along the posterior aspect of the spine, the vertebrae communicate with one another through the lumbar zygo-epophyseal joint (facet joint) bilaterally. With age, the spine undergoes degenerative changes marked by dehydration of the intervertebral disc. This in combination with the body's weight on the vertebral bodies creates stress on the facet joints. Over time there is also development of calcifications along the edges of the disc spaces (disc osteophyte changes). The calcifications, joint arthritis, and dehydration of the discs create arthritic changes of the spine called lumbar spondylosis. Thus spondylosis is a broad term describing arthritic changes of the spine.

What is a lumbar strain?

Lumbar strain is the most common cause of lower back pain. Over 85% of patients will have nonspecific low back pain. Statistics suggest that 80% to 90% of all back pain improves. A majority of these cases fall under this type of injury. Strains can be caused by overuse, misuse, or trauma to the lower back. Injury occurs to the soft tissue causing micro trauma to the muscle, tendon, or ligament. Pain is localized without nerve injury. Since this is a soft tissue injury, no imaging (x-ray, computed tomography [CT] scan, magnetic resonance imaging [MRI]) is necessary for workup. Treatments include 1 to 2 days of relative rest followed by a return to normal activity. Nonsteroidal antiinflammatory drugs (NSAIDs), heat or ice as well as manual treatment may provide supportive improvement to assist with pain relief. Strains tend to improve over the course of several weeks. Prolonged rest, which was thought to be helpful, has now been found to prolong recovery.

Tell me about lumbar radiculopathy?

Lumbar radiculopathy is caused by direct injury to the nerve roots in the lumbar spine, most often when these nerves exit the neural foramina. Estimated lifetime prevalence is approximately 3% to 5% of adults, with equal amounts among men and women. The most common sources of this injury are due to disc herniation and arthritic overgrowth of the spine. It is rare that radiculopathy is caused by infection, inflammation, neoplasm, or vascular disease. Each nerve root will provide a predominant area of sensation in the leg. This is called a *dermatome*. Each nerve root will also provide predominant innervation to muscles in the leg; this motor assignment is called a *myotome*. The L5 nerve root is the most common nerve affected in lumbar radiculopathies. An L5 radiculopathy will present as pain along a dermatomal distribution, along the lateral leg to the top of the foot. Strength is diminished with foot dorsiflexion, toe extension, and both foot inversion and eversion. When nerve damage progresses, there is hip abduction weakness. The second most common nerve affected is the S1 nerve root. Examination suggesting S1 involvement will include sensory changes along the posterior leg and bottom of foot, with weakness on plantar flexion and possibly hip extension and knee flexion. Ankle reflexes may be absent. Lumbosacral myotomal and dermatomal distributions are noted in Chart 1. Radiculopathy is diagnosed clinically, although it may be recommended to perform imaging such as an MRI or CT scan to confirm this diagnosis. A noncontrast MRI or CT myelogram provides good visualization of the nerve roots. It is strongly recommended imaging be performed if there is suspicion of neoplasm, neurologic deficits, urinary changes, saddle anesthesia, severe lower extremity weakness, or abscess/inection. An electromyography (EMG) can be performed if there is any question regarding the specific nerve root involvement. With EMG testing, typically the nerve conduction testing is normal with abnormal insertional activity in muscles predominantly innervated by a specific nerve root. For severe S1 radiculopathies, the H reflex will be absent.

Most cases of lumbar radiculopathy are self-limiting. Nonetheless radiculopathy can be extremely painful. NSAIDs and activity modification are typically recommended. If severe pain continues despite NSAIDs use, short-term (3 days to 2 weeks) opioid medication can be considered. Systemic glucocorticoids can be considered. Although activity modification is recommended during acute presentation, physical therapy can be considered if pain persists over 3 weeks. Epidural steroid injections provide modest temporary benefits, lasting approximately 3 months. Surgery may be an option if disabling pain persists for 6 weeks or there is profound weakness. Presentation of cauda equina syndrome is an emergent indication for surgery.

What is spondylolysis? How must one evaluate and treat this injury?
Spondylolysis describes a fracture of the pars interarticularis, which is located along the posterior arch of the bony spine. These fractures can be unilateral or bilateral; a bilateral presentation makes 80% of the cases. These fractures are caused by activity fatigue or acute overload. More than 90% of these fractures occur at the L5 vertebrae. Spondylolysis is the common cause of back pain in young athletes. Gymnasts, football players, wrestlers, dancers, and any young athletes who perform repetitive twisting and extension motions are at risk for back injury. Fatigue fractures in athletes commonly occur during growth spurts. Stress along the pars interarticularis will cause underlying spondylolysis (also known as "pars defect"). Spondylolysis is commonly asymptomatic, with diagnosis commonly found incidentally. Pain is often intermittent and can refer to the buttock or posterior thigh. Extension and rotation of the lumbar spine will commonly reproduce the pain. Tight hamstrings can usually be found on examination.

AP and lateral x-rays are the initial visual modality to rule out fracture. If the x-rays are clear but there is still clinical suspicion of a fracture, an MRI or single-photon emission computed tomography (SPECT) bone scan can be performed. A CT scan can be performed but it encompasses exposure to high doses of radiation. Those with bilateral spondylolysis may also develop spondylolisthesis, or shifting of the one lumbar vertebra over the other. With uncomplicated cases (without radiculopathy, factures, etc.) it is advised to limit inciting activity for 2 to 4 weeks. This simple plan is very effective for most cases. For athletes unwilling to rest, bracing during activity can be utilized. NSAIDs are recommended for pain management. Those with nerve injury must receive a consultation with a spine specialist. On physical exam, testing for hypermobility should be strongly considered. Patients with a grade 2 or higher (spondylolisthesis is scored at grade 1 to 5) should be evaluated by a surgeon. After treatment, once the patient is pain free, slow reintegration back into sports should be undertaken.

What are common sources of spinal infection?
Vertebral osteomyelitis and discitis typically occurs from transmission of infection from an outside focus. Infection can also spread through adjacent tissue, from a spinal surgery, injections, direct invasive diagnostic procedures, or spread through the blood stream. Infection of the disc and bony vertebrae are, for the most part, treated similarly. The incidence of osteomyelitis increases with age. Risk factors include degenerative discs, endocarditis, history of spine surgery, diabetes, steroid exposure, immune-compromised states, and history of drug use. Staph aureus accounts for more than 50% of the bacterial infections. Pain is typically localized at the site of infection. Fever is not a good predictor of whether or not an infection is present. Erythrocyte sedimentation rate (ESR) and C-reactive protein (CRP) lab work is advised. Blood cultures and MRI of the spine should also be considered. Diagnosis is made with a CT guided biopsy and culture of infected tissue. Diagnosis may be inferred even if cultures and Gram stain are negative, but clinical suspicion exists. Antibiotic therapy is the mainstay of treatment. This treatment can last from 6 to 12 weeks with weekly ESR and CRP levels drawn. If there is evidence of abscess, nerve injury, or cord compression, a surgery may be considered. Relative rest and opioid pain management is recommended for the focal pain.

Tell me about epidural abscesses?

Epidural abscesses are most often found in the thoracolumbar spine. Bacteria can travel hematogenously into the epidural space, by adjacent tissue or from contamination postspinal procedure. Risk factors include diabetes, HIV infection, trauma, alcoholism, IV drug abuse, tattooing, neighboring infection, or hemodialysis. Staph aureus makes up 63% of all infections. Methicillin-resistant *Staphylococcus aureus* (MRSA) makes up roughly one-fourth of all Staph infections. Fever may or may not be present. Symptoms include severe, focal pain. Based on the extent of compression along the nerves and spinal cord, nerve injury ranges from radicular pain to paralysis. WBC, ESR, CRP, and blood cultures can be drawn. MRI should be performed if there is clinical suspicion of abscess. CT with IV contrast may be an alternative image modality. Abscess fluid culture is recommended. Treatment includes direct incision and drainage as well as antibiotic therapy. Empiric antibiotics following collection of two sets of cultures should start once the suspicion of infection is made. Treatment lasts for 4 to 8 weeks. Repeat MRI should be performed between 4 and 6 weeks. Serial WBC, ESR, and CRP values should be performed.

Please explain what a vertebral compression fracture is?

Osteoporosis is the most common cause of vertebral compression fractures, followed by trauma. The most common levels of compression fractures are at T7-8 and T12-L1. Osteoporosis causes low trauma fractures that can be asymptomatic. On the other hand, acute, fairly severe compression fractures can be painful. This pain is fairly localized. If there is retropulsion of bony elements, this can narrow the central canal, causing nerve-related pain. Back pain can be reproduced with sitting, spinal extension, movement, or bearing down. There is often tenderness to palpation on examination. Neurologic examination should be performed to rule out nerve injury. Typically acute pain subsides after 3 to 6 weeks, although it may take longer for others to heal. It usually takes 3 months for full healing to occur. Multiple fractures in the thoracic spine can lead to thoracic kyphosis. If severe pain persists, this may indicate an additional compression fracture. There is a 19% risk of recurrent fracture over a year. Women are 4 times more likely to get another compression fracture. Diagnosis can be made with plain radiographs, which will show anterior wedging of the vertebrae due to vertebral collapse. An MRI of the lumbar spine can be performed to determine the acuity, evaluate neurologic compromise, and rule out infection or malignancy (if there is a high suspicion of either metastatic disease or infection). First line of treatment for pain includes Tylenol or NSAIDs. Intranasal calcitonin (200 units daily) can also be considered if over-the-counter treatment is not enough for mild to moderate pain. If severe pain is present, short-term opioids may be considered during the acute phase. Physical therapy can work on core strengthening and ambulation once activity can be tolerated. Exercise is also beneficial to improve bone density. Aquatic therapy is a great alternative exercise strategy for pain sufferers. Bracing has not been proven to be effective, but can be used as a kinesthetic reminder to limit flexion. If severe pain persists for over 6 weeks, opioids are poorly tolerated, and activities of daily living are compromised, vertebral augmentation (vertebroplasty and kyphoplasty) may be considered. The difference between vertebroplasty and kyphoplasty is that kyphoplasty uses a balloon mechanism to expand the vertebral space before cement is injected in the collapsed space. Vertebroplasty is easier to perform and more cost effective.

CHRONIC PAIN

This is a type of pain that can last for 3 months or longer. Similar to acute pain, the time frame can be somewhat arbitrary. While acute pain is clearly related to direct trauma to the musculoskeletal system, this is more of an "adaptive" or protective mechanism to safeguard from injury. Chronic pain tends to occur as either part of a disease process (arthritis, malalignment), or it can be a maladaptive transmission through the neurologic pathway. This syndrome of pain will be present despite completing the anticipated time frame of healing. This refers to more of an unidentifiable pain with no clear pain generator. This pain signal is generated and controlled by the central nervous system. This type of pain is modified by factors outside the scope of physical trauma. Modifiers include mood, sleep, physically deconditioned states, or even medications. While one can argue that acute pain serves a biological purpose to protect humans from further damage, there is unfortunately no biological purpose for some chronic pain. Treatment objective is focused on modifying this pain response for sufferers to function effectively in their daily lives.

What is facet arthritis?

Facet-mediated pain is a relatively localized back pain that can be caused by lumbar facet arthritis. Facet-mediated pain without clear arthritic change can also be present. This presentation is marked by pain across the back, with radiation occasionally down the buttock or posterior thighs. Discomfort is reproduced with lumbar extension and rotation (facet loading). Plain films can be performed to confirm arthritis and to rule out bone trauma. Techniques to correct leg and pelvic posture, NSAID administration, and lumbar facet injections or radiofrequency ablation can be performed for treatment.

What is lumbar stenosis? How does is present?

This type of pain presentation is commonly noted in the aging population (those over the age of 60) who develop degenerative changes in the spine. Nonetheless lumbar stenosis can be created by a large central disc herniation. A combination of factors, including disc bulging, facet capsular hypertrophy, ligamentum flavum hypertrophy, and osteophyte formation, can all contribute to narrowing of the central canal. Spondylolisthesis can also contribute to central canal narrowing. Due to this narrowing, the spinal nerve roots that make up the cauda equina can be compressed and ischemic. Any of the potential nerve roots traveling distally can be affected by this tight squeeze. Also, the increase in intrathecal pressure, decrease in arterial flow, and venous congestion can additionally affect these nerve structures. A flexed posture will traditionally open the canal, while standing erect or extending the spine will promote increased intrathecal pressure. Manifestation of neurologic symptoms is described as neurogenic claudication. Sitting and lying flat provides symptomatic relief. Upright postures tend to narrow the canal; standing and walking are uncomfortable. Pain can be nonspecific, depending on the predominant nerve root(s) affected. A wide-based gait is the most common examination finding, followed by absent ankle reflexes (noted in less than half of sufferers). Diagnosis is made based on clinical findings in conjunction with neuroimaging. Noncontrast MRI of CT myelogram of the lumbar spine is recommended, since the soft tissue elements (ligament, joint capsule, disc) causing stenosis can be visualized, as well as the bony factors. Area in the canal less than 76 mm^2 marks severe stenosis; less than 100 mm^2 for moderate stenosis. Because spinal stenosis is most often due to degenerative changes, symptoms often persist long term. About 20% to 30% of those with stenosis are asymptomatic. On the other hand, those with lumbar stenosis can present with progressive disability. Conservative care includes physical therapy, NSAIDs or analgesic administration, and epidural injections. Should conservative approaches fail, surgery can be considered.

What is sacroiliac joint dysfunction?

Sacroiliac joint dysfunction may present as pain along the superior aspect of the buttock adjacent to the L5 vertebrae. Pain is reproduced with lumbar flexion and extension. Atrophy of the lumbar extensors muscles or disuse often predisposes those to sacroiliac joint instability. Provocative testing on physical exam to confirm sacroiliac joint dysfunction includes pelvic distraction, compression, Gaenslen's, FABERs (Flexion ABduction External Rotation), and thigh thrust. Treatment includes relative rest, NSAIDs, physical therapy, and joint injections.

How does diabetic amyotrophy present?

This will occur in those with type 2 diabetes. Common presentation is acute, asymmetric, and focal onset of pain and weakness usually in the proximal leg. This will progress over the course of a few months and then partially or fully resolve over time. As this pain progresses, symptoms may become symmetric. Weight loss may be associated with onset of diabetic amyotrophy. Electrodiagnostic testing, namely nerve conduction studies, show significant reduction in motor amplitudes and sensory action potentials but mild slowing of conduction velocities. EMG testing will show fibrillation potentials as well as decreased recruitment, with motor units demonstrating high amplitude and long duration. Lumbar imaging may be used to rule out other sources of nerve injury stemming from the spine. Symptomatic management with neuropathic pain agents and consideration of opioid pain management may be considered.

KEY POINTS

1. 85% of low back pain sufferers will present with nonspecific pain.
2. 80% to 90% of low back pain will resolve over time.
3. The L5 nerve root is the most common nerve injured in a lumbar radiculopathy; the S1 nerve root is the second most common nerve root affected.
4. 80% of lumbar spondylolysis occurs bilaterally.

BIBLIOGRAPHY

1. Woolf AD, Pfleger B. Burden of major musculoskeletal conditions. *Bull World Health Organ.* 2003;81:646.
2. Deyo RA, Tsui-Wu YJ. Descriptive epidemiology of low-back pain and its related medical care in the United States. *Spine.* 1987;12:264.
3. Chou R. In the clinic. Low back pain. *Ann Intern Med.* 2014;160:ITC6.
4. Tarulli AW, Raynor EM. Lumbosacral radiculopathy. *Neurol Clin.* 2007;25:387.
5. Cho SC, Ferrante MA, Levin KH, Harmon RL, So YT. Utility of electrodiagnostic testing in evaluating patients with lumbosacral radiculopathy: an evidence-based review. *Muscle Nerve.* 2010;42:276.
6. Roelofs PD, Deyo RA, Koes BW, Scholten RJ, van Tulder MW. Non-steroidal anti-inflammatory drugs for low back pain. *Cochrane Database Syst Rev.* 2008;(23):CD000396.
7. Chou R, Hashimoto R, Friedly J, et al. Epidural corticosteroid injections for radiculopathy and spinal stenosis: a systematic review and meta-analysis. *Ann Intern Med.* 2015;163:373.
8. Chou R, Loeser JD, Owens DK, et al. Interventional therapies, surgery, and interdisciplinary rehabilitation for low back pain: an evidence-based clinical practice guideline from the American Pain Society. *Spine.* 2009;34:1066.
9. Sakai T, Sairyo K, Suzue N, Kosaka H, Yasui N. Incidence and etiology of lumbar spondylolysis: review of the literature. *J Orthop Sci.* 2010;15:281.
10. McTimoney CA, Micheli LJ. Current evaluation and management of spondylolysis and spondylolisthesis. *Curr Sports Med Rep.* 2003;2:41.
11. Berbari EF, Kanj SS, Kowalski TJ, et al. 2015 Infectious Diseases Society of America (IDSA) clinical practice guidelines for the diagnosis and treatment of native vertebral osteomyelitis in adults. *Clin Infect Dis.* 2015;61:e26.
12. Markus HS. Haematogenous osteomyelitis in the adult: a clinical and epidemiological study. *Q J Med.* 1989;71:521.
13. Genant HK, Cooper C, Poor G, et al. Interim report and recommendations of the World Health Organization Task-Force for Osteoporosis. *Osteoporos Int.* 1999;10:259.
14. Papaioannou A, Watts NB, Kendler DL, et al. Diagnosis and management of vertebral fractures in elderly adults. *Am J Med.* 2002;113:220.
15. Classification of chronic pain. Descriptions of chronic pain syndromes and definitions of pain terms. Prepared by the International Association for the Study of Pain, subcommittee on taxonomy. *Pain Suppl.* 1986;3:S1.
16. Katz JN, Harris MB. Clinical practice. Lumbar spinal stenosis. *N Engl J Med.* 2008;358:818.
17. Garland H. Diabetic amyotrophy. *BMJ.* 1955;2:1287.

CHAPTER 22

ACUTE AND CHRONIC NECK AND ARM PAIN

Sarah Narayan and Andrew Dubin

Neck pain is not as common as low back pain. Cervicalgia is experienced by 10% of all adults.

One must appreciate the cervical anatomy to better appreciate areas of potential injury. The neck is made up of seven bony vertebrae.

What are certain features of the cervical spine? Tell about common injuries affecting the cervical spine?

The integration of the occiput with C1 and the atlantooccipital joint, provide one-third of flexion-extension and 50% of lateral bending. The atlantoaxial joint and articulation between C1 and C2 provide 50% of rotation. The joints of the C2-C4 vertebrae contribute to two-thirds of flexion-extension, 50% rotation, and 50% of lateral bending. Typically most degenerative changes occur at the C2-C7 segments of the cervical spine. The cervical spine has a normal lordotic curvature. This curve flattens or reverses with arthritic changes or muscle spasm. Accentuated curvature may be a secondary postural adjustment that can occur with thoracic kyphosis or poor posture. Average rotational capability is 90 degrees; lateral bending is 45 degrees, flexion at 60 degrees, and extension at 75 degrees.

Injuries to the cervical spine can cause localized neck pain (axial) versus pain that is referred into the upper extremities.

Cervical strain describes irritation to the muscles or ligaments of the neck. This pain can be attributed to overuse, poor posture, and positioning. The pain will typically last for several weeks but will improve if the source of the pain is avoided.

Myofascial neck pain is described as pain in areas of the neck and shoulders. This is more of a chronic pain marked by tight bands of both muscle and tissue, called *trigger points*. Palpation of trigger points can refer pain to a different location of the upper body. Myofascial pain can be modified with various stressors, including physical, emotional, or psychological.

Whiplash injury occurs from abrupt, forceful flexion-extension of the cervical spine. This can occur quite often on impact during a motor vehicle collision. The violent movement of the neck will often stress the surrounding joints, muscles, discs, nerves, and ligaments of the cervical spine. Pain will occur nonspecifically along the neck and shoulders. Although this injury is common, the nature of the pain is poorly understood. In one meta-analysis it was found that 50% of adults with whiplash will still have pain after 1 year. Microvascular bleeding and soft tissue inflammation explain the acute source of soft tissue pain. The cause of the chronic pain is not quite understood. It is theorized injury to the alar ligaments may explain the chronic nature of the pain.

Cervical radiculopathy refers to injury of the cervical nerve root. The common injury to a cervical nerve root can be caused by direct compression from a disc herniation, from degenerative changes narrowing the neuro-foramina, or from central stenosis. The C7 nerve root is the most common site of injury, making up 70% of all cervical radiculopathy injuries. The C6 nerve root makes up 20% of cervical nerve root injuries. Radicular pain is marked by paresthesias and/or numbness along a dermatomal distribution down the neck, arm, and hand. Some will experience weakness along a myotomal distribution or will have reflex changes, depending upon the nerve affected. Diagnosis is made based on history and physical examination. On examination, the Spurling's maneuver (cervical extension and ipsilateral rotation) can reproduce cervical nerve root compression. This examination maneuver is highly specific but carries a low sensitivity. Neuroimaging or electromyography (EMG) testing can be confirmatory but not necessarily diagnostic. An MRI or CT myelogram can confirm nerve compression or central stenosis. An EMG can confirm the location and general timing of the cervical radiculopathy. A short period of high-dose glucocorticoids can provide good temporary relief. Nonsteroidal antiinflammatory drugs may also be an option for management of neck pain. Both tricyclic and reuptake inhibitor antidepressants as well as gabapentin have been prescribed for radicular pain. Cervical traction can be used to expand the intervertebral disc spaces and decompress the area of neck pain. Physical therapy can be performed in conjunction with the traction. Epidural steroid injections have been shown to provide good improvement of radicular pain for up to 6 months of relief. Surgery can be performed if pain persists for 6 to 8 weeks despite conservative care, or for signs of weakness and/or cervical myelopathy.

What are common presentations of cervical radiculopathy?

C5: May have weakness with shoulder abduction and external rotation. Muscles affected may be the rhomboid, deltoid, biceps, and infraspinatus muscles. This may affect the biceps reflex.

C6: Weakness with shoulder external rotation and elbow flexion. Muscles affected include the infraspinatus, biceps, brachioradialis, triceps, and pronator teres muscles. Affects biceps and brachioradialis reflexes. Affects sensation down the lateral extremity to the first and second digits of the hand.

C7: Affects elbow extension and forearm pronation. Weakness of the triceps, pronator teres, and flexor carpi radialis. Will affect the triceps reflex. Affects sensation along the posterior extremity to the second and third digits.

C8: May weaken finger abduction and grip strength. Muscles affected may include the flexor digitorum profundus, opponens pollicis, flexor pollicis longus, and hand intrinsics. Can affect sensation along the medial upper extremity and fourth and fifth digits of the hand.

Cervical myelopathy is marked by mechanical compression of the spinal cord. This compression produces spinal cord ischemia when the venous and arterial distribution is compromised. Common causes of compression include degenerative narrowing, disc herniation, or trauma. Spondylosis, or cervical spondylotic myelopathy, is the most common cause of myelopathy in those 55 and older. Cervical myelopathy can present as vague weakness or sensory changes in the arms or legs. Hyperreflexia/hyporeflexia, gait disturbance, bowel or bladder changes may all occur. Some may experience a positive Lhermitte sign, which is described as a shock-like sensation down the spine or into the arms with cervical flexion. This positive sign confirms cord injury. If there is clinical suspicion of cervical myelopathy, then an MRI or CT myelogram should be ordered to confirm. Central canal diameter less than 14 mm can be attributed to myelopathic changes of the spinal cord. Nonsurgical treatment includes rest, bracing, activity restriction, and pharmacologic pain management. Surgical decompression is a more invasive means of treatment if all else is ineffective

Although the most common source of neck pain is related to musculoskeletal complaints, other diagnoses to account for neck discomfort should not be excluded. Tumors, arterial dissections (carotid and vertebral arteries), infection (herpes zoster, Lyme disease), abscess formation or meningitis, and migraines should also be considered.

Please go over some changes that may be seen on physical examination

On inspection, observation of the neck and shoulder posture can be helpful. Flattening of the cervical spine could suggest degenerative change or muscle tightness. Neck stiffness can also allude to the severity of the patient's pain as well. Limitation in range of motion can suggest soft tissue and muscle stiffness or arthritic changes that limit movement of the neck. Palpation of the cervical spinous processes or specific muscle groups can occur depending upon the injury. Manual muscle testing of strength should be performed to determine if there is any weakness along a myotomal distribution. Reflex testing is recommended. Provocative testing (Spurlings, Lhermitte), evaluation of gait, Hoffman's testing, ankle clonus, and Babinski testing should be performed in neurologic testing.

Please go over common imaging and testing modalities for neck pain

Depending on presentation of pain, evaluation with imaging can be useful. Plain films or x-ray seems to be most useful when evaluating a patient who is 50 years of age or older. Lateral views can help evaluate facet arthritis and foraminal narrowing, related to arthritic change. Oblique views can also show a better view of the foraminal spaces. Also flattening of the normal lordotic curvature may be present in those with arthritis or muscle spasm. AP views will assess for abnormal rotational changes such as torticollis. Odontoid view will determine if there is any major proximal fracture or vertebral displacement. Flexion-extension views will determine if there is any instability of the spine or dynamic spondylolisthesis. X-ray can grossly assess bony integrity, as an initial evaluation for fractures.

MRI or CT imaging is recommended to be performed in those neck pain sufferers with a history of infection and/or malignancy. Those with clinical findings of cervical radiculopathy should also be imaged if these findings persist for 6 weeks or more. Those with signs and symptoms of cervical myelopathy should receive this imaging modality immediately. MRI imaging better views soft tissue structures that may contribute to pain and nerve injury such as disc herniation, ligament hypertrophy, tumor, and infection. MRI also can show nerve root compression and myelopathic changes to the spinal cord. It can also show capsular changes of the facet joints. CT scan and CT myelogram can show bony changes such as fracture. It can show stenosis, degenerative change, nerve compression, tumors, and disc herniation.

EMG and nerve conduction testing is another good confirmatory tool to determine the timing (acute or chronic) and location of radiculopathy. The needle EMG becomes most useful for diagnosis. If motor axonal injury is present, there will be abnormal findings in the muscles predominantly innervated by a particular nerve root. Nonetheless, radiculopathy can be present in some cases without abnormal findings. For example, if the sensory afferent fibers are injured at the dorsal root ganglia and no motor innervations are lost, EMG will be normal. Electrodiagnostic testing should be performed 2 to 3 weeks after initial presentation of radicular signs and/or symptoms.

Please go over common treatment options for neck pain

When treating axial neck pain, one must differentiate between a muscle/soft tissue injury versus bone/joint-related injury. Soft tissue injury may include whiplash injury, muscle strain, or myofascial pain. In these cases, conservative strategies are emphasized. Postural correction while sitting, at work, or in bed is recommended. Physical therapy working on strength and dynamic exercise has been helpful for neck pain, to some degree. Manual therapy can be beneficial.

Nonetheless, in a study involving whiplash injury sufferers, those who sought medical and/or alternative treatment had a longer recovery time. This may suggest that treatment may enable behaviors or perception of disability.

For mild-to-moderate neck pain, acetaminophen and nonsteroidal antiinflammatories may be administered. For management of facet-mediated pain, medial nerve branch blocks or steroid joint injections can be performed. Radiofrequency neurotomy can be performed for more sustained relief. Epidural injections can be performed for radicular pain. For chronic pain, cognitive behavioral therapy has proven to be beneficial.

KEY POINTS

1. The C7 nerve root is the most common nerve root injured in a cervical radiculopathy.
2. Indications for MRI or CT scan include radicular pain lasting at least 6 weeks, motor weakness, history of malignancy, and concern about spinal infections. Neurogenic findings suggesting stenosis, bowel/bladder changes, and gait imbalance should be indications for imaging.
3. Those seeking medical care for whiplash injury are slower to recover.
4. Fifty percent of those with whiplash injury will still experience pain after 1 year.

BIBLIOGRAPHY

1. Hadler NM. Illness in the workplace: the challenge of musculoskeletal symptoms. *J Hand Surg Am*. 1985;10:451.
2. Monahan JJ, Waite RJ. Cervical spine. In: Steinberg GG, Akins CM, Baran DT, eds. *Orthopaedics in Primary Care*. Baltimore: Lippincott Williams and Wilkins; 1999.
3. Bron C, Dommerholt JD. Etiology of myofascial trigger points. *Curr Pain Headache Rep*. 2012;16:439.
4. Carroll LJ, Holm LW, Hogg-Johnson S, et al. Course and prognostic factors for neck pain in whiplash-associated disorders (WAD): results of the Bone and Joint Decade 2000–2010 Task Force on Neck Pain and Its Associated Disorders. *Spine*. 2008;33:S83.
5. Krakenes J, Kaale BR. Magnetic resonance imaging assessment of craniovertebral ligaments and membranes after whiplash trauma. *Spine*. 2006;31:2820.
6. Yoss RE, Corbin KB, Maccarty CS, Love JG. Significance of symptoms and signs in localization of involved root in cervical disk protrusion. *Neurology*. 1957;7:673.
7. Ellenberg MR, Honet JC, Treanor WJ. Cervical radiculopathy. *Arch Phys Med Rehabil*. 1994;75:342.
8. Montgomery DM, Brower RS. Cervical spondylotic myelopathy. Clinical syndrome and natural history. *Orthop Clin North Am*. 1992;23:487.
9. Viikari-Juntura E, Porras M, Laasonen EM. Validity of clinical tests in the diagnosis of root compression in cervical disc disease. *Spine*. 1989;14:253.
10. https://acsearch.acr.org/docs/69426/Narrative/.
11. Cohen SP. Epidemiology, diagnosis, and treatment of neck pain. *Mayo Clin Proc*. 2015;90:284.
12. Ylinen J, Takala EP, Nykänen M, et al. Active neck muscle training in the treatment of chronic neck pain in women: a randomized controlled trial. *JAMA*. 2003;289:2509.

13. Hoving JL, Koes BW, de Vet HC, et al. Manual therapy, physical therapy, or continued care by a general practitioner for patients with neck pain. A randomized, controlled trial. *Ann Intern Med.* 2002;136:713.

14. Côté P, Hogg-Johnson S, Cassidy JD, et al. Initial patterns of clinical care and recovery from whiplash injuries: a population-based cohort study. *Arch Intern Med.* 2005;165:2257.

15. Manchikanti L, Singh V, Falco FJ, Cash KM, Fellows B. Cervical medial branch blocks for chronic cervical facet joint pain: a randomized, double-blind, controlled trial with one-year follow-up. *Spine.* 2008;33:1813.

16. Lord SM, Barnsley L, Wallis BJ, Mcdonald GJ, Bogduk N. Percutaneous radio-frequency neurotomy for chronic cervical zygapophyseal-joint pain. *N Engl J Med.* 1996;335:1721.

17. Aker PD, Gross AR, Goldsmith CH, Peloso P. Conservative management of mechanical neck pain: systematic overview and meta-analysis. *BMJ.* 1996;313:1291.

18. Deyo RA. Drug therapy for back pain. Which drugs help which patients? *Spine.* 1996;21:2840.

19. Monticone M, Cedraschi C, Ambrosini E, et al. Cognitive-behavioural treatment for subacute and chronic neck pain. *Cochrane Database Syst Rev.* 2015;(5):CD010664.

20. Dillingham TR, Lauder TD, Andary M, et al. Identification of cervical radiculopathies: optimizing the electromyographic screen. *Am J Phys Med Rehabil.* 2001;80:84.

CHAPTER 23

ABDOMINAL PAIN

Emily K. Stern and Darren Brenner

1. **What are the three afferent relays that mediate perception of abdominal pain?**
   - Visceral, or splanchnic, pathway
   - Somatic, or parietal, pathway
   - Referred pathway

   Visceral abdominal pain is produced by stimulation of nociceptors located in the walls of the abdominal viscera. Somatic abdominal pain is produced by stimulation of nociceptors located in the parietal peritoneum and intraabdominal supporting structures. Referred pain occurs when strong visceral impulses enter the spinal cord at the same level as afferents from other areas; this is mistakenly "read" as pain arising from the second area (e.g., shoulder pain in a gallbladder disorder).

2. **How does the perceived pain differ between the three pain pathways?**
   Visceral pain is more vague in onset and location than the other types of pain. It is typically perceived as a dull pain. Somatic pain is often sharp, intense, and localized. Referred pain is perceived at a location that is distant from the inciting disorder.

3. **Can abdominal pain be caused by extra abdominal disorders?**
   Pain felt in the abdomen can be generated by distant structures. Just as abdominal pathology can cause pain to be referred elsewhere in the body, irritation of distant structures can cause pain to be referred to the abdomen. For example, pathology of the thoracic vertebra can be referred to the abdomen, giving the mistaken impression that an intraabdominal problem exists. If the causal lesion is midline, then pain can be referred to both sides of the abdomen. Similarly, irritation of thoracic nerves can cause radiation of neuropathic pain to the abdomen. For example, intercostal neuralgia will produce pain in a dermatomal distribution of the involved nerve. If a lower intercostal nerve is involved, the pain will be felt in the abdomen. Because allodynia is one of the features of neuropathic pain, care must be taken to ensure that intense pain on palpation of the abdomen is not in fact allodynia.

4. **List some of the well-recognized thoracic disorders that can present as abdominal pain.**
   Thoracic disorders that can cause abdominal pain include:
   - Myocardial infarction or ischemia
   - Myocarditis
   - Pneumonia
   - Emphysema
   - Pulmonary embolism
   - Pneumothorax
   - Esophagitis

5. **What are some diagnostic considerations in women with abdominal pain?**
   A full history and physical is required of all women with lower abdominal pain, including a detailed sexual and menstrual history, pelvic examination, and pregnancy test (for women of childbearing age). Diagnostic considerations include pelvic inflammatory disease, endometriosis, ectopic pregnancy, uterine obstruction, ovarian cyst torsion, ovulatory pain (mittelschmerz), and ruptured ovarian cyst. Pain occurring at monthly intervals suggests endometriosis or ovulatory pain.

6. **Can the location of abdominal pain be useful in determining the etiology of the pain?**
   The location of abdominal pain can be very helpful in determining the cause of the pain. The abdomen can be easily divided into four quadrants—right upper, right lower, left upper, and left lower (Table 23.1). Focal abdominal pain is often related to a disorder of the underlying organ. Individuals may manifest pain differently, however, so it is important to keep a broad differential.

Table 23.1. Abdominal Pain by Location

RIGHT UPPER QUADRANT	LEFT UPPER QUADRANT
Biliary colic	Splenic infarct, abscess, or rupture
Cholecystitis—acute or chronic	Gastric ulcer
Hepatic distension or inflammation	Gastric outlet obstruction
Hepatic infarct or abscess	Pancreatitis or pancreatic pseudocyst
Right lower lobe pneumonia	Small bowel obstruction
Myocardial infarction	Left lower lobe pneumonia
	Myocardial infarction
RIGHT LOWER QUADRANT	**LEFT LOWER QUADRANT**
Appendicitis	Diverticulitis
Infectious, inflammatory, or ischemic colitis	Infectious, inflammatory, or ischemic colitis
Irritable bowel syndrome	Irritable bowel syndrome
Ectopic pregnancy	Ectopic pregnancy
Tuboovarian disorders	Tuboovarian disorders
Pyelonephritis	Pyelonephritis
Renal stones	Renal stones

7. List common gastrointestinal causes of pain in the right upper quadrant:
   - Biliary colic
   - Acute and chronic cholecystitis
   - Gallstone ileus
   - Acute hepatitis
   - Hepatic infarct
   - Hepatic abscess
   - Hepatic mass

8. What are common causes of left upper quadrant pain, and which abdominal organs are often involved?
   - Spleen—splenic infarct, splenomegaly, splenic abscess
   - Stomach—peptic ulcer disease, gastritis, gastric outlet obstruction, gastroparesis
   - Pancreas—pancreatitis, pancreatic pseudocyst
   - Small bowel—obstruction, ileus, inflammatory bowel disease

9. What are common causes of lower abdominal pain? What organ systems are commonly involved?
   Pain in the lower quadrants can be due to a number of causes from multiple organ systems.
   - Gastrointestinal—diverticulitis (classically left sided), appendicitis (classically right sided), infectious, ischemic or inflammatory colitis, irritable bowel syndrome (IBS)
   - Genitourinary—ureteral or kidney stones, pyelonephritis, ovarian or testicular torsion, pelvic inflammatory disease, tuboovarian abscess, ruptured ectopic pregnancy
   - Musculoskeletal—muscular strain or sprain, rectus sheath hematoma, retroperitoneal hematoma

10. What historical attributes must always be asked about when obtaining the history from a patient with abdominal pain?
    The mnemonic PQRST provides a framework that ensures a full exploration of a given patient's abdominal pain:

    P: Factors that *p*alliate or *p*rovoke abdominal pain. For example, pain from pancreatitis is improved with sitting forward. Pain from kidney stones is worsened with movement

Q: *Q*ualities of the pain (burning, sharp, crampy, dull)
R: *R*adiation of pain. For example, biliary tract pain radiates to the right periscapular region; pancreatic pain radiates to the back; and subdiaphragmatic pain may be referred to the shoulder tips.
S: *S*everity of the pain. This is often rated on a scale from 1 to 10.
T: *T*emporal events associated with the pain (duration of pain, constant or intermittent, new or chronic)

Another commonly used mnemonic is OLDCARTS. Physicians often prefer this mnemonic as it includes an assessment of the significance of the pain:

O: *O*nset of pain
L: *L*ocation of pain
D: *D*uration of pain
C: *C*haracteristics of the pain
A: *A*ggravating and alleviating factors
R: *R*adiation of the pain
T: *T*reatments already tried for the pain
S: *S*ignificance of the pain to the patient

11. What is dyspepsia, and how is it classified?
Dyspepsia is a broad term used to describe persistent or recurrent upper gastrointestinal symptoms. It is characterized by sensations of abdominal fullness, epigastric pain, or burning. It is also commonly associated with other gastrointestinal (GI) symptoms including nausea, vomiting, bloating, distention, early satiety, and weight loss. Dyspepsia is commonly divided into two categories: investigated and uninvestigated. Functional dyspepsia refers to the persistence or recurrence of these symptoms subsequent to an adequate evaluation for other organic, systemic, or metabolic disorders. The Rome IV Consensus Committee currently defines functional dyspepsia as the presence of one or more of the following in the absence of structural disease:
1. Bothersome postprandial fullness
2. Early satiation
3. Epigastric pain
4. Epigastric burning

12. What is the most common organic cause of dyspepsia?
Peptic ulcer disease (PUD) is the most common organic cause of dyspepsia. PUD is a term used to describe ulcerations and erosions in the stomach and duodenum. PUD can be due to a number of causes, but the most common include infection with *Helicobacter pylori* (Hp) bacteria or the use of aspirin or nonsteroidal antiinflammatory drugs (NSAIDs).

13. What "alarm features" should be elicited in patients with dyspepsia?
Alarm signs may be manifestations of a serious underlying organic pathology. Examples of alarm signs include unintentional weight loss, persistent vomiting, bleeding (hematemesis or melena), dysphagia, and family history of gastric cancer. Patients with alarm signs should have a thorough medical workup prior to being diagnosed with functional dyspepsia.

14. What tests may be used to diagnose common causes of dyspepsia?
PUD is commonly evaluated with upper endoscopy. If an endoscopy is performed, identification of Hp can be obtained via biopsies and visualization under a microscope. In addition to endoscopy, Hp can be diagnosed with breath, stool, or blood testing. Hp breath testing is based upon the fact that these organisms break down urea, a metabolic by-product, into carbon dioxide and ammonia. Patients consuming a radiolabeled urea excrete elevated levels of carbon dioxide, which can be quantified and used to detect the presence of the organism. Stool antigen testing is also available and both of these tests have high sensitivity and specificity. Blood tests to detect the presence of Hp are much less accurate and are best utilized for their ability to rule out Hp infection in low risk populations. They should not be used to assess confirmation of Hp eradication subsequent to treatment.

15. How is dyspepsia treated?
Treatment of dyspepsia depends on the underlying cause. If Hp is present, treatment is directed against the pathogenic organism. Common drug regimens include 10- to 14-day courses of triple

(proton pump inhibitor [PPI], clarithromycin and amoxicillin) or quadruple therapy (PPI, bismuth subsalicylate, metronidazole and tetracycline). If there is no evidence of concurrent PUD, the likelihood of symptom resolution is 10% to 15%. If ulcers are identified, treatment includes a course of antisecretory drug therapy with either a PPI (preferred) or a second-generation antihistamine. These medications alleviate symptoms and promote mucosal healing. If no abnormalities are identified, and the patient is diagnosed with functional dyspepsia, standard therapies include PPIs, pro-kinetic agents, and anti-depressants.

16. Name three complications of untreated peptic ulcer disease.
The most common complication of PUD is gastrointestinal blood loss. Occasionally, asymptomatic patients are found to be anemic on routine blood work. Other times, patients may present to the emergency room with significant GI tract bleeding. GI bleeding from PUD is treated with PPI therapy and removal of the underlying cause, such as Hp or NSAIDs. Endoscopic intervention may also be required.
    A rare but serious complication of PUD is perforation. Patients with a perforation present with acute abdominal pain, guarding, and rebound tenderness. Emergency surgery may be required to close the defect in the intestinal wall. Occasionally, this is the initial manifestation of PUD.
    Infrequently, patients with PUD may present with symptoms of gastric outlet obstruction. This is an increasingly rare complication of PUD given the widespread use of PPI therapy. Symptoms of gastric outlet obstruction include pain, nausea, vomiting, abdominal fullness, and early satiety. Patients may also note gastric distension and bloating.

17. What complications can arise from chronic *Helicobacter pylori* infection?
Although most patients are asymptomatic, approximately 10% to 15% of patients with chronic Hp infection will develop ulcers, gastric adenocarcinoma, or gastric lymphoma ("MALT lymphoma"). Early stages of MALT lymphoma may be cured by antibiotic and antisecretory therapy alone. More advanced stages, however, often require chemotherapy, radiation, or surgery.

18. What is acute pancreatitis? How is acute pancreatitis diagnosed?
The term "pancreatitis" literally means inflammation of the pancreas. Acute pancreatitis, as the name implies, presents with sudden, severe, and persistent epigastric pain. Classically, pancreatitis pain radiates to the back, is worse after eating, and is relieved by sitting forward. The diagnosis of acute pancreatitis requires the presence of two of the following three criteria:
* Acute onset severe, persistent epigastric pain, often radiating to the back
* Elevation in serum lipase or amylase, greater than three times the laboratory upper limit of normal
* Characteristic findings of acute pancreatitis on computed tomography, magnetic resonance imaging, or abdominal ultrasound

19. What are the two most common causes of acute pancreatitis? Name some additional causes of pancreatitis.
The two most common causes of acute pancreatitis are gallstones and chronic alcohol abuse. Other causes of pancreatitis include hypertriglyceridemia, pancreatic cancer, medication side effects, genetic mutations, ischemia, and complications after an endoscopic retrograde cholangiopancreatography (ERCP).

20. Name two physical exam findings that are characteristic of severe acute pancreatitis.
* Grey Turner's sign: flank bruising (can be unilateral or bilateral)
* Cullen's sign: periumbilical bruising
    Both findings are due to the presence of hemorrhagic pancreatic fluid that has tracked into these regions. The presence of these signs often portends a poor prognosis.

21. What is chronic pancreatitis? How is chronic pancreatitis diagnosed?
Chronic pancreatitis refers to progressive inflammation of the pancreas leading to irreversible structural damage. Similar to acute pancreatitis, the pain of chronic pancreatitis is typically epigastric, radiates to the back, is worse after eating and is improved with sitting forward. Early in the disease course, the pain may be intermittent, but as the process progresses, the pain may become constant. In addition to pain, patients with chronic pancreatitis often have evidence of pancreatic dysfunction such as hyperglycemia and fat malabsorption complicated by diarrhea.

The diagnosis of chronic pancreatitis is not as straightforward as the diagnosis of acute pancreatitis. It often involves the combination of clinical history, laboratory findings, and imaging studies. Occasionally, special pancreatic function testing is used to support the diagnosis.

22. **Name three differences between acute and chronic pancreatitis.**
    - Acute pancreatitis is almost always painful, whereas pain is not always present with chronic pancreatitis.
    - Patients with acute pancreatitis tend to have elevated amylase and lipase, whereas pancreatic enzyme levels are often normal in patients with chronic pancreatitis.
    - Pancreatic endocrine dysfunction, including diabetes and steatorrhea (diarrhea due to fat malabsorption), is seen almost exclusively with chronic pancreatitis.

23. **How do patients with biliary pain typically describe their symptoms?**
    Pain arising from the biliary tree is often localized to the epigastric or right upper quadrant. It may be precipitated by eating—classically by a fatty meal. The pain often radiates to the scapula, right shoulder, or lower abdomen. Patients may describe nausea and vomiting.

24. **Why is the commonly used term *biliary colic* a misnomer?**
    Biliary tract pain is not colicky but is typically a pain that steadily rises to a peak that may be sustained for several hours before subsiding (crescendo/decrescendo). Although biliary tract pain may fluctuate in intensity and severity, it is not generally intermittent as the term colic implies.

25. **What are the differences between cholelithiasis, cholecystitis, choledocholithiasis, and cholangitis? How are patients with these disorders managed?**
    - *Cholelithiasis* is the term used to describe gallbladder stones. Patients with symptomatic cholelithiasis often note episodic abdominal pain, which is due to a gallstone obstructing the cystic duct. Patients with asymptomatic cholelithiasis require no intervention. Those with symptoms may undergo elective cholecystectomy.
    - *Cholecystitis* implies inflammation of the gallbladder wall. This syndrome is associated with abdominal pain, fever, and an elevated white blood cell count. Ninety percent of cases are due to gallbladder outlet obstruction by a gallstone, although a subset of cases can occur without gallstones ("*acalculous cholecystitis*"). Patients are treated with antibiotics and surgical removal of the gallbladder.
    - *Choledocholithiasis* is the term that describes stones in the bile ducts. This can be painful or asymptomatic. Complications of choledocholithiasis, such as pancreatitis and cholangitis (discussed later), can have significant morbidity and mortality. Therefore, patients with choledocholithiasis often require intervention such as ERCP (to dislodge a stone) and cholecystectomy (to minimize the formation and passage of additional stones).
    - *Cholangitis* describes an infection due to obstruction of the bile ducts. The infection can be mild or life threatening. Treatment of cholangitis includes urgent stone removal (often by ERCP) and antibiotics. Patients with cholangitis from an obstructed gallstone also require cholecystectomy to prevent recurrence.

26. **What is Charcot's triad? Reynolds' pentad?**
    - *Charcot's triad* refers to the classic presenting signs of acute cholangitis: fever, abdominal pain, and jaundice. Rarely do patients have all three of these findings.
    - Reynolds' pentad includes hypotension and confusion in addition to fever, abdominal pain, and jaundice. Patients with all the symptoms in Reynolds' pentad are critically ill.

27. **How is pain originating from the small bowel usually characterized? What are common causes of small bowel pain?**
    Pain related to the small bowel is often felt in the midline or periumbilical region. Occasionally, it is felt in the flank or back. Classically, small intestine pain is worse after food intake. Depending on the underlying etiology, the severity can range from mild discomfort to severe acute pain. Intermittent "colicky" pain is often seen in the setting of small bowel obstruction (SBO), when the bowel wall smooth muscle contracts vigorously proximal to the obstruction. Mucosal inflammation or ulcerations may result in a vague soreness and ache. An inflammatory or neoplastic process that extends through to the serosa and adjacent parietal peritoneum will stimulate somatic pain pathways and manifest as more sharply localized pain at the site of the lesion.

28. **What are the most common causes of small bowel obstruction? What mnemonic can be used to remember them?**
The following are common causes of small bowel obstruction:
- Adhesions secondary to prior abdominopelvic surgery (60% to 85%)
- Crohn's disease (5% to 7%)
- Malignancy (2% to 5%)
- Hernia (2% to 3%)
     The "ABC" mnemonic can be used to remember these causes:

  A—Adhesions
  B—Bulge (hernia)
  C—Cancer/Crohn's

29. **What term describes the group of gastrointestinal disorders related to inadequate blood flow?**
The term "intestinal ischemia" describes GI tract disorders due to insufficient blood flow. Both the small and large bowel can be involved. Intestinal ischemia can be caused by both arterial and venous insufficiency.

30. **What is the difference in presentation between acute and chronic mesenteric ischemia? How is this difference explained by the underlying pathophysiology?**
Acute mesenteric ischemia (AMI) typically presents with sudden-onset abdominal pain. The pain is classically "out of proportion to findings on physical exam," because early in the presentation of AMI the patient may have a normal abdominal exam. AMI is caused by hypoperfusion of the small intestine, which can be due to embolization, thrombosis, or nonocclusive mesenteric ischemia (NOMI) due to low flow to the superior mesenteric artery or celiac artery. Acute mesenteric vein thrombosis causes a similar presentation.
     Unlike AMI, chronic mesenteric ischemia may be asymptomatic or have an insidious onset. Patients often note recurrent episodes of pain during the first hour after eating, which typically subsides over the course of several hours. Patient may therefore develop *sitophobia*, meaning fear of eating, and present with weight loss and nutritional deficiencies. Symptoms often are progressive. With a careful history, patients who present with AMI often give a history consistent with chronic mesenteric ischemia. This disorder is classically associated with occlusion of two of three major braches from the aorta that feed the intestinal tract: celiac, superior, and inferior mesenteric arteries.

31. **When is treatment indicated for chronic mesenteric ischemia? Why is treatment important?**
All patients with symptomatic chronic mesenteric ischemia should be treated. The goal of treatment is both to improve symptoms and to prevent future complications. Treatment options include open and endovascular repair of the involved vascular structures. After blood flow to the small bowel is improved, patients are often able to gain weight and improve their nutritional status. The prevention of AMI is of paramount importance, because bowel necrosis has an extremely high morbidity and mortality.

32. **What causes liver-related abdominal pain? Do patients with chronic liver disease typically have liver-related abdominal pain?**
Most chronic liver diseases, such as viral hepatitis, alcoholic cirrhosis, and fatty liver disease, do not cause abdominal pain. Instead, they may present with complications such as jaundice, variceal bleeding, or ascites. Liver-related pain is caused by stretching of the liver capsule, called Glisson's capsule. The hepatic parenchyma is insensitive to pain.
     Disorders that cause stretch on Glisson's capsule and thus cause liver-related abdominal pain include:
- Acute viral hepatitis—Inflammation and swelling of the liver can cause capsular stretch.
- Budd-Chiari syndrome—A blood clot in the hepatic vein or inferior vena cava (IVC) obstructs venous outflow from the liver, which can cause engorgement of the hepatic venous system and stretch on Glisson's capsule.
- Masses—A rapidly growing hepatic lesion can cause distortion of the normal liver architecture and stretch Glisson's capsule.

33. **What are the two subtypes of inflammatory bowel disease, and how does pain typically present in inflammatory bowel disease patients?**
Inflammatory bowel disease can be subdivided into Crohn's disease and ulcerative colitis (UC). Both of these diseases can present with abdominal pain, change in bowel habits, and weight loss. Pain is usually a more predominant symptom in patients with Crohn's disease.
   Crohn's disease affects all layers of the gastrointestinal tract, whereas ulcerative colitis only affects the inner walls of the gastrointestinal tract. Due to the transmural nature of Crohn's disease, patients often develop strictures, which can cause intermittent colicky pain due to obstruction. Patients with Crohn's also develop intraabdominal abscesses, which may present with pain and fevers. Other common manifestations of Crohn's disease include diarrhea, anemia, and extraintestinal changes such as arthritis, uveitis, and skin rashes and ulcerations. Ulcerative colitis also presents with abdominal pain, often in context of bloody diarrhea and urgency. Extraintestinal manifestations are less common in UC than in Crohn's.

34. **What is irritable bowel syndrome, and how is it subcategorized?**
Irritable bowel syndrome is a disorder characterized by abdominal pain associated with changes in stool frequency and/or texture. It is categorized into four major subgroups dependent on the predominant stool consistency. These include IBS-C (constipation predominant), IBS-D (diarrhea predominant), IBS-M (alternate between diarrhea and constipation), and the much less common IBS-U (does not meet criteria of a predominant stool texture).

35. **What criteria are used to diagnose irritable bowel syndrome?**
IBS is classically diagnosed by the Rome criteria, which were recently updated. IBS is defined as abdominal pain associated with at least two of the following: (A) the pain is temporally related to defecation, or (B) the pain is associated with a change in the patient's stool frequency and/or (C) stool texture. These symptoms should be present, on average, 1 day/week for the past 3 months with symptom onset more than 6 months prior to making the diagnosis. Other associated symptoms include nausea, bloating, abdominal distention, borborygmi, and the increased passage of flatus.

36. **What treatment options are available for patients with irritable bowel syndrome?**
Many different treatment modalities exist for treating IBS and the choice is determined by the predominant stool type(s) (constipation, diarrhea, mixed). Treatment options include diet modification, behavioral therapy, probiotics, antibiotics, antidepressants, laxatives, antidiarrheals, secretagogues, antispasmodics, serotonin antagonists, and bile-acid binding agents. Treatments should be individualized and based on patient preference.

37. **How can abdominal pain caused by disorders of the abdominal wall be distinguished from pain of intraabdominal origin?**
Carnett's test can help make this distinction. First, the site of maximum tenderness is identified. The patient is then asked to assume a partial seated position with arms crossed, which causes the abdominal wall muscles to generate increased tension. Carnett's test is positive if increased tenderness on repeat palpation is noted. The differential diagnosis of chronic abdominal wall pain includes rectus sheath hematoma, rib tip syndrome, abdominal wall hernia, myofascial pain syndrome, and cutaneous nerve entrapment syndromes.

38. **Patients who are immunocompromised by virtue of disease or immunosuppressive therapy may present with abdominal pain. What are some diagnostic considerations?**
The immunocompromised individual with acute intraabdominal pathology may have few abdominal signs and symptoms, blunted systemic manifestations, and minimal change in biochemical and hematologic parameters. The differential diagnosis includes any of the disorders that can occur in the general population as well as problems unique to the immunocompromised host. Specific considerations include neutropenic enterocolitis (typhlitis), graft versus host disease, opportunistic infections (e.g., cytomegalovirus infection, atypical mycobacterial infection, fungal infection), and tumors arising from immune deficiency (e.g., lymphoma, Kaposi's sarcoma).

39. **What are some of the caveats about atypical presentations of abdominal pain?**
In certain circumstances, such as in older or immunosuppressed patients, common abdominal disorders may present in an atypical fashion. Fever may be absent or low grade, signs of peritoneal irritation may be blunted, and an altered mental status (e.g., dementia) may modify the history and physical examination.

Acknowledgments

The current authors would like to acknowledge the contributions of the previous authors, Drs. Ronald E. Greenberg and Charles E. Argoff.

KEY POINTS

1. Abdominal pain can be visceral, somatic, or referred in nature.
2. Abdominal pain is not always caused by intraabdominal pathology: it may be caused by problems at a distant site and referred to the abdomen.
3. The location of the abdominal pain can often be used to help guide the differential diagnosis.
4. *H. pylori* infection and NSAID use are the most common causes of peptic ulcer disease.

BIBLIOGRAPHY

1. Cartwright SL, Knudson MP. Evaluation of acute abdominal pain in adults. *Am Fam Physician*. 2008;77(7):971-978.
2. Cartwright SL, Knudson MP. Diagnostic imaging of acute abdominal pain in adults. *Am Fam Physician*. 2015;91(7):452-459.
3. Chen EH, Mills AM. Abdominal pain in special populations. *Emerg Med Clin North Am*. 2011;29(2):449-458, x.
4. Clair DG, Beach JM. Mesenteric Ischemia. *N Engl J Med*. 2016;374(10):959-968.
5. Feldman M, Friedman LS, Brandt LJ. *Sleisenger and Fordtran's Gastrointestinal and Liver Disease: Pathophysiology, Diagnosis, Management*. 10th ed. Philadelphia: Elsevier/Saunders; 2016.
6. Kruszka PS, Kruszka SJ. Evaluation of acute pelvic pain in women. *Am Fam Physician*. 2010;82(2):141-147.
7. Lacy BE, Mearin F, Chang L, et al. Bowel disorders. *Gastroenterology*. 2016;150(6):1393-1407.
8. Majumder S, Chari ST. Chronic pancreatitis. *Lancet*. 2016;387(10031):1957-1966.
9. Stanghellini V, Chan FK, Hasler WL, et al. Gastroduodenal disorders. *Gastroenterology*. 2016;150(6):1380-1392.
10. Talley NJ, Ford AC. Functional dyspepsia. *N Engl J Med*. 2015;373(19):1853-1863.
11. Weinberg DS, Smalley W, Heidelbaugh JJ, Sultan S, Association AG. American Gastroenterological Association Institute Guideline on the pharmacological management of irritable bowel syndrome. *Gastroenterology*. 2014;147(5):1146-1148.
12. Yamada T, Alpers DH. *Principles of Clinical Gastroenterology*. Chichester, West Sussex; Hoboken, NJ: Wiley-Blackwell; 2008.

CHAPTER 24

CHRONIC PELVIC PAIN

Andrew Dubin

What is chronic pelvic pain? By definition, it is pain that is located in the lower abdominal or groin region. It is noncyclical in nature. It has been present for more than 3 to 6 months and is not exclusively associated with intercourse or menstruation. Twenty-five percent of adult-community-living women have issues of chronic pelvic pain, and in the majority of women the etiology is never fully elucidated.

The limitations of the above definition are obvious. It does not address the male population. Men also have issues of chronic pelvic pain; however, they are less likely to seek out medical evaluation.

Establishing the diagnosis presents a challenge. Many times the interplay between the urological, gynecological, as well as gastrointestinal systems can complicate the presentation. Additionally neurological, endocrinologic, and psychological issues can all add confounding layers to the presentation and pain. Lastly the musculoskeletal system can have dramatic impact on pelvic pain or can be the primary source generator for pelvic pain.

Unfortunately the musculoskeletal system is not typically thought of as a source of pelvic pain until many providers have been seen, multiple tests have been performed, and in many instances many procedures have been done. In essence it becomes the default organ system.

COMMON PRESENTING COMPLAINTS AND SYMPTOMS

Chronic pelvic pain (CPP) patients commonly present with complaints of pain with Valsalva type activities, such as straining to have a bowel movement. They may note pain with ambulation, prolonged sitting, lumbar flexion, and/or extension. A quick look at the following complaints leads one to realize the lack of specificity of these complaints. They can be seen in lumbar degenerative disc disease, disc herniation, as well as in posterior element dysfunction, such as facet joint arthritis. Pain with extension and ambulation can be seen in spinal stenosis. Groin pain with ambulation may be secondary to degenerative joint disease of the hip. Patients may additionally complain of urinary urgency, frequency, as well as sensory dysesthesias in the perineum. Males can complain of erectile dysfunction. The complaints of urinary urgency and frequency can be seen not only in primary urological issues such as benign prostatic hypertrophy, but are frequently noted in patients with cervical or thoracic level myelopathy. Sensory dysesthesias can be seen in myelopathies as well as cauda equine level dysfunction. Erectile dysfunction can be seen in both upper motor neuron and lower motor neuron dysfunction. Realizing that pelvic pain can arise from multiple pathologies, the criticality of the history and physical cannot be overemphasized.

This section will focus primarily on the musculoskeletal system as the source generator for pelvic pain, as it is the most frequently overlooked system.

The physical exam starts with observation. Note how the patient ambulates. Do they walk with a compensated Trendelenburg gait pattern? Primary hip pathology, as well as a possible profound L5 radiculopathy, needs to be explored. In the setting of an L5 radiculopathy that is severe enough to cause a compensated Trendelenburg, an associated foot drop should also be noted. If one is not present, the diagnosis of L5 radiculopathy is highly unlikely, as nerve function recovers proximal to distal. However, isolated superior gluteal nerve neuropathy, gluteus medius muscle tear, or primary hip pathology all remain in the differential. Observe sitting posture. Patients that are comfortable sitting or sitting forward flexed may have facet joint arthritis, or spinal stenosis. Patients that prefer to stand or sit with lumbar support may have issues of discogenic pain.

A complete pelvic pain workup must include a thorough examination of the musculoskeletal system. It should include an assessment of lumbosacral spine motion and gait evaluation. Additionally, manual muscle testing should be performed on both lower extremities to compare side to side, and should include assessment of strength of the hip flexors, knee extensors, as well as ankle toe dorsiflexors and plantar flexors. Given the strength of the ankle plantar flexors, having the patient perform multiple calf raises will sometimes elucidate subtle weakness of S1 innervated musculature not appreciated on manual muscle testing. In addition, heel walking may bring out slight weakness of ankle dorsiflexors not appreciated on physical exam.

Evaluation of reflexes is critical. Notation of hyperreflexia, ankle clonus, crossed adductors, and positive Babinski raises the specter of a central nervous system level dysfunction. Abnormal findings in the upper extremities manifesting with overflow reflex activity and hyperreflexia, Hoffmann's sign, with associated sensory symptoms in the hands, and concomitant cervical radicular distribution of weakness raise the specter of cervical level dysfunction. Brain level dysfunction needs to be considered in the setting of diffuse upper and lower extremity hyperreflexia, with long tract signs without a clear-cut cervical radicular pattern of weakness that localizes a cervical root level issue in concert with cervical cord compression. A clear radicular level of weakness in the upper extremities on manual muscle testing with hyperreflexia below is classic for a radiculo-myelopathy and warrants magnetic resonance imaging (MRI) of the cervical spine. Diffuse hyperreflexia, with associated weakness in a more diffuse or patchy nonradicular distribution, especially in young women with appropriate historical data, including changing neurological symptoms over time in addition to issues of vision loss, transient foot drop, or wrist drop, should raise an index of suspicion for multiple sclerosis. At that point, MRI of the brain and spinal cord both with and without contrast would be very reasonable. Diffuse lower extremity hyporeflexia can be seen in peripheral neuropathies, or polyradiculopathies. Unilateral sensory dysesthesias involving the perineum should raise the question of a symptomatic Tarlov cyst. It is important to remember that not all Tarlov cysts are asymptomatic or incidental findings, and their symptomatic presentation is commonly limited to the perineum, with sensory complaints noted. Additionally, males may note erectile dysfunction, and women may note changes in clitoral sensitivity. In this scenario, detailed physical exam to assess sensation in the perineum as well as reflex testing of the bulbocavernosus reflex in men and the clitoral-anal reflex in women is critical. Workup for a suspected Tarlov cyst should include sacral MRI as well as needle electromyography (EMG) of the right and left anal sphincter musculature looking for denervation, as well as changes in typical motor unit morphology. Needle EMG of the anal sphincter should only be done by people with significant experience in evaluating this muscle as the normal anal sphincter motor units look abnormal in comparison to typical motor units seen in appendicular skeletal muscles. Work by Podnar et al. revealed that in males, abnormal penile sensation in concert with an abnormal or absent bulbocavernosus reflex on physical exam was highly correlative to abnormal electrodiagnostic testing. Unfortunately in women, the clitoral-anal reflex can be difficult to obtain on physical exam, and as such in this group, electrophysiologic testing, including reflex testing and anal sphincter EMG, may have great utility. Normal reflexes in the upper extremities with loss of reflexes in the lower extremities can be seen in patients with peripheral neuropathy. The history will be critical at that point to determine whether or not this is potentially a hereditary neuropathy that has now progressed to the point where it is becoming symptomatic versus an acquired neuropathy. Causes of acquired neuropathies can range from cryptogenic to toxic metabolic to autoimmune, inflammatory mediated, and require detailed workup to avoid missing treatable causes. Other causes of lower motor neuron findings isolated to the lower extremities can include cauda equina, but this will typically manifest with marked lower extremity weakness in a polyradicular pattern weakness, as well as marked sensory dysfunction in the perineum. While myopathies are not a common cause of pelvic pain, patients who note that their symptoms worsen throughout the day and note cramping pelvic pain, especially after straining during a bowel movement, may be exhibiting findings of muscle fatigue of proximal musculature with prolonged activity. Physical examination and detailed manual muscle testing may reveal a proximal to distal gradient of motor weakness or possibly patterns of weakness such as scapula humeral peroneal or facial scapula humeral peroneal. In these instances, preexercise and postexercise creatine phosphokinase (CPK) levels may be very illustrative, as the patient may have a normal to minimally elevated CPK at rest only to have it rise markedly 24 to 36 hours postregular and routine exercise. This group of patients may note on direct questioning that they are always sore in their muscles after they exercise, but assume it is normal, as they have always felt this way. In most instances, the complaints of pelvic level pain in patients with myopathy is secondary to altered gait mechanics, with subsequent overload of the SI joint of lumbar facet joints in patients who stand and walk with excessive lumbar lordosis as a result of manifest proximal weakness. Typically in adults this would be seen in limb girdle dystrophies or adult onset myopathies.

Hip joint pathology can be a common source of pelvic region pain. True intraarticular hip joint pathology will classically cause groin pain. Patients will complain of pain with weight bearing and walking. Pain will improve when they are sedentary. Additionally, use of a cane in the contralateral hand will ease their pain. Startup pain is a common phenomenon, but unfortunately is not unique to hip joint pathology. Physical exam findings will classically include replication of groin pain with internal rotation of the affected hip. Proxy referral patterns of pain include radiating anterior thigh pain or referral to the knee with internal rotation of the hip. Intraarticular hip joint pathology can present many challenges when it becomes part of the differential diagnosis for the workup for pelvic pain. It is not an uncommon finding in an aging population, and as such can also be associated with degenerative changes in the lumbar spine. The physical exam may help delineate the driver of the patient's pain, but if doubt persists as to the role the hip is playing in the patient's pain complaints, a diagnostic and potentially therapeutic intraarticular hip joint injection, done either under fluoroscopic guidance or ultrasound, can easily be done. A markedly positive response to the injection will quickly confirm the clinical suspicion, and a negative response efficiently removes the joint from the equation and allows the physician to turn his or her attention to other potential source generators.

Anterior groin pain and associated pelvic level pain in younger patients may be due to labral pathology. Patients may note that their pain worsens with standing and walking. Unlike hip pain from degenerative joint disease (DJD), patients with femoral acetabular impingement (FAI) with labral pathology may also complain of pain while seated. Additionally, FAI may also have replication of groin pain with external rotation of the hip as well as hip abduction. Complaints of sudden sharp pain with clicking and a sensation of give way weakness can also be seen with FAI. The differential diagnosis is rather extensive when FAI is entertained and includes such entities as iliopsoas impingement, subspine impingement, and ischiofemoral impingement. Iliopsoas impingement, more common in women than men, may be secondary to repetitive traction injury to the tendon with subsequent scarring and adherence of the tendon to the capsule-labrum complex of the hip. This can be seen in younger patients involved in sports and activities that place the patient in positions of extreme hip extension or rapid eccentric loading of the hip flexors. Subspine impingement, more common in men than women, is thought to be the result of a prominent anterior superior iliac spine (ASIS) abnormally contacting the distal femoral neck. Symptoms in this case are typically seen with attempts at deep hip flexion (catchers in softball and baseball). The etiology of the prominent ASIS may be secondary to repetitive avulsion type injury to the ASIS during repetitive knee flexion with hip extension type activities (soccer players). Ischiofemoral impingement is typically more commonly seen in women than men. It results from a tight space between the ischial tuberosity and the lesser trochanter, causing repetitive impingement and trapping of the quadratus femoris muscle. This is typically a congenital issue, but can develop after hip fracture, or in association with early superior and medial migration of the femoral head in early hip DJD. While imaging studies clearly have a role and place in the workup of anterior groin and pelvic level pain, all findings need to be placed into context. The context grows from the physical exam. Previous work by Silvis et al. revealed a high prevalence of abnormal findings on MRI of pelvis, hip, and groin regions on a cohort of asymptomatic college and professional hockey players. These abnormalities included common adductor and rectus abdominus tendonitis, with associated bone edema in the symphysis pubis. Additionally, partial tears as well as complete tears of the above muscles off the pubis were noted. Finally, hip abnormalities including labral tears, as well as osteochondral lesions of the femoral head, were noted. To further cloud the picture, similar findings have been noted on lumbar MRIs in asymptomatic patients (Brandt-Zawadz et al).

As one can see, hip joint pathology and its associated groin level pain can present unique challenges as part of the workup for pelvic pain. The physical exam is critical in helping delineate the driver of the patient's pain. Sometimes, even after detailed physical exam, it may still be difficult to determine if intraarticular or extraarticular sources are the primary source generator for the patient's groin and pelvic level pain. In these scenarios where doubt persists as to the role intraarticular joint pathology is playing in the patient's pain complaints, a diagnostic and potentially therapeutic intraarticular hip joint injection, done either under fluoroscopic guidance or ultrasound, can easily be done. A markedly positive response to the injection will quickly confirm the clinical suspicion, and a negative response efficiently removes the joint from the equation and allows the physician to turn his or her attention to other potential source generators.

In summary, pelvic pain presents many unique challenges for the treating physician. Many of these patients have seen multiple providers and have had multiple procedures performed. These patients not uncommonly present with a high level of frustration as well as a degree of mistrust for the medical community, as they have often been shuffled from provider to provider. Obtaining a detailed history and performing a thorough physical can go a long way to elucidating the problem. Sometimes just getting the patient to understand why they have their pain goes a long way in helping them manage their pain. It all starts with the history and physical and the trust that develops over time as the patient grows to realize that you as the treating physician are taking a measured, thoughtful approach to their pain.

KEY POINTS

1. Chronic pelvic pain may result from a variety of etiologies, including intrapelvic sources and pain that is referred from nonpelvic sources.
2. Numerous medications may contribute to chronic lower abdominal pain; thus, this needs to be considered when evaluating a patient with chronic pelvic pain.
3. Chronic pelvic pain does not only occur in women.
4. EDX specifically needle EMG of the anal sphincter is highly sensitive for evaluation of S2-S4 nerve function.
5. Physical examination of the pelvic pain patient must include assessment of lower extremity strength and reflexes.

BIBLIOGRAPHY

1. Mui J, Allaire C, Williams C, Yong PJ. Abdominal wall pain in women with chronic pelvic pain. *J Obstet Gynaecol Can.* 2016;38(2):154-159.
2. Ploteau S, Cardaillac C, Perrouin-Verbe MA, Riant T, Labat JJ. Pudendal neuralgia due to pudendal nerve entrapment: warning signs observed in two cases and review of the literature. *Pain Physician.* 2016;19(3):E449-E454.
3. Speer LM, Mushkbar S, Erbele T. Chronic pelvic pain in women. *Am Fam Physician.* 2016;93(5):380-387.
4. Podnar S. Utility of sphincter electromyography and sacral reflex studies in women with cauda equina lesions. *Neurourol Urodyn.* 2014;33(4):426-430.
5. Podnar S. Cauda equina lesions as a complication of spinal surgery. *Eur Spine J.* 2010;19(3):451-457.

CHAPTER 25

FIBROMYALGIA AND MYOFASCIAL PAIN

David McLain, MD, FACP, FACR

1. What are the chronic pain syndromes that involve muscle and fascia?
   Myofascial pain syndrome and fibromyalgia are chronic pain syndromes that involve the muscle and soft tissues. Myofascial pain syndrome is regional in distribution, whereas fibromyalgia involves the entire body. These diagnoses may represent two points in a spectrum of disease, as subgroups of fibromyalgia have been identified on the basis of differing clinical findings and prognoses.

2. Describe the myofascial pain syndrome.
   The myofascial pain syndrome is a chronic, regional pain syndrome that involves muscle and soft tissues. It is characterized by trigger points and taut bands (see Questions 7 and 8). Originally described by Travell and later elaborated on by Travell and Simons, myofascial pain syndrome occurs in most body areas, most commonly in the cervical and lumbar regions.

3. What is fibromyalgia?
   Fibromyalgia is a clinical syndrome characterized by chronic, diffuse pain and multiple tender points at defined points in muscle and other soft tissues. Periosteal tender points are frequently present. Widespread pain can be felt both above and below the waist and bilaterally. Other characteristic features of the syndrome include fatigue, sleep disturbance, irritable bowel syndrome, interstitial cystitis, stiffness, paresthesias, headaches, depression, anxiety, and decreased memory and vocabulary.

4. What are the latest criteria for the diagnosis of Fibromyalgia?
   The latest criteria are 2016 revisions to the 2010/2011 fibromyalgia diagnostic criteria.
   - Generalized pain, defined as pain in at least 4 of 5 regions, is present.
   - Symptoms have been present at a similar level for at least 3 months.
   - Widespread pain index (WPI) ≥ 7 and symptom severity scale (SSS) score ≥ 5 OR WPI of 4–6 and SSS score ≥ 9.
   - A diagnosis of fibromyalgia is valid irrespective of other diagnoses. A diagnosis of fibromyalgia does not exclude the presence of other clinically important illnesses.
   Note that the tender point examinations were removed in the 2010/2011 criteria. They were part of the 1990 criteria.

   WPI definition: note the number of areas in which the patient has had pain over the last week. In how many areas has the patient had pain? Score will be between 0 and 19.

Left upper region (Region 1) Jaw, left Shoulder girdle, left Upper arm, left Lower arm, left	Right lower region (Region 4) Hip (buttock, trochanter), right Upper leg, right Lower leg, right
Right upper region (Region 2) Jaw, right Shoulder girdle, right Upper arm, right Lower arm, right	Axial region (Region 5) Neck Upper back Lower back Chest Abdomen
Left lower region (Region 3) Hip (buttock, trochanter), left Upper leg, left Lower leg, left	

Symptom severity scale (SSS) score
Fatigue
Waking unrefreshed
Cognitive symptoms
For the each of the 3 symptoms *above,* indicate the *level* of severity over the past week using the following scale:

0 = No problem
1 = Slight or mild problems, generally mild or intermittent
2 = Moderate, considerable problems, often present and/or at a moderate level
3 = Severe: pervasive, continuous, life-disturbing problems

The symptom severity scale (SSS) score: is the sum of the severity scores of the 3 symptoms (fatigue, waking unrefreshed, and cognitive symptoms) (0-9) plus the sum (0-3) of the number of the following symptoms the patient has been bothered by that occurred during the previous 6 months:

(1) Headaches (0-1)
(2) Pain or cramps in lower abdomen (0-1)
(3) And depression (0-1)

The final symptom severity score is between 0 and 12.
The fibromyalgia severity (FS) scale is the sum of the WPI and SSS.

5. Do all fibromyalgia patients have the same symptoms?
   No. There is a high degree of variability in the presentation of fibromyalgia. Subgroups of the syndrome have been identified based on the number of active tender points, sleep quality, and cold pain threshold. These subgroups have different prognoses. Patients may also be grouped according to related disease. Of patients with irritable bowel syndrome (IBS), 20% demonstrate findings consistent with fibromyalgia. Fibromyalgia is more common in diabetics than in the general population, and the severity of pain correlates with the duration of diabetes. These may constitute additional subgroups of fibromyalgia. Fibromyalgia is also common in autoimmune diseases, such as Sjögren's Syndrome, systemic lupus erythematosus, Hashimoto's thyroiditis, and rheumatoid arthritis.

6. Name syndromes that are associated with fibromyalgia.
   - Chronic fatigue syndrome
   - Irritable bowel syndrome
   - Restless leg syndrome
   - Interstitial cystitis
   - Temporomandibular joint dysfunction
   - Sicca syndrome
   - Raynaud's phenomenon
   - Autonomic dysregulation with orthostatic hypotension
   - Mood disorder
   - Hypermobility syndrome

7. What are trigger points?
   Trigger points are sites in muscle or tendon that, when palpated, produce pain at a distant site. These occur in consistent locations with predictable patterns of pain referral. Trigger points are often associated with prior trauma, "near falls," or degenerative osteoarthritis.

8. What are "taut bands"? How are they associated with trigger points?
   In patients with myofascial pain, deep palpation of muscle may reveal areas that feel tight and bandlike. Stretching this band of muscle produces pain. This is a taut band. Trigger points are characteristically found within taut bands of muscle. Despite the muscle tension, taut bands are electrophysiologically silent (i.e., the electromyogram [EMG] is normal). Rolling the taut band under the fingertip at the trigger point (snapping palpation) may produce a local "twitch" response.

9. Describe the prevalence and typical demographics of the fibromyalgia patient
   In most reported series, 80% to 90% of patients with fibromyalgia are female, with a peak incidence
   in middle age and a prevalence of 0.5% to 5% of the general population.

10. What laboratory investigations are useful in fibromyalgia?
    All laboratory values in fibromyalgia are used for exclusionary purposes. There are no characteristic
    chemical, electrical, or radiographic laboratory abnormalities. However, several consistent
    investigational serum markers of the disease have been reported in the literature. An increase in
    cytokines, with a direct relationship between pain intensity and interleukin-8, has been reported.
    Other investigational findings include a decrease in circulating cortisol (this may play a role in
    decreased exercise tolerance), a decrease in branched-chain amino acids (perhaps correlating with
    muscle fatigue), and decreased lymphocyte G protein and Cyclic adenosine monophosphate (cAMP)
    concentrations. Four studies have shown an increase in Substance P in the cerebrospinal fluid in
    fibromyalgia. At present, these findings are not clinically useful for the diagnosis, prognosis, or
    monitoring of the treatment response of fibromyalgia patients. Sleep studies are often abnormal
    ("alpha-delta," nonrestorative sleep), but the abnormalities are also seen in other chronic painful
    conditions. Functional magnetic resonance imaging (MRI) studies have shown augmented responses
    in the insula and anterior lingual gyrus to nonpainful sensory stimuli in fibromyalgia patients, but not
    in controls.

11. What treatments are commonly used for fibromyalgia and for myofascial pain?
    A combination of physical, anesthesiologic, and pharmacologic techniques are employed. Some of
    the most common treatments involve lidocaine injection or dry-needling of trigger points. These
    approaches are based on the concept that trigger points represent areas of local muscle spasm.
    However, the efficacy of trigger point injections has never been fully substantiated, although they do
    offer transient relief to some patients. Physical techniques, such as stretching, spray, and stretch
    (see Question 19), massage, and heat and cold application, have all been advocated, but none are
    fully validated by well-controlled studies.

12. Describe the role of physical therapy modalities in the treatment of myofascial
    pain.
    Most studies documenting the efficacy of physical therapy modalities are anecdotal and include
    relatively small subject numbers. They suggest the efficacy of transcutaneous electrical nerve
    stimulation (TENS), balneotherapy, ice, massage, ischemic compression (acupressure), and
    biofeedback in the treatment of myofascial pain. Low-power laser has been studied for its effect on
    myofascial pain associated with fibromyalgia. This modality seems to significantly reduce pain,
    muscle spasm, stiffness, and number of tender points.

13. Which medications are commonly used in the treatment of fibromyalgia and
    myofascial pain syndrome?
    Tricyclic antidepressants are widely used drugs for these disorders. They are used because they
    have the potential to regularize sleep patterns, decrease pain and muscle spasm, and because of
    their mood-enhancing properties. However, many tricyclic antidepressants are on the Beers List of
    drugs that are potentially inappropriate for the elderly and not allowed by Medicare. Selective
    serotonin-reuptake inhibitors (SSRIs) are used to elevate mood, but have little analgesic effect.
    Serotonin-norepinephrine reuptake inhibitors (SNRIs), such as duloxetine and milnacipran, have
    recently been shown to have pain-reducing properties in patients with fibromyalgia and can also
    improve mood. Pregabalin, milnacipran, and duloxetine have received an indication for the treatment
    of fibromyalgia in the United States. Nonsteroidal antiinflammatory drugs (NSAIDs), opioids, and
    nonnarcotic analgesics are also frequently used, but their role is also unclear and not evidence
    based. Many medications, such as cyclobenzaprine, baclofen, tizanidine, and chlorzoxazone, have
    been used to achieve symptom relief. However, a treatment effect has not been consistently
    supported. Medications that target associated symptoms are often employed. Among the most
    common of these are sleep medications such as zolpidem and fludrocortisone to treat postural
    hypotension and adynamia.

14. What are some other interventions that have been studied for the treatment of
    fibromyalgia?
    There is a large series investigating the role of diet in treating fibromyalgia. Some studies promote a
    raw vegetarian diet; others tout *Chlorella pyrenoides* (algae) as a dietary supplement. Monosodium

glutamate and aspartame have both been implicated in producing symptoms common to fibromyalgia and may play a role in pathogenesis for certain fibromyalgia subgroups.

Botulinum toxin injection and acupuncture (and dry needling) have also been studied. They appear to be helpful in certain instances, but consistent efficacy has not been proven.

15. **Is exercise useful in the treatment of fibromyalgia and myofascial pain syndrome?**
Yes. The most consistent improvement in fibromyalgia and myofascial pain syndrome occurs with exercise. The exercise hormonal response is abnormal in patients with fibromyalgia (increase in growth hormone concentration, the opposite of normal response), so the frequency and intensity of exercise needs to be carefully adjusted to the patient's tolerance. Although strengthening (progressive resistive or isokinetic) exercise can be helpful, the best outcome appears to result from conditioning, or aerobic, exercise.

16. **What are the proposed pathophysiologic mechanisms for fibromyalgia?**
Fibromyalgia is associated with an augmentation of sensation. Pathophysiologic explanations for fibromyalgia have ranged from primarily central, to a combination of central and peripheral, to primarily peripheral. Here are some examples:
- Fibromyalgia is a variation of an affective disorder. This idea was based on its common association with depression, IBS, and chronic fatigue syndrome.
- A sleep abnormality is the main disturbance, leading to altered pain perception.
- Peripheral factors, such as small fiber neuropathy, are most important.
- Travell and Simons believed that the muscle problem was primary.

It remains unclear whether there is one pathological mechanism for fibromyalgia or a variety of etiologic factors. Nevertheless, current hypotheses under investigation hold some promise that the pathogenesis and pathophysiology of fibromyalgia may soon be clarified:
- The cause is neuroendocrine in origin. This concept is largely based on the observation of decreased circulating cortisol levels and abnormal 5-HT metabolism.
- Peripheral C-fiber and central nociceptive sensitization occurs following a painful stimulus (wind-up). This sensitization is ameliorated by N-methyl-D-aspartate (NMDA) receptor blockade. NMDA activation causes release of Substance P, which has been found to be elevated in the CSF in fibromyalgia patients. Thus fibromyalgia represents "central sensitization."
- Association with infection: High levels of circulating immunoglobulin M (IgM) in response to an enteroviral infection have been demonstrated in some fibromyalgia patients. Hepatitis C has been associated with fibromyalgia.
- A Chiari I malformation, with brainstem compression, leads to an altered autonomic response, orthostasis, and fibromyalgia syndrome.
- Glial cell activation, which includes neuroinflammation, glial cell dysfunction (GCD), cellular destruction, hyperarousal of the sympathetic nervous system, and stimulation of the hypothalamic-pituitary complex. Neurogenic neuroinflammation due to glial cell activation leads to production of proinflammatory cytokines, nitric oxide, prostaglandin E2, and reactive oxygen and nitrogen species. This is an active area of current fibromyalgia research.

17. **How is sleep disturbance related to fibromyalgia?**
Sleep disturbance is one of the most common complaints of patients with fibromyalgia. It was initially described as "nonrestorative sleep." Some patients were shown to have an intrusion of alpha rhythms into their stage-IV sleep ("alpha-delta" sleep). However, the same electroencephalographic pattern is often seen in other chronically painful conditions. Moreover, other disorders frequently found in association with fibromyalgia, such as restless leg syndrome, can contribute to a sleep disorder. The incidence of sleep disturbance seems more related to the duration of chronic pain than to the specific diagnosis of fibromyalgia.

18. **What is the "spray and stretch" technique?**
The spray and stretch technique is based on the theory that trigger points located in taut muscle bands are the principal cause of pain in fibromyalgia and in myofascial pain syndrome. A taut band in the muscle is identified, and then a vapo-coolant spray (ethylchloride or fluoromethane) is applied directly along the muscle band. Once cooled, the muscle is stretched along its long axis. This helps to relax muscle tension (via muscle spindle and Golgi tendon organ stimulation), improve local circulation, decrease the number of active trigger points, and reduce the amount of pain.

19. Are there any factors that can precipitate the onset of fibromyalgia?

Fibromyalgia can occur without any identifiable precipitating factors. However, it seems that it can also be initiated by trauma (e.g., surgery, childbirth, accident, severe infection, severe emotional strain, sexual abuse) and can then be classified as "posttraumatic fibromyalgia."

20. What drugs have recently been added to the list of medications used in the symptomatic treatment of fibromyalgia?

Although only pregabalin, milnacipran, and duloxetine have received a specific indication for use in the treatment of fibromyalgia, a number of others have recently been used in increasing volumes. These include centrally acting α_2 adrenergic agonists such as the muscle relaxant/analgesic tizanidine and the 5-HT3 antagonists such as ondansetron, granisetron, and tropisetron. Low-dose naltrexone (LDN) has been shown in a small double-blind study to be effective in fibromyalgia. It is a microglial modulator and has to be compounded.

21. Are there any alternative therapeutic options for the treatment of myofascial syndrome?

Pregabalin and duloxetine are examples of oral drugs, indicated for other disease states, that can be used with benefit in the treatment of myofascial syndrome. A number of topical options also exist. These include topical capsaicin, glyceryl trinitrate (which has a localized antiinflammatory effect), lidocaine (Lidoderm patch), and doxepin (a tricyclic antidepressant with localized analgesic effects). Injection of local anesthetic into tender points can be used, as well as injection with corticosteroid. Corticosteroids stabilize nerve membranes, reduce ectopic neural discharge, and have a specific effect on dorsal horn cells as well as their well-known antiinflammatory effects.

22. Are there any acute treatments that can be used to lessen the pain of fibromyalgia during a flare-up of this condition?

It has recently been shown that parenteral injection of the 5-HT3 antagonist tropisetron can reduce the pain of fibromyalgia.

KEY POINTS

1. Myofascial pain syndrome is regional in distribution, whereas fibromyalgia is bodywide.
2. Fibromyalgia is more common in females.
3. Laboratory investigations cannot be used to diagnose fibromyalgia but can be used to exclude other conditions.
4. The cause of fibromyalgia is not known.

BIBLIOGRAPHY

1. Arnold LM, Rosen A, Pritchett YL, et al. A randomized, double-blind, placebo-controlled trial of duloxetine in the treatment of women with fibromyalgia with or without major depressive disorder. *Pain.* 2005;119:5-15.
2. Bergman S, Herrstrom P, Jacobsson LTH, Peterson IF. Chronic widespread pain: a three-year follow-up of pain distribution and risk factors. *J Rheumatol.* 2002;29:818-825.
3. Bohr WT. Fibromyalgia syndrome and myofascial pain syndrome. Do they exist? *Neurol Clin.* 1995;13(2):365-384.
4. Clark SR, Jones KD, Burckhardt CS, Bennett R. Exercise for patients with fibromyalgia: risks versus benefits. *Curr Rheumatol Rep.* 2001;3(2):135-146.
5. Criscuolo CM. Interventional approaches to the management of myofascial pain syndrome. *Curr Pain Headache Rep.* 2001;5(5):407-411.
6. Garland EM, Robertson D. Chiari I malformation as a cause of orthostatic intolerance symptoms: a media myth? *Am J Med.* 2001;111(7):546-552.
7. Gowans SE, deHueck A, Voss S, et al. Effect of a randomized, controlled trial of exercise on mood and physical function in individuals with fibromyalgia. *Arthritis Rheum.* 2001;45(6):519-529.
8. Gur A, Karakoc M, Nas K, et al. Cytokines and depression in cases with fibromyalgia. *J Rheumatol.* 2002;29(2):358-361.
9. Hurtig IM, Raak RI, Kendall SA, Gerdle B, Wahren LK. Quantitative sensory testing in fibromyalgia patients and in healthy subjects: identification of subgroups. *Clin J Pain.* 2001;17(4):316-322.
10. Moldofsky H. Fibromyalgia, sleep disorder and chronic fatigue syndrome. In: Bock C, Whelan J, eds. *Chronic Fatigue Syndrome.* CIBA Foundation Symposium 173. Chichester: Wiley; 1993:262-271.
11. Muller W, Stratz T. Results of the intravenous administration of tropisetron in fibromyalgia patients. *Scand J Rheumatol.* 2000;113(suppl):59-62.

12. Offenbacher M, Stucki G. Physical therapy in the treatment of fibromyalgia. *Scand J Rheumatol.* 2000;113(suppl):78-85.

13. Park DC, Glass JM, Minear M, Crofford LJ. Cognitive function in fibromyalgia patients. *Arthritis Rheum.* 2001;44(9):2125-2133.

14. Parker AJ, Wessely S, Cleare AJ. The neuroendocrinology of chronic fatigue syndrome and fibromyalgia. *Psychol Med.* 2001;31(8):1331-1345.

15. Simons DG, Travell JG, Simons LS. *Myofascial Pain and Dysfunction: The Trigger Point Manual.* 2nd ed. Baltimore: Williams & Wilkins; 1999.

16. van West D, Maes M. Neuroendocrine and immune aspects of fibromyalgia. *Biodrugs.* 2001;15(8):521-531.

17. West SG. *Rheumatology Secrets.* Philadelphia: Hanley & Belfus; 1997.

18. White KP, Harth M. An analytical review of 24 controlled clinical trials for fibromyalgia syndrome. *Pain.* 1996;64:211-219.

19. White KP, Harth M. Classification, epidemiology, and natural history of fibromyalgia. *Curr Pain Headache Rep.* 2001;5(4):320-329.

20. Gedalia A, Press J, Klein M, Buskila D. Joint hypermobility and fibromyalgia in schoolchildren. *Ann Rheum Dis.* 1993;52(7):494-496.

21. Acasuso DM, Collantes-Estevez E. Joint hypermobility in patients with fibromyalgia syndrome. *Arthritis Care Res.* 1998;11:39-42.

22. Russell IJ, Orr MD, Littman B, et al. Elevated cerebrospinal fluid levels of substance P in patients with the fibromyalgia syndrome. *Arthritis Rheum.* 1994;37(11):1593-1601.

23. Liu Z, Welin M, Bragee B, Nyberg F. A high-recovery extraction procedure for quantitative analysis of substance P and opioid peptides in human cerebrospinal fluid. *Peptides.* 2000;21(6):853-860.

24. Vaeroy H, Helle R, Forre O, Kass E, Terenius L. Elevated CSF levels of substance P and high incidence of Raynaud phenomenon in patients with fibromalgia: new features for diagnosis. *Pain.* 1988;32(1):21-26.

25. Bradley LA, Alberts KR, Alarcon GS, et al. Abnormal brain regional cerebral blood flow (rCBF) and cerebrospinal fluid (CSF) levels of substance P (SP) in patients and non-patients with fibromyalgia (FM). *Arthritis Rheum.* 1996;39(suppl): S212.

26. The American Geriatrics Society 2012 Beers Criteria Update Expert Panel. American Geriatrics Society updated Beers criteria for potentially inappropriate medication use in older adults. *J Am Geriatr Soc.* 2012;60:616-631.

27. Mclain DA. An open label dose finding trial of Tizanidine [Zanaflex™] for treatment of fibromyalgia. *J Musculoskel Pain.* 2002;10(4):7-18.

28. Younger J, Noor N, Mccue R, Mackey S. Low-dose naltrexone for the treatment of fibromyalgia: findings of a small, randomized, double-blind, placebo-controlled, counterbalanced, crossover trial assessing daily pain levels. *Arthritis Rheum.* 2013;65(2):529-538.

29. Younger J, Parkitny L, Mclain D. The use of low-dose naltrexone (LDN) as a novel anti-inflammatory treatment for chronic pain. *Clin Rheumatol.* 2014;33(4):451-459.

30. Liu H, Mantyh PW, Basbum AI. NMDA-receptor regulation of substance P release from primary afferent nociceptors. *Nature.* 1997;386:721-724.

31. Graven-Nielsen T, Sorensen J, Henriksson KG, Bengtsson M, Arendt-Nielsen L. Central hyperexcitability in fibromyalgia. *J Musculoskel Pain.* 1999;7:261-271.

32. Buskila D, Shnaider A, Neumann L, et al. Fibromyalgia in hepatitis C virus infection. Another infectious disease relationship. *Arch Intern Med.* 1997;157:2497-2500.

33. López-Solà M, Pujol J, Wager TD, et al. Altered functional magnetic resonance imaging responses to nonpainful sensory stimulation in fibromyalgia patients. *Arthritis Rheumatol.* 2014;66(11):3200-3209.

34. Littlejohn G. Neurogenic neuroinflammation in fibromyalgia and complex regional pain syndrome. *Nat Rev Rheumatol.* 2015;11(11):639-648. http://dx.doi.org/10.1038/nrrheum.2015.100.

POSTOPERATIVE PAIN MANAGEMENT

Andras Laufer

CHAPTER 26

1. Discuss the pathophysiology of postoperative pain.

   Surgery produces tissue injury with consequent release of histamine and inflammatory mediators, such as bradykinin, substance P, prostaglandins, neurotransmitters (e.g., serotonin), and neurotrophins (e.g., nerve growth factor). Noxious stimuli are transduced by peripheral nociceptors and transmitted by A-delta and C nerve fibers from peripheral visceral and somatic sites to the dorsal horn of the spinal cord. These stimuli are transmitted to higher centers through the spinothalamic and spinoreticular tracts, where they induce suprasegmental and cortical responses to ultimately produce the perception of and affective component of pain.

2. Describe the phenomenon of peripheral and central sensitization.

   Sensitization of peripheral nociceptors may occur upon noxious stimuli and is marked by a decreased threshold for activation. This may lead to functional changes in the dorsal horn of the spinal cord that may later cause postoperative pain to be perceived as more painful than it would otherwise have been, and result in central sensitization.

3. What are the predictors of postoperative pain?

   Preoperative pain, anxiety, young age, obesity, surgical fear, catastrophizing, and type of surgery (abdominal, orthopedic, and thoracic surgery, long duration), age, and psychological distress have been identified as predictors of postoperative pain. Intensity of perioperative pain, old age, obesity, depression, psychological vulnerability, stress, and duration of disability (time to return to work) are the best predictors of persistent postoperative pain.

4. What is preventive analgesia?

   The focus of preventive analgesia is not on the relative timing (preemptive analgesia) of analgesic interventions, but on attenuating the impact of the peripheral nociceptive barrage associated with noxious preoperative, intraoperative, and/or postoperative stimuli. By interrupting the transmission of the peripheral nociceptive barrage to the spinal cord throughout the perioperative period, a preventive approach aims to block the induction of central sensitization, resulting in less intense postoperative pain and lower analgesic requirements. Preventive analgesia is demonstrated when postoperative pain and/or analgesic use are reduced beyond the duration of action of the target drug, and the observed effects are not direct analgesic effects of the target drug.

5. Describe your options using nonsteroidal antiinflammatory drugs in the perioperative period.

   Perioperative administration of COX-2 inhibitors for total joint arthroplasty has been shown to result in a reduction in perioperative pain and improvement in outcomes without the added risk of increased perioperative bleeding. Currently available nonsteroidal antiinflammatory drugs (NSAIDs) for parenteral administration in United States are ketorolac and diclofenac. The apprehension about ketorolac stems from the fact that it is a reversible cyclooxygenase inhibitor. Postoperative bleeding was not significantly increased with using low-dose ketorolac, and the incidence of adverse events, including postoperative nausea and vomiting, was significantly lower.

6. Describe the benefit of intravenous, patient controlled (IV PCA) versus intravenous, intramuscular, and transdermal iontophoretic pain medication administration.

Advantages and Disadvantages of Modes of Drug Administration

	IV PCA	Intermittent IV	Intramuscular	Transdermal Iontophoretic System
Access for the patient:	Readily available when needed	Needs trained personnel	Needs trained personnel	Easy, noninvasive
Bioavailability:	Good	Good	Depends on tissue perfusion	Depends on tissue perfusion
Risk of significant side effects:	Less likely of overdose	Overdose more likely	Overdose more likely, painful, risk of infection	Less likely overdose
Expense:	Expensive machine, low cost of maintenance	Potentially high administration cost	Potentially high administration cost	Only device cost

IV PCA, Intravenous patient controlled analgesia.

7. **How do local anesthetics block nerve function?**
   Local anesthetics block voltage-gated sodium channels, thereby interrupting the initiation and propagation of action potential in axons. Based on this mechanism of action, local anesthetics provide a wide variety of biologic actions, both desirable and unwanted, and have side effects through other mechanisms. In addition to blockade of the action potential, local anesthetics can inhibit various receptors, enhance release of glutamate, and depress the activity of certain intracellular signaling pathways. Toxicity may be local or systemic. The central nervous and cardiovascular systems are most commonly the targets for acute clinical toxicity caused by local anesthetics.

8. **What is the role of local anesthetics in postoperative pain management?**
   When a local-anesthesia-based regimen is used in epidural analgesia, peripheral nerve block catheters, or local infiltration, it allows continuous analgesia, which is superior to systemic opioids. The beneficial effect of the infiltration of the surgical wound may be extended up to 2 days with available liposomal bupivacaine. Perioperative lidocaine infusion reduces the intraoperative and postoperative opioid need.

9. **Does regional analgesia influence surgical outcome?**
   Epidural analgesia: Lower pain scores with epidural analgesia than with systemic opioids. It reduces risk of myocardial infarction and dysrhythmias (thoracic epidural analgesia [TEA] in high-risk patients). It facilitates earlier return of bowel function after major abdominal surgical procedures. The beneficial effect of reduced risk of postoperative pulmonary complications in case of utilizing TEA is well established.
   Peripheral nerve block analgesia: Lower pain scores with peripheral nerve analgesia than with systemic opioids, allowing significant opioid sparing effect. It facilitates earlier rehabilitation goals, reduced length of stay and enhanced recovery after surgery (ERAS).

10. **What could be examples of appropriate regional analgesia for perioperative pain management in shoulder arthroplasty, thoracotomy, inguinal hernia repair, laparotomy, hip arthroplasty, and knee arthroplasty?**
    Shoulder arthroplasty—interscalene brachial plexus block; Thoracotomy—thoracic epidural or thoracic paravertebral analgesia; inguinal hernia repair—transverse abdominis plane (TAP) block; laparotomy—TAP or TEA; hip arthroplasty—lumbar plexus/sciatic plexus block or lumbar epidural analgesia; knee arthroplasty—femoral nerve block or lumbar epidural analgesia.

11. What does multimodal analgesia mean? What are its benefits?
    Multimodal techniques for pain management include the administration of two or more drugs that act by different mechanisms for providing analgesia, and regional analgesia techniques. The drugs may be administered via the same route or by different routes, and the choice of medication, dose, route, and duration of therapy should be individualized. Dosing regimens should be administered to optimize efficacy while minimizing the risk of adverse events.

12. When should the postoperative pain management treatment start?
    Preoperative patient evaluation and planning is integral to perioperative pain management. Proactive individualized planning, premedication, and regional techniques are anticipatory strategies for postoperative analgesia that integrate pain management into the perioperative care of patients. Patient factors to consider in formulating a plan include type of surgery, expected severity of postoperative pain, underlying medical conditions (e.g., presence of respiratory or cardiac disease, allergies), the risk–benefit ratio for the available techniques, and a patient's preferences or previous experience with pain.

13. Describe the role of ketamine in postoperative pain management.
    Ketamine is traditionally recognized as an intraoperatively administered anesthetic; however, small-dose ketamine can facilitate postoperative analgesia because of its N-methyl-D-aspartate receptor (NMDA)-antagonistic properties, which may be important in attenuating central sensitization and opioid tolerance. Pain therapy can be improved using intravenous subanesthetic ketamine (0.05 to 0.2 mg/kg per hour), when added as an adjunct to general anesthesia, reduced postoperative pain, and opioid requirements.

14. Describe the negative effects of the untreated or undertreated postoperative pain.
    Acute effect: Increased sympathetic tone, increased catecholamine and catabolic hormone secretion, and decreased secretion of anabolic hormones. The effects include sodium and water retention and increased levels of blood glucose, free fatty acids, ketone bodies, and lactate. A hypermetabolic, catabolic state occurs as metabolism and oxygen consumption are increased and metabolic substrates are mobilized from storage depots, hypercoagulability, and immunosuppression. Hyperglycemia from the stress response may contribute to poor wound healing and depression of immune function.
    Chronic effect: Persistent postsurgical pain (PPP) is a largely unrecognized problem that may occur in 10% to 65% of postoperative patients (depending on the type of surgery), with 2% to 10% of these patients experiencing severe PPP.

15. What is the current concept of background continuous infusion with intravenous patient controlled analgesia?
    Findings from meta-analyses indicate more analgesic use when IV PCA with a background infusion of morphine is compared with IV PCA without a background infusion; findings were equivocal regarding pain relief, nausea and vomiting, pruritus, and sedation in opioid naïve patients.

16. What are the special considerations of opioid use for postoperative pain control when using in geriatric patients?
    Elderly patients suffer from conditions such as arthritis or cancer that render them more likely to undergo surgery. Their pain is often undertreated, and elderly individuals may be more vulnerable to the detrimental effects of such undertreatment. The physical, social, emotional, and cognitive changes associated with aging have an impact on perioperative pain management. These patients may have different attitudes than younger adult patients in expressing pain and seeking appropriate therapy. Altered physiology changes the way analgesic drugs and local anesthetics are distributed and metabolized, and frequently requires dose alterations.

17. What are the special considerations of opioid use for postoperative pain control with children?
    The emotional component of pain is particularly strong in infants and children. Absence of parents, security objects, and familiar surroundings may cause as much suffering as the surgical incision. Children's fear of injections makes intramuscular or other invasive routes of drug delivery aversive. Even the valuable technique of topical analgesia before injections may not lessen this fear. In the absence of a clear source of pain or obvious pain behavior, caregivers may assume that pain is not present and defer treatment. Safe methods for providing analgesia are underused in pediatric patients for fear of opioid-induced respiratory depression.

18. **Which opioid neuraxial administration has higher chances of resulting in delayed respiratory depression? Why?**

    Neuraxial administration of lipophilic opioids, such as fentanyl and sufentanil, provides a rapid onset of analgesia, and their rapid clearance from cerebrospinal fluid (CSF) may limit cephalic spread and the development of certain side effects such as delayed respiratory depression. On the other hand, hydrophilic opioids (i.e., morphine and hydromorphone) tend to remain within the CSF and produce a delayed but longer duration of analgesia, along with a generally more frequent incidence of side effects because of the cephalic or supraspinal spread of these compounds.

19. **How would you treat opioid related pruritis?**

    Pruritus is one of the most common side effects of epidural or intrathecal administration of opioids, with an incidence of approximately 60% versus about 15% to 18% for epidural local anesthetic administration or systemic opioids. Many drugs have been evaluated for the prevention and treatment of opioid-induced pruritus, which can be difficult to manage and quite bothersome for some patients. Low doses of intravenous naloxone, naltrexone, nalbuphine, and droperidol appear to be efficacious for the pharmacologic control of opioid-induced pruritus. Poor opioid receptor antagonists are not ideal therapeutic agents against pruritus, because opioid analgesia is also reversed by these agents.

20. **What are your options to treat opioid-induced nausea and vomiting?**

    Nausea is a highly distressing symptom that may occur with or without vomiting and can affect overall outcome. Opioid-induced nausea and vomiting (OINV) may be due to multiple opioid effects, including (a) enhanced vestibular sensitivity (symptoms may include vertigo and worsening with motion), (b) direct effects on the chemoreceptor trigger zone, and (c) delayed gastric emptying (symptoms of early satiety and bloating, worsening postprandially). The treatment may target different receptors: 5-HT3 receptor antagonists (i.e., ondansetron), dopamine receptor antagonists (i.e., promethazine, droperidol), and modulation of opioid signaling (i.e., subcutaneous methylnaltrexone).

21. **How would you treat opioid related constipation?**

    Strong evidence for efficacy has been established for stimulant (senna, bisacodyl) and osmotic laxatives (milk of magnesia). Opioid-induced constipation is predominantly mediated by gastrointestinal μ-opioid receptors. Selective blockade of these peripheral receptors might relieve constipation without compromising centrally mediated effects of opioid analgesia or precipitating withdrawal. Treat with peripherally restricted μ-opiate receptor antagonists if conservative treatment failed (subcutaneous methylnaltrexone or alvimopan).

22. **How would you treat opioid-related respiratory depression in the postoperative setting?**

    Opioids activating the μ receptor cause dose-dependent depression of respiration, primarily through a direct action on brainstem respiratory centers. Naloxone was introduced into clinical practice in the late 1960s. Side effects (increases in heart rate and blood pressure) and more serious complications (e.g., pulmonary edema) have been reported. The initial dose recommendations for naloxone in adults is 0.4 mg to 2 mg and is 0.1 mg/kg in pediatrics. Recent recommendations rather suggest titrating even lower doses in order to reverse the severe postoperative respiratory depression due to opioids, but not fully reverse its analgesic effect.

23. **What are the specific goals of postoperative pain management after total knee arthroplasty?**

    The goals extend beyond simply improving patient comfort and satisfaction. It is essential to enable patients to ambulate and move their joints soon after surgery and, where appropriate, to shorten the length of stay, in many cases allowing patients to be discharged within 1 or 2 days. For balanced multimodal analgesia an effective preoperative regimen may include COX2 inhibitor (celecoxib), acetaminophen, gabapentinoids, regional analgesia, and opioids. Perioperative intraarticular injections have been shown to be an effective alternative to femoral nerve blockade.

24. **Is the thoracic paravertebral block superior to thoracic epidural analgesia?**

    TEA has been traditionally regarded as the "gold standard." A growing body of evidence supports that thoracic paravertebral block (TPVB) is at least comparable to TEA for postoperative analgesia in thoracic and abdominal surgeries with a superior side effect profile, avoiding epidural hematoma and abscess, injury to neuroaxis, postdural puncture headache, and intrathecal injection. It decreases the rate of pulmonary complications, incidences of hypotension, urinary retention, and block failure. Application of continuous TPVB needs special training, while the TEA has been the gold standard and part of training curricula for decades.

25. What is your postoperative pain management strategy treating patients with opioid tolerance due to chronic pain and chronic opioid use?

Several patient variables predict poorer pain control and increased analgesic requirements in the postoperative period. These variables include preexisting pain conditions and the preoperative use of opioids. An adequate opioid dose needs to be maintained to prevent opioid withdrawal. Patients should be informed about the potential for aggravated pain, increased opioid requirements, and alternative methods complementing opioid therapy. Use of adjuvant agents like ketamine, NSAIDs, acetaminophen, gabapentinoids, and regional analgesia (single shot or continuous) has significant opioid sparing effect.

26. What is opioid-induced hyperalgesia?

Patients receiving opioids to control their pain somewhat paradoxically may become more sensitive to pain (i.e., hyperalgesic) and may aggravate their preexisting pain as a direct result of opioid therapy. The disappearance of opioid treatment effects, particularly if coupled with the unexplained expansion of pain complaints, may signal the expression of OIH. In this setting, the use of alternative analgesics, multimodal approach, and detoxification from opioids may need to be considered. The prevalence of clinically significant OIH is currently unknown.

27. How does preoperative buprenorphine treatment influence postoperative pain management strategies?

Buprenorphine is a partial mu-agonist and kappa-antagonist. Clinically, however, it behaves as a full mu-opioid agonist for analgesia and may have antihyperalgesic properties. It also has high opioid receptor affinity and slow offset kinetics, leading to concerns that the resultant blockade could interfere with effective acute pain management using other full mu-opioid agonists. As a result, conflicting recommendations exist as to whether high-dose buprenorphine should be continued or ceased in the perioperative period. The recommendations are (a) stop taking buprenorphine at least 72 hours prior the expected surgery, or (b) continue the buprenorphine therapy and administer significantly higher doses of opioid, as needed. Multimodal analgesia with adjuvants and regional techniques have important role in treating opioid tolerant patients.

KEY POINTS

1. Surgery predictably will result in pain, and untreated postoperative pain negatively influences surgical outcome.
2. Multimodal postoperative pain management utilizes adjuvants and regional analgesia techniques besides opioid pain medications with optimized benefits and decreased side effects.
3. Preventive analgesia starts at the preoperative visit. Its benefit lasts longer than the multimodal therapy expected effect.
4. Postoperative pain influenced by not only the nature of the surgery, but the patient age, gender, medical, psychological, and social history, as well.

BIBLIOGRAPHY

1. Alford DP, Peggy Compton RN, Samet JH. Acute pain management for patients receiving maintenance methadone or buprenorphine therapy. *Ann Intern Med.* 2006;144(2):127-134.
2. Cohen NH. *Miller's Anesthesia.* 8th ed. Philadelphia: Elsevier/Saunders; 2015.
3. Gobble RM, Hoang HL, Kachniarz B, Orgill DP. Ketorolac does not increase perioperative bleeding: a meta-analysis of randomized controlled trials. *Plast Reconstr Surg.* 2014;133:741-755.
4. Himmelseher S. Ketamine for perioperative pain management. *Anesthesiology.* 2005;102(1):211-220.
5. Huxtable C, Roberts LJ, Somogyi AA, MacIntyre PE. Acute pain management in opioid-tolerant patients: a growing challenge. *Anaesth Intensive Care.* 2011;39:804-823.
6. Katz J. Preventive analgesia: quo vadimus? *Anesth Analg.* 2011;113(5):1242-1253.
7. Practice Guidelines for Acute Pain Management in the Perioperative Setting: an updated report by the American Society of Anesthesiologists Task Force on Acute Pain Management. *Anesthesiology.* 2012;116(2):248-273.
8. Scuderi GR. The challenges of perioperative pain management in total joint arthroplasty. *Am J Orthop (Belle Mead NJ).* 2015;44(10 suppl):S2-S4.
9. Smith HS, Laufer A. Opioid-induced nausea and vomiting. *Eur J Pharmacol.* 2014;722:67-78.
10. Wu CL, Raja SN. Treatment of acute postoperative pain. *Lancet.* 2011;377(9784):2215-2225.

CHAPTER 27

CANCER PAIN

Katherine Galluzzi

1. **What causes pain in patients with cancer?**

   A diagnosis of cancer is feared not only because of possible mortality but also due to the morbidity caused by pain and potential loss of functional capacity. Malignancies cause nociceptive effects in the form of visceral, somatic/inflammatory pain, and can also result in neuropathic pain. More than one of these types of cancer-mediated pain may coexist in a patient; in addition, patients with cancer may have pain due to preexisting comorbidities (diabetes, arthritis, migraine), or they may have pain due to treatment effects. Furthermore, nociceptive pain may be amplified by psychological suffering, whereby the experience of pain or discomfort causes additional distress in the form of existential issues such as changes in role, identity, quality of life, and spiritual concerns.

2. **Which common types of cancer cause inflammatory pain?**

   Commonly occurring cancers such as prostate, breast, and lung frequently metastasize to bone. Bone metastases cause painful pathological and/or compression fractures; the metastatic lesions themselves can incite significant pain due to the release of pain-signaling substances such as prostaglandins, endothelins, and bradykinin. Gastrointestinal malignancies such as colon, pancreatic, and hepatocellular carcinoma can progress to increased tumor burden; the resulting abdominal pain may be due to ascites, visceral capsular stretching, and/or extrinsic pressure on intraabdominal structures. Central nervous system tumors typically cause headache, visual pain, and/or blindness, and possible loss of sensory or motor function.

3. **What causes neuropathic pain in patients with cancer?**

   Neuropathic pain represents a derangement of central and peripheral nervous system pain signaling, which is a consequence of nerve injury/destruction, disease (acquired, viral, or congenital), or toxins (drugs, ingested/inhaled substances). Malignancies may cause neuropathic pain due to tumor infiltration that invades and destroys neural tissue or through tumor spread that impinges on nerve structures. Neuropathic pain caused by tumor invasion usually presents as a plexopathy (injury to nerve fibers in a specific distribution)—typically brachial, thoracic, or lumbosacral. Neuropathic pain may also arise from treatment side effects such as surgery, radiation-induced injury to peripheral nerves or spinal cord, drug-induced neuropathy, or chemotherapy. Several commonly used chemotherapeutic agents (cisplatin, vincristine, procarbazine) can cause painful peripheral neuropathy, typically in a stocking-glove distribution. Motor neuropathies may also occur, such as the peroneal palsy (foot-drop) that results from chemotherapeutic agents.

4. **How common is nociceptive pain in cancer?**

   The prevalence of cancer pain ranges from 14% to 100% based on several large epidemiologic surveys. In advanced disease it is estimated that two-thirds of cancer patients will have pain due to tumor invasion into bone, viscera or other soft tissue, nerves, ligaments, or fascia. Almost one-fourth will experience pain as a direct consequence of treatment for cancer.

5. **How common is neuropathic pain in patients with cancer?**

   Neuropathic pain has been estimated to occur in up to 90% of patients receiving chemotherapy with agents that are neurotoxic. It can also occur from tumor infiltration of neural structures or as a result of surgery or radiation-induced nerve damage. About one-third of patients with cancer have a neuropathic component to their pain.

6. **How does cancer treatment cause pain?**

   The fact that treatment effects can themselves cause pain is well documented. Postoperative pain (e.g., surgical resection, postthoracotomy, or mastectomy chest wall pain) and acute amputation pain followed by "phantom" pain are common problems. Chemotherapeutic agents cause toxic side effects (e.g., chemotherapy-induced mucositis). Chemotherapeutic agents that can cause neuropathy include cisplatin, oxaliplatin, paclitaxel, thalidomide, vincristine, and vinblastine. External beam radiation may also be a pain generator (e.g., painful neuropathy).

7. Is it common for patients with cancer to have more than one painful site?
Yes, several large studies indicate that more than a quarter of patients with cancer report pain in more than one site. For example, a patient with lung cancer may experience chest wall pain (costochondritis) from the effort of breathing or coughing, and also have significant back pain from vertebral metastasis. As already noted, effects of surgery, radiation, and/or chemotherapy can cause additional pain; many patients with cancer have preexisting pain from degenerative arthritis, painful diabetic neuropathy, fibromyalgia, migraine, or other chronic nonmalignant painful conditions. Patients with cancer also have evolving pain with tumor progression. Thus careful ongoing evaluation of all potential and changing sources of pain is needed.

8. Which types of malignancies are least likely to be painful?
In general, leukemias are not physically painful but instead cause debility and extreme fatigue.

9. Which neuropathic pain syndromes are commonly seen in patients with cancer?
Lumbosacral plexopathy may be caused by lymphoma or colon cancer. Injury to the intercostobrachial nerve during radical mastectomy may result in pain or numbness distal to the axilla on the inner aspect of the arm. The neuropathy that develops from chemotherapy with cisplatin or vinca alkaloids is dose-related and usually affects the extremities; sensory as well as motor neuropathies can occur (e.g., peroneal palsy). Cancer patients appear predisposed to developing herpes zoster (shingles) that can progress to postherpetic neuralgia (PHN; pain that persists >6 weeks after complete resolution of the shingles lesions). Complex Regional Pain Syndromes Type I and II, postradiation plexopathy, radiculopathy, and neuroma formation are other neuropathic syndromes seen in cancer patients.

10. What is the postthoracotomy pain syndrome?
The pain from thoracotomy encompasses the acute postoperative pain that resolves (usually within 3 months) and pain that persists longer than 3 months or recurs at the surgical site. The latter either is of neuropathic origin (as seen in postmastectomy axillary numbness) or may represent tumor recurrence. When pain recurs after a pain-free interval, infection or tumor recurrence should be ruled out.

11. Why do women treated with radical mastectomy have a numb area just distal to the axilla on the upper part of the arm?
Surgical injury to the intercostobrachial nerve causes numbness along its distribution, a condition referred to as *postmastectomy syndrome*.

12. What is the most common site for tumor infiltration of the brachial plexus?
The type of tumor will determine where infiltration is likely to occur, but most commonly the lower brachial plexus is involved, leading to pain and hand weakness in a C7 to T1 distribution. This is typically caused by a tumor located in the superior sulcus (Pancoast tumor) or at the thoracic inlet adjacent to the eighth cervical nerve roots, the first and second thoracic trunk distribution, the sympathetic chain, and the stellate ganglion. Horner syndrome may also be present.

13. What are the clinical differences between radiation injury to the brachial plexus and tumor involvement of the plexus?
Although clinically similar, radiation of the brachial plexus (nerve network that supplies innervation to upper extremity and shoulder extending from spinal cord to axilla) is more likely to cause involvement of all three trunks of the plexus, whereas tumor involvement more commonly affects smaller branches of the brachial plexus and/or specific nerves (e.g., axillary, musculocutaneus, median, radial, or ulnar nerve).

14. Is phantom limb sensation common after amputation?
Most, if not all, patients who undergo amputation, either traumatic or surgical, will experience sensation at the site of the missing part. This is because, despite disruption and removal of neural tissue, sensory pathways in the peripheral and central nervous system persist and continue to signal aberrantly. These neuropathic sensations can manifest as electric shock-like pain, numbness, burning, tingling, or other unpleasant sensory effects. Preemptive analgesia may prevent or limit the extent and intensity of postamputation phantom pain.

15. **What is the most common cause of lumbosacral plexopathy?**
The most common cause of pain in a lumbosacral distribution is colorectal carcinoma with local extension, although metastasis from any source that impinges upon or causes destruction of neural structures may be involved.

16. **What are the pain-sensitive structures in bones and joints?**
The periosteum and all intraarticular components with the exception of cartilage are pain sensitive; articular cartilage lacks innervation and is not a pain-sensitive structure. The annulus fibrosus of the intervertebral discs has nociceptors, but the nucleus pulposus does not.

17. **Do nonsteroidal antiinflammatory drugs have direct tumor effects?**
Nonsteroidal antiinflammatory drugs (NSAIDs) are useful for tumor-induced pain, partially because of their effects on the inflammatory substrate at the tumor margins. Bone metastases require prostaglandin E2 for growth; NSAIDs inhibit prostaglandin synthesis and thus may decrease osteoblastic tumor proliferation. The use of NSAIDs is, however, limited by its potential effect of reducing renal function and gastrotoxicity, as well as the class-wide black box warning regarding cardiovascular risk, including myocardial infarction (MI) and stroke.

18. **What are paraneoplastic syndromes and do they cause pain?**
Paraneoplastic syndromes are relatively rare clinical symptom complexes due to nonmetastatic effects of cancer. They may manifest as remote effects on the nervous system (e.g., sensorimotor peripheral neuropathy, mononeuritis multiplex, brachial neuritis, and painful peripheral neuropathy resulting from islet cell tumors or paraproteinuria). The painful symptoms result from disturbances of the immunologic system and/or from substances (toxins, hormones, electrolyte imbalance) produced by the tumor but occurring remotely from the site of the tumor. The most common paraneoplastic syndrome is fever, but presentation can vary from dermatomyositis-polymyositis to Cushing syndrome or the malignant carcinoid syndrome.

19. **What other pain syndromes occur in patients with cancer?**
PHN, defined as persistence of pain for weeks or months after complete resolution of the herpes zoster (shingles) rash, can follow an episode of shingles in a cancer patient. While advanced age (related to waning cell-mediated immunity) is the most common factor associated with development of PHN, those with immunosuppression or cancer are most likely to develop PHN. The Shingles Prevention Study showed that immunization against herpes zoster decreased overall incidence of shingles and reduced the incidence of PHN by 65% in individuals over age 60. The Advisory Council on Immunization Practice recommends that all individuals receive zoster immunization at age 60. Patients newly diagnosed with cancer should receive zoster immunization as soon as possible prior to initiation of chemotherapy. A recent study of the new herpes zoster subunit vaccine (HZ/su) showed that vaccine efficacy against herpes zoster was 91.3%, and vaccine efficacy against PHN was 88.8%.

In addition to the risk for shingles/PHN, many common chemotherapeutic agents cause mucositis and some therapies (e.g., everolimus, sorafenib, regorafenib) cause painful stomatitis. Frequency and severity are both drug- and dose-dependent. Three commonly used cytotoxic agents associated with oral mucositis are doxorubicin, fluorouracil, and methotrexate. Mucositis develops in nearly all patients receiving radiation treatment (RT) to the head and neck region. RT-induced mucositis is similar to that induced by chemotherapy, usually developing 2 to 3 weeks after starting treatment. Incidence and severity of RT-induced mucositis depend on the field, total dose and duration of RT, and the use of concomitant chemotherapy. Anticipatory treatment may include oral lubricants and mouthwash containing antihistamine or local anesthetic to reduce pain and discomfort, antibiotic (bactericidal), antifungal, corticosteroid (antiinflammatory), and an antacid to ensure the other ingredients adequately coat the buccal mucosa. Most pharmacies compound such a substance, known as Magic Mouthwash.

20. **Are opioids known to increase the risk for acute herpes zoster? Are they associated with risk for subsequent postherpetic neuralgia?**
The answer to both questions is no. In addition to vaccination against zoster, studies have demonstrated that early (within 72 hours of symptom or rash onset) initiation of antiviral therapy and assiduous pain management, including opioids if indicated, may prevent the development or reduce the severity of PHN.

21. Are additional symptoms common in patients with cancer who are experiencing pain?

Yes, patients with cancer pain report significant rates of anhedonia, fatigue, low energy levels, trouble falling or staying asleep, cognitive impairment, dyspnea either at rest or with minor exertion, dry mouth, indigestion, nausea/vomiting, and drowsiness or excessive somnolence. Dysphoria is a common comorbid problem in cancer patients, both as preexisting or new-onset depression. Debility and impaired mobility coupled with potent analgesics (especially opioids) make constipation a very common symptom in cancer patients. A multimodal approach that takes into account all potential sources of distress is therefore recommended for patients with cancer pain.

22. What is meant by "incident pain?"

Incident pain is the term used to describe pain precipitated by movement such as repositioning, deep respiration, or ambulation. It may also be caused by procedures such as venipuncture, cannula insertion, or physical therapy. Pretreatment with appropriate pain medications or adjuvants prior to procedures, dressing changes, personal care, toileting, or ambulating are useful for mitigating incident pain.

23. How is "incident pain" different from "breakthrough pain"?

Incident pain is a nociceptive response to an activity (wound care, toileting). Breakthrough pain is defined as pain that occurs when the threshold of pain relief afforded by scheduled, around-the-clock analgesics is breached. Typically, patients who are on long-acting analgesics who experience breakthrough pain benefit from up-titration of the analgesic and/or immediate administration of a short-acting analgesic to mitigate the acute pain.

24. What are the oncologic emergencies that cause pain?

The most common painful emergencies associated with cancer are fracture of a weight-bearing bone, neuraxial metastasis with threatened neural injury (e.g., cauda equina syndrome), bacterial infection/sepsis, and obstructed or perforated viscus. Treatment for these conditions includes pain management as well as immediate treatment of the medical emergency.

25. Are there recommended guidelines or protocols for management of cancer pain?

Yes, several consensus panels have established guidelines for cancer pain management. They include (but are not limited to) protocols developed by the National Comprehensive Cancer Network (NCCN) and The Joint Commission. American Pain Society guidelines for assessment and treatment of cancer pain in adults and children were published in 2004 and await an update.

26. What are the initial National Comprehensive Cancer Network recommendations for cancer pain screening and assessment?

NCCN recommends the following: Screen all patients with cancer for pain. If no pain is present, rescreen at each visit. If pain is present, use a pain intensity rating scale to determine rates of current, usual, worst, and least pain in the past 24 hours. Treat severe, uncontrolled pain immediately. Conduct a comprehensive pain assessment to determine the cause of pain, pathophysiology of pain, presence of specific cancer pain syndrome(s), and patient goals for comfort and function. Anticipate anxiety about painful events and procedures and offer analgesics (topical, local, or systemic) and anxiolytics for procedures causing pain or anxiety.

In nonverbal patients, use alternative methods for evaluating the level of pain—for example, observe patient behavior (withdrawal, grimacing), obtain family/caregiver input on the patient's behavior and its meaning, and evaluate the patient's response to pain medication and nonpharmacological treatments.

27. Summarize the National Comprehensive Cancer Network approach to management of cancer pain that is not related to oncologic emergency.

The first step is to determine whether the patient is opioid naïve or opioid tolerant (see Question 29). In opioid naïve patients, consider titration of appropriate pharmacologic analgesics such that the dose relieves pain throughout the dosing interval but does not cause unmanageable adverse events. Titration must utilize caution in patients with risk factors: decreased hepatic or renal function, chronic lung disease, upper airway compromise, obstructive sleep apnea, or compromised cognitive and/or physical function.

Oral routes of administration are preferred; however, consider alternate routes (topical, transdermal, subcutaneous, or intravenous) to maximize comfort. Patient referrals should be considered for those who may benefit from nerve block, in those in whom adequate analgesia cannot be obtained or who are experiencing intolerable side effects. Consider interventional strategies (regional infusions such as epidural, intrathecal, or regional plexus blocks, as well as kyphoplasty, neurodestructive procedures, neurostimulation procedures, or radiofrequency ablation) if it is determined that they may provide sufficient benefit.

28. **Summarize the Joint Commission Standards for Pain Management.**
The Joint Commission on Accreditation of Hospitals recommends the following six standards:
- Recognize the right of individuals to appropriate pain management.
- If pain exists, determine this and also assess the nature and intensity.
- Establish policies and procedures to support ordering safe, effective pain medication.
- Educate patients and families about effective pain management.
- Consider pain management needs in the discharge planning process.
- Incorporate pain management in the organization's performance improvement process.

29. **What is "opioid tolerance"?**
In general, tolerance to a drug occurs when, with continuous administration over time, greater amounts of that drug are required to achieve the original degree of its desired therapeutic effect. Patients will develop tolerance to both the analgesic effect as well as the side effects of opioids.

    To avoid the adverse drug reaction of fatal respiratory depression, minimum opioid dosages that assure tolerance have been defined. The minimum dosage at which a patient is deemed "opioid tolerant" is oral morphine 60 mg/day, or oxycodone 30 mg/day, or an equi-analgesic (morphine mg equivalent) dose of another opioid for at least 1 week. Patients are considered "opioid naïve" if they have not taken opioids at these specific dosages for a week or longer.

30. **What non-opioid analgesics are appropriate for patients with cancer pain?**
The selection of a nonopioid analgesic as a first-line agent for opioid naïve patients is encouraged, and if well-tolerated, that analgesic may be continued during initiation and up-titration of opioids. Consider NSAIDs or acetaminophen for mild to moderate pain, utilizing caution in patients with renal or hepatic impairment. There is good medical evidence for the efficacy of NSAIDs in patients following surgery or other painful procedures; they are considered first-line treatment for inflammatory pain such as that caused by bone metastasis. The use of NSAIDs for cancer pain may be limited by their adverse effect on renal function and by potential gastric mucosal irritation or ulceration as well as cardiovascular risk.

    Bisphosphonates have some efficacy for treatment of bone metastasis, possibly through stabilization of the metastatic focus. Corticosteroids are effective for management of bone as well as brain metastases and for nerve compression, but their use may be limited by tolerance issues such as sodium and water retention, hyperglycemia, or gastric ulceration.

    Acetaminophen, while a useful antipyretic at therapeutic doses, is a relatively weak analgesic whose use may be limited due to hepatotoxicity, which can occur at dosages of 3 to 4 g/day.

    Topical analgesic options may be useful for patients who can pinpoint a localized focus of pain. These include topical NSAIDs, capsaicin, or lidocaine, among others. Anticonvulsants and antidepressants are considered to be first-line treatment for neuropathic pain.

31. **What complementary and alternative therapies are useful for cancer pain?**
Fifty percent to 83% of cancer patients report the use of at least one type of complementary and alternative medicine (CAM) modality. CAM therapies include osteopathic manipulative treatment or other manual medicine technique (e.g., chiropractic, traditional Chinese and Ayurvedic medicine, naturopathy, and homeopathic medicine). Acupuncture, herbs, supplements, and aromatherapy may be effective adjunctive treatments for cancer pain. Manual medicine techniques include physical therapy for bracing or splinting. Relaxation, mindfulness, and stress management programs; movement modalities such as yoga or Pilates; meditation and prayer as well as expressive arts; and support groups are all potential CAM therapies. Patients may embrace CAM as a way of imbuing their cancer treatment with a more integrated and holistic approach.

32. **What is the role for palliative care in management of patients with cancer pain?**
Recognizing that approximately 70% of patients will experience severe pain some time during their illness, as well as the unfortunate fact that up to a quarter of cancer patients continue to die in severe pain, it is imperative that care embracing a "mind-body-spirit" approach be initiated early in the course of disease. While many patients with cancer are not ready to elect the hospice Medicare benefit, most—if not all—will benefit from an interdisciplinary approach (e.g., pain specialists,

radiation oncologists, mental health professionals, neurosurgeons) to multiple symptom management, psychosocial/spiritual support, and pain management.

33. **Who are the members of a palliative care interdisciplinary team?**
Palliative care interdisciplinary team (IDT) members include a medical director (palliative care physician), registered nurses, social workers, psychologists, pastoral care counselors, volunteer coordinators, and others who assist with formulating and delivering the plan of care to patients receiving palliative or hospice care. The IDT meets regularly to discuss the patients under their care, and assess pain and symptom burden, as well as psychosocial concerns; the team can intervene at many levels to support that patient with cancer and his family and caregivers. The goal is to provide comprehensive, supportive care, as well as to utilize appropriate pharmacologic, nonpharmacologic, or CAM treatments.

34. **When are opioids prescribed for cancer pain? How do they work?**
Opioids are prescribed for cancer pain when other modalities (procedural, pharmacologic, and nonpharmacologic) fail to provide analgesia sufficient to allow achievement of realistic patient goals, including maintenance of function (activities of daily living) and overall quality of life. Opioids are pharmaceutical agents with morphine-like effects; they are opioid-receptor (mu, kappa, delta, etc.) agonists that will reliably provide analgesia at therapeutic dosages. Opioid analgesics are available in several formulations for oral, subcutaneous, intravenous, and transdermal administration, which makes them a mainstay of the armamentarium against cancer pain.

35. **Are long-acting opioid preparations preferred over short-acting types?**
Theoretically, extended release, long-acting (ER/LA) opioids afford cancer pain relief over a longer period of time (8 to 72 hours based on the product properties), whereas the duration of action of immediate release (IR) opioids is limited to about 4 to 6 hours. There is little evidence that ER/LA opioids provide pain relief that is superior to IR opioids, but it must be stressed that all pain patients benefit from scheduled, around-the-clock dosing schedules, as opposed to their use on an as-needed (prn) basis.

36. **Should patients with cancer who receive opioid therapy undergo the same screening and monitoring procedures as patients with chronic noncancer pain?**
Yes, there is the same incidence of opioid abuse, misuse, and diversion among cancer pain patients, as in noncancer patients. While the risk of addiction in patients with life-limiting illness may be less of a concern, it is also true that cancer patients who have the disease of addiction or opioid abuse disorder deserve assiduous pain management that may include referrals to pain management experts to assure safe use and careful monitoring of opioid therapy.

37. **Comment on the population of patients who have been successfully treated for cancer with respect to ongoing problems with pain.**
The burden of pain in cancer survivors (i.e., the posttreatment population) is as prevalent as that among cancer patients in general. Cancer survivors deserve pain management that takes into account the persistent, potentially long-term sequelae of disease—that is, they warrant ongoing multimodal therapy just as is recommended for those with ongoing, progressive malignant disease.

38. **What is the role for radiation therapy in cancer pain?**
Palliative radiation is most useful for pain related to bone metastases. There is evidence that single fraction radiation is as effective as multiple fractions for relieving bone pain during the final 3 months of life. Bear in mind that other modalities, such as are those needed to mitigate radiation effects and/or ongoing pain therapy regimens, should be continued concomitant with radiation therapy.

39. **What other therapies are available to treat pain from bone metastasis?**
Percutaneous image-guided cryoablation, radiofrequency ablation, and radioisotopes may be helpful in patients with unrelieved pain from vertebral and/or axial bone metastasis.

40. **Are interventional procedures necessary for most patients with cancer pain?**
No, there is good evidence to suggest that pharmacologic treatment coupled with appropriate multimodal, interdisciplinary therapy is effective for pain management in 95% of patients with cancer pain. Thus it appears that only 5% of cancer pain sufferers will require interventional procedures as part of their pain treatment plan.

KEY POINTS

1. Patients with cancer develop pain as a direct result of the malignancy, but they may also have pain due to nonmalignant causes, including comorbid conditions and psychological/existential distress.
2. Interventional procedures (surgical, radiologic, chemotherapeutic) directed at curing or reducing cancer burden may themselves result in pain, such as phantom pain, neuropathy, mucositis, or neuritis.
3. New onset pain (e.g., back pain) in a cancer patient should arouse suspicion of tumor progression such as vertebral metastasis or epidural tumor formation.
4. Opioid analgesics are a mainstay in the armamentarium of pain management for cancer patients; their use may be combined with other medications and/or nonpharmacologic therapies aimed at maintenance of function and improved quality of life.
5. An interdisciplinary approach that utilizes multiple modalities spanning medical, nursing, psychologic, and other disciplines is most desirable for addressing the complex and often coexisting types of cancer pain.

BIBLIOGRAPHY

1. Fisch MJ, Burton AW, eds. *Cancer Pain Management.* New York: McGraw-Hill, Medical Pub. Division; 2007.
2. Foley KM. How well is cancer pain treated? *Palliat Med.* 2011;25(5):398-401.
3. Mercadante S, Portenoy RK. Breakthrough cancer pain: twenty-five years of study. *Pain.* 2016;157(12):2657-2663.
4. Pergolizzi JV, Gharibo C, Ho KY. Treatment considerations for cancer pain: a global perspective. 2014 World Institute of Pain. *Pain Pract.* 2015;15(8):778-792.
5. Portenoy RK, Lesage P. Management of cancer pain. *Pain.* 1999;353:1695-1700.
6. Smith TJ, Saiki CB. Cancer pain management. *Mayo Clin Proc.* 2015;90(10):1428-1439.

PAIN ASSOCIATED WITH RHEUMATOID ARTHRITIS AND OSTEOARTHRITIS

Andrew Dubin

This chapter will focus on aspects of rheumatoid as well as osteoarthritis (OA). Given the complexity of each disorder, they will be addressed as separate sections within the chapter.

Rheumatoid arthritis (RA) is a common chronic inflammatory disease. While many of its manifestations present as musculoskeletal in nature, the involvement of extraarticular structures and organs should make one view it as more of a syndrome.

The incidence of RA is 0.5% to 1%. It is more common in northern climes and in urban versus rural areas. A positive family history for RA increases the risk by approximately three- to fourfold, with seropositive RA patients demonstrating a 40% to 60% hereditability rate, as opposed to 20% for seronegative patients.

While classically RA is thought to be an autoimmune antibody mediated disorder, the presence of auto antibodies (seropositive) is more accurately a marker for more severe symptoms such as joint damage, extraarticular manifestations, and increased mortality.

The focus of this manuscript will be on the articular manifestations of RA and the associated pain and dysfunction.

Joint swelling is a hallmark finding in patients with RA and can be followed as a marker for disease response to interventions. The etiology of the joint swelling in RA patients is as a result of synovial membrane inflammation mediated by immune activation. This active synovitis ultimately leads to a dramatic tissue response with synovial fibroblast proliferation, resulting in inflammation and invasion. This in turn leads to increased chondrocyte catabolism and synovial osteoclastic activity resulting in articular surface destruction.

Complicating the management of RA patients is that no true diagnostic criteria exist for RA. While the typical RA patient will commonly complain of morning joint stiffness, in addition to multiple tender and swollen small joints, these are nonspecific findings. A clue in the history that may be helpful is asking the patient how long the morning stiffness lasts. In patients with RA as well as other inflammatory arthropathies, the stiffness will tend to last for greater than 30 minutes, as opposed to the patient with OA where the stiffness will typically last less than 30 minutes and not uncommonly no more than 15 minutes. Laboratory studies can be helpful as well, but again increased erythrocyte sedimentation rate (ESR) and/or C reactive protein are nonspecific and can be seen in other inflammatory arthropathies, including reactive arthritis, OA, psoriatic arthritis, as well as infectious etiologies. In addition, rarer connective tissues disorders need to be included in the differential if there are other historical, physical, or serologic markers present. Findings of Raynaud's, mouth ulcers, historical complaints consistent with Sicca syndrome, elevated ANA and elevated muscle enzymes (CPK, LDH, Aldolase) can be seen in patients with connective tissue disorders. Given the diagnostic conundrum facing the clinician when working up a patient for possible RA, newer diagnostic criteria have been established. New criteria from the American College of Rheumatology now incorporate aspects of chronicity and poor prognosis. The new criteria now include the finding of a single clinically swollen joint as entry criteria, where no other diseases would explain the joint swelling. Additional factors include serological markers such as rheumatoid factor (RF), long symptom duration, and other lab markers of systemic inflammation. The major change has been the addition of there just needing to be one clinically swollen joint. This has increased the sensitivity of detecting RA by 21% compared with the older criteria. However, the specificity has decreased by 16%.

While this may seem more like an academic exercise, understanding the diagnostic criteria to raise the index of suspicion for the diagnosis of RA is critical. Early detection and treatment offers the best chance for modifying the disease and preventing a downstream cascade of events, resulting in joint destruction, extraarticular organ involvement, and chronic pain.

The underlying unifying pathophysiologic event in RA is inflammation. Understanding the role that inflammation plays in the disease is critical. It drives joint destruction, clinical symptoms such as pain, morning stiffness, and so on, and in the end in part determines disability and potential comorbidities.

In many instances pain is the major complaint that the RA patient has. Many older RA patients, before the development of potent disease-modifying antirheumatic drugs (DMARDs), had significant joint damage and yet were highly functional despite this. In many instances the lack of pain allowed them to be active and productive, despite polyarticular joint involvement. This underscores the need to manage the RA patient with pain. Nonsteroidal antiinflammatory drugs (NSAIDs) are interesting drugs. While their name implies they are antiinflammatory drugs, they do not modify the progression of joint damage and as such cannot be considered DMARDs. However, they have a role in the management of the RA patient as they do improve pain, decrease complaints of joint stiffness, and overall are associated with an improvement in function. Glucocorticoids have a long history in the management of RA. They are extremely potent modifiers of the disease with a rapid onset of action; however, their well-documented long-term serious adverse side effect profile markedly limits their role in management of RA.

While the in depth discussion of DMARDs is beyond the scope of this chapter, an appreciation of the broad classes is needed and an appreciation for some of the potential side effects is appropriate.

One major category of DMARDs is the family of conventional synthetic DMARDs. These would include such agents as methotrexate, sulfasalazine, leflunomide, and hydroxychloroquine. All of these agents have been around for years and have a documented track record of utility; however, all come with side effects.

Methotrexate (MTX) can cause folate deficiencies and as such requires supplemental folate dosing. As a folate antagonist, MTX is associated with side effects (e.g., stomatitis, gastrointestinal (GI) toxicity, and anemia) that are a consequence and mimic the clinical scenario of primary folate deficiency. The anemias can be associated with fatigue, lack of energy, and decreased tolerance for activity, all of which can impact on quality of life. The issue of stomatitis can be functionally significant, as it can impair speech, eating, and in severe enough cases even impact on sleep secondary to pain.

Sulfasalazine is generally well tolerated but is not uncommonly associated with increased skin sensitivity to sunlight. It can also be associated with bone marrow toxicity, and as such can be associated with anemias and increased risk for infection.

Leflunomide is an immunomodulatory drug. While its exact mechanism of activity is not fully known, it appears that it may exert its effect by inhibiting the mitochondrial enzyme dihydroorotate dehydrogenase (DHODH). The inhibition of human DHODH by A77 1726, the active metabolite of leflunomide, prevents the expansion of activated and autoimmune lymphocytes by interfering with the cell cycle. The most common drug-related adverse events associated with leflunomide in clinical trials were diarrhea, abnormalities in liver enzymes, rash, and hypertension. The side effect of hypertension needs to be considered when other medications are utilized for management of painful RA flares. NSAIDs can be very helpful in the management of the RA patient's pain but may potentiate the issue of hypertension, particularly in a patient with baseline essential hypertension. This issue can be further complicated in the patient with underlying chronic kidney disease (CKD) secondary to long-term NSAID use.

Hydroxychloroquine is an old antimalarial medication. It has efficacy in treating mild arthritis or as part of combination therapy. Its most worrisome side effects relate to ocular issues. It can be associated with visual blurring with loss of accommodation. This is usually dose related and reversible. Corneal changes are typically reversible with drug cessation; the retinal issues can be more severe and are not as predictably reversible.

The next class of medications that physicians treating patients with RA and their associated pain issues need to be familiar with are the broad category of biological DMARDs. This would include the subclasses of tumor necrosis factor (TNF) inhibitors, anti–B-cell, anti–T-cell, and anti–IL-6R medications. While the subclass of anti-TNF agents generally has a good side effect profile, there have been reports of the development of a distal acquired demyelinating symmetric neuropathy or distal acquired demyelinating symmetric (DADS) neuropathy in patients treated with adalimumab. The immunogenicity of the various anti-TNF agents is not fully understood, but various theories have been postulated, including either the induction of or unmasking of demyelination as a class effect of anti-TNF inhibiting agents. As such, physicians need to be aware that patients complaining of new onset distal sensory symptoms with or without significant distal motor findings may be having side effects of their medication, and discontinuation needs to be contemplated.

Common reactions to anti–B-cell medications can include muscle spasms, myalgia, and arthralgia. Clearly this needs to be appreciated when treating an RA patient who notes these symptoms, as this may be due to the disease but may also be a side effect of the treatment. Once again, the issue of hypertension and NSAID use becomes a potential issue, as anti–B-cell therapy medications can independently be associated with hypertension and can be exacerbated with NSAID use.

Common reactions to anti–T-cell medications include hypertension as well as back pain. Clearly the issue of back pain as well as extremity pain can complicate the pain management of the RA patient on this class of medications.

Anti–IL-6R medications can cause hypertension as well as headaches as common reactions and side effects.

The class of targeted synthetic DMARDs can be associated with common reactions, including headache as well as an increase in serum creatinine. The increase in serum creatinine is potentially an issue when and if NSAIDs are being used either concomitantly or as an adjuvant rescue medication in the case of flares.

Physical therapy can be very useful in aiding in the management of the patient with RA. Many patients are reluctant to exercise out of fear of injuring themselves. PT allows the patient to start a program of conditioning, including aerobic as well as light strength training in a structured supervised environment. Over time the supervision is decreased; activity levels are increased with the ultimate goal of the patient being able to safety and successfully continue in an unsupervised setting such as a home exercise program or through utilization of equipment at a gym. Patients with RA need to be educated about the importance of maintaining aerobic fitness as well as muscular strength. They also need to understand how certain activities of daily living may in fact increase their symptoms by increasing deforming forces across joints. As such, a close collaboration between physical therapy (PT) and occupational therapy (OT) can be very helpful for this group of patients.

Many times the pain associated with RA can be a direct result of underlying joint damage or joint deformity. In these instances the use of appropriate bracing or orthotic devices can be very helpful. Before one contemplates bracing or other intervention, sometimes something as simple as the use of elevated seating surfaces can facilitate mobility, independence, and safety. The use of canes can also be very helpful to help improve patients' sense of balance and stability. However, the cane should have a built up handle to decrease stress on the wrist and hand, and should also be a J style cane, as opposed to the more commonly seen hook cane. The J cane will allow for more in line force transmission for weight bearing and actually allow for improved weight-bearing mechanics through the cane. Crutches can also be useful for painful lower extremity issues, but care needs to be taken to make sure they have built up well-padded handgrips, to avoid exacerbating painful hand and wrist joints. Caution and close observation is needed in patients who are frequent utilizers of canes and/or crutches, as both of these devices can increase the risk for development of carpal tunnel syndrome by increasing loading through the wrist joint.

Painful feet can be due to structural issues such as progressive flat foot deformity, secondary to damage to surrounding ligamentous structures during disease activity. In an acute flare, a period of rest and off-loading of the foot with utilization of ice as a local antiinflammatory agent may be quite helpful. Once the acute flare has been resolved, the addition of a custom shoe insert to support the medial longitudinal arch and reconstitute the arch if the deformity is still flexible can prove very efficacious. A point to remember is that when adding an insert to the shoe, one must recognize that there is the potential for the foot to now be crowded within the shoe, placing the patient at risk for further pain and possibly skin breakdown. As such, in these cases one should make sure the patient also secures a pair of shoes that are extra depth and have a wide toe box. This will ensure adequate room for the foot and the show insert. Over time a flexible flat foot deformity may progress to a rigid fixed deformity with varying degrees of a rocker bottom deformity noted. In this case, trying to reconstitute the arch not only is going to result in more pain but also is actually contraindicated. Attempting to force the rigid foot into a new position will only result in further orthopedic issues and expose the foot to the high risk of skin breakdown, as forces will be focalized over very discrete points—namely, the apex of the rocker bottom deformity. Treatment for this issue revolves around understanding the biomechanics of the deformity and appreciating that this is no longer a reducible or correctable deformity. Once the rigid nature of the deformity has been confirmed on physical exam of the foot, the development of a fully accommodating orthotic to support and stabilize the foot becomes obvious. These inserts need to be snug fitting to stabilize the deformity and supply support of the structures, and also need to be well padded to off-load areas of potential high pressure.

Ankle pain with or without deformity can also be commonly seen in patients with RA. The pain can be very debilitating and profoundly impact on the patient's quality of life. For the patient with ankle joint pain without deformity, the use of a lace-up ankle gauntlet with or without the removable lateral stays may be very helpful. The device will allow for support without dramatically limiting range of motion in ankle plantar and dorsiflexion. The addition of the lateral stays will further augment the support and increase medial/lateral stability without impacting on plantar/dorsiflexion motion. In addition, the lace-up feature of the ankle gauntlet will allow for adjustability if the patient experiences any issues with edema or joint swelling. With disease progression, one can experience issues of ankle pain with associated deformity. These can present challenges, but the thoughtful use of an orthotic device can be very helpful. Ankle foot orthoses (AFO) can be very helpful. These are custom-designed and custom-fitted devices typically fabricated out of plastic. They can have a rigid fixed ankle angle or have a joint to allow for varying degrees of ankle plantar and dorsiflexion. These devices can be custom fabricated to accommodate a fixed ankle deformity and supply support to the ankle. Depending on their design features, either they can be fully accommodating of a deformity, or if there is some degree of flexibility to the deformity, they can partially correct the deformity and then stabilize and support the residual fixed deformity. An additional feature that can be incorporated into the design of the AFO is a patellar tendon bearing (PTB) bar and cuff. This allows one to move weight-bearing forces proximally and unload the painful ankle if need be. The degree of unloading can be very minimal, all the way up to 100% of loading of the ankle if the PTB is designed and manufactured to mimic the bearing characteristics of the PTB used in a below-knee amputation prosthesis. This type of AFO, namely a PTB bypass AFO, can allow the patient to walk while resting and unloading an inflamed active ankle joint.

Knee pain and deformity can also be a challenge. The typical deformities seen at the knees are a valgus deformity or knock-kneed posture. This relates to the primary pathophysiology of RA. Remember that in RA the inciting event is an overactive hyperemic synovium. This leads to secondary ligamentous damage and subsequent deformity of the joint through a combination of joint mechanics, joint loading during activity, and late bony involvement. The normal position of the knee is a mild degree of valgus. The involvement of ligamentous structures, the major stabilizers to prevent excessive valgus (namely the medial collateral ligament), is compromised. As a result, the normal weight-bearing alignment of the joint now drives the knee into further valgus, creating and worsening the deformity over time. Knee orthoses can be used but may be of limited utility. One of their limitations relates to basic body habitus. A typical complaint patients have when using a knee orthosis is that the device has a tendency to slide down such that it is no longer appropriately situated. This renders the device less useful and can also result in pain secondary to incongruity of the orthosis and the patient knee anatomy. In early easily reducible cases of valgus posturing of the knee, the custom molded plastic AFO with a well-developed medial buttress along the tibial shank can work quite well. The force application of the medial buttress will counter the valgus posture of the knee by keeping the tibia more vertically aligned. This device will not slide about, as it is fixed in place and anchored into the shoe through the foot plate that slides into the patient's set of extra depth shoes. A fixed deformity and or a marked degree of knee joint instability is best managed with a knee ankle foot orthosis (KAFO). These devices are custom-made and can be designed with knee joints that limit degrees of flexion. They can also supply stability during weight bearing in patients with a knee flexion contracture. Knee joints can be designed to lock upon weight bearing and unlock during swing phase. Depending upon the design characteristics, these devices can allow for full weight bearing through the knee and ankle or can unload the knee, ankle, or both joints, with weight now being transferred to the thigh through the thigh cuff, as well as to the patella tendon via a PTB. As one can see, the design options for KAFOs are quite broad and do require close partnership among the brace maker, patient, and ordering physician.

Upper extremity involvement with RA can significantly impact on quality of life. Painful hands and metacarpal phalangeal (MCP) joints can limit one's ability to comfortably perform activities of daily living (ADLs).

Simple interventions such as the use of electric can openers in place of mechanical can openers can be very helpful. Built-up handles can make grasping pots and pans less problematic. Replacing round door knobs with door knob handles can ease opening and closing doors. Sometimes just adding a rubberized door knob cover over a round door knob to improve grip can be very helpful. Conversion of laced shoes to Velcro closure can make donning and doffing footwear much less problematic. Various orthoses can be prescribed and fabricated for the RA patient with upper extremity involvement, but many of these are poorly tolerated, as they tend to get in the way of performance of ADLs, and as such long term are rejected by the patient. That being said, there are various devices that do not dramatically impact on the patient from a cosmetic standpoint or impede their ability to perform functional tasks, and as such have a fairly high degree of acceptance. Lumbrical splints, which help maintain the MCP joint arch, are well tolerated, do improve function, and as such do have utility. Spring loaded finger splints to treat issues of extensor lag can also be helpful and are well tolerated. Thumb Spica splints can be very useful for the patient with a painful unstable thumb. A wrist gauntlet can supply a degree of support to allow for improved ADLs. Reachers can also be helpful to facilitate light ADLs, such as reaching for light items up on a shelf or picking up light items from a floor. In general, patients will tolerate upper extremity orthoses so long as they are not overly restrictive and do not negatively impact on performance of ADLs. The conundrum is that sometimes the performance of the ADLs hastens the development of the deformity. As such, in managing patients with RA, patient education is paramount. Getting the patient to understand why a particular device may be helpful is critical to increase patient compliance.

Osteoarthritis (OA) has been classically thought of as wear and tear arthritis. Newer information does indicate that inflammation may also play a role in the pathogenesis of OA. Unlike RA, where the initial pathology is at the level of the synovium, in OA the primary pathology is at the level of the articular cartilage. As a disorder, OA will progress over time to encompass all aspects of the joint. Ultimately cartilage, synovium, as well as bone are all involved in the progression of OA and the debility that can be associated with it. Understanding the pathogenesis of OA is essential when considering the various options potentially available to treat the symptoms.

Realizing that the pathology in OA is at the level of the cartilage, an understanding of the primary function of the articular cartilage needs to be appreciated. The major function of cartilage is to allow for the smooth movement of many joints in the body. Cartilage is a highly dynamic structure, and its maintenance is dependent upon the balance of cartilage matrix turnover. Anything that throws the balance between synthesis and normal degradation into disequilibrium ultimately leads to deterioration in cartilage. Multiple factors can lead to alterations in this normal balance. Mechanical trauma to the joint, progressive joint instability, as well as production of inflammatory cytokines can all trigger the development of OA. A consistent feature of osteoarthritic joints is the development of osteophytes, which represent new development of both cartilage and bone. While the exact function of osteophyte formation is unclear, it may serve to stabilize the joint, as it is seen in non-weight-bearing joints, and may also be an attempt to increase the weight-bearing surface of load-bearing joints such as the hip and knee to help disperse the load over a broader surface area.

The management of OA typically depends upon the stage of the disease. In early OA the use of exercise and weight control are of paramount importance. Exercise should be encouraged and is typically well tolerated. Patients may be reticent to engage in a walking program if they have early knee OA; however, the data do indicate that the aerobic conditioning obtained through walking is of great benefit. Failure to participate in regular routine aerobic activity is actually associated with greater debility. Aerobic activity helps control issues of weight gain, and helps maintain muscle mass and decrease both joint and soft tissue stiffness. Taken as a whole, aerobic activity also helps decrease risk for fall and associated orthpedic trauma. As such, the benefits clearly outweigh the risks. In addition, research indicates that lack of regular routine exercise may be associated with accelerated cartilage degradation by altering the dynamics of the cartilage matrix. The importance of controlling pain from soft tissue stiffness cannot be overemphasized, as this becomes a predictable problem in the population of patients with lower extremity joint OA who assume a sedentary lifestyle. This group of patients not uncommonly find themselves faced with the conundrum of worsening pain as their activity level declines, and not realizing that the way out of the cycle of pain and immobility is to in fact increase their activity level, not restrict it further. In general, in early OA walking, cycling and even light jogging are typically well tolerated. Patients may express concern about walking and light jogging. It should be noted that biomechanical studies consistently reveal that the compressive and tensile loads that the articular cartilage is exposed to are well below the threshold for cartilage damage. Cycling is an excellent form of exercise, and is well tolerated even at high intensity. Given its high degree of tolerance, it may have particular utility for aerobic conditioning and weight control above and beyond that of walking or jogging. Swimming has been touted as an excellent form of exercise for OA patients, but in general the aerobic benefits are limited by the patient's expertise as a swimmer. In addition, since it is not associated with weight bearing, it will not help maintain bone mass, which is critical in the older OA patient. Swimming is probably best thought of as a bridge activity between water-based exercises and ultimately land-based activities. An additional possible drawback to swimming is availability of swimming facilities, local climate, and the potential increased risk of slipping and falling on a slick wet poolside surface.

Strength training has reliably been shown to decrease pain scores and increase function in multiple studies of patients with knee OA. Individualization of the strengthening program cannot be overemphasized. A common mistake is telling the patient to just go out and exercise, only to have the patient return with more knee pain. While quadriceps strengthening is clearly important, as most patients with knee OA have some element of quadriceps weakness, the knee jerk reaction of placing the patient with knee OA on a regimen of quadriceps strengthening needs to be avoided in patients with structural malalignment issues. This group of patients not uncommonly will note that quadriceps strengthening increases the compressive forces across the knee joint and increases pain. In this group, avoidance of open chain kinetic quadriceps strengthening is key, and alternative modes of quadriceps strengthening should be explored. Referral to a physical therapist well versed in closed kinetic chain lower extremity strengthening exercises can be very rewarding to the patient. In addition, in this population, hamstring as well as hip abductor and lower leg muscle strengthening may actually be of more benefit than quadriceps strengthening.

Balance training in patients with OA has also been associated with improvements in balance and proprioception. Whether this is due to increases in strength that occur with balance training type activities or is as a direct result of the focused balance training is unclear, but the correlation has been clearly noted and is reproducible. Improvements in balance decrease the risk to fall, which decreases the risk for orthopedic trauma. In addition, improved balance may also increase a patient's sense of well-being, as well as improve their ability to manage their activities of daily living and navigate their community. All of these benefits result in increased independence and a decrease in caregiver burden.

Obesity has a great impact on joint OA development. This, along with a history of prior joint trauma, constitutes major risk factors for the development of OA, particularly in weight-bearing joints. Maintenance of appropriate body weight may be one of the most significant interventions that can be taken to decrease the risk for development of OA in weight-bearing joints. As rates of childhood obesity rise, this point needs to be emphasized. Early control of weight and optimization of body weight is of paramount importance in impacting on a modifiable risk for the development of OA in weight-bearing joints. Even in obese patients, a relationship between reduction in weight and reducing the risk for developing OA in weight-bearing joints has been demonstrated. Aerobic conditioning should be an integral component of a weight reduction program. Initially activities such as cycling may be the preferred form of aerobic exercise by patients with obesity and OA of the hips and or knees, as it is well tolerated. As weight loss progresses, walking as an additional form of exercise may be more easily tolerated and can also be incorporated into the regimen, as can balance training activities.

Physical therapy can be very useful in aiding in the management of the patient with OA. Many patients are reluctant to exercise out of fear of injuring themselves. PT allows the patient to start a program of conditioning, including aerobic as well as strength training activities in a structured supervised environment. Over time, the supervision is decreased and activity levels are increased, with the ultimate goal of the patient being able to safely and successfully continue in an unsupervised setting such as a home exercise program or through utilization of equipment at a gym.

As with RA, simple adaptive equipment can have significant positive impacts. Reachers to ease reaching overhead can be very helpful for the patient with OA of the shoulder. Elevated seat heights can ease getting into and out of chairs.

For patients with issues of OA involving the foot, fabrication of supportive shoe inserts to spread load over a larger surface area may dramatically reduce pain and increase walking tolerance. Ankle braces from simple lace-up style ankle gauntlets all the way to formal AFOs can be utilized in patients with OA of the ankle and subtalar joint. The degree of bracing will typically depend upon the extent of joint involvement and the degree of motion control that is needed.

Knee OA can be a particularly frustrating issue for the patient. The typical deformity in knee OA is one of a varus knee deformity or bowlegged deformity. This is a result of early wearing and ultimate loss of the media joint space. Patients will note pain with weight bearing and with walking. Various options are available to manage this deformity and the associated pain. A lateral shoe wedge affixed to the sole of the foot applies a counterforce to the knee, taking it out of its varus posture to a more neutral to slightly valgus posture. This reduces the stress on the stretched lateral collateral knee ligament and partially unloads the painful medial joint space. The lateral wedge can be augmented with the addition of a lateral flare to further counter the varus moment at the knee. This combined effect has been shown to result in decreased knee pain. A medial unloader brace, which is a more aggressive form of intervention to unload the medial knee joint, can be of utility in more advanced cases of knee OA. Medial unloading or varus correction braces may not be well tolerated, as significant force is placed through the knee and patients may find the brace straps uncomfortable and restrictive. The use of a lateral wedge with or without lateral flare is a good first line intervention and is generally well tolerated and accepted. When compared with medial unloader braces, walking tolerance in the appropriate patient population is more variable and less pronounced in patients using lateral wedges as opposed to medial unloader braces, but compliance is better for lateral wedges. In cases of more severe knee OA where multiplanar instability becomes an issue, a knee ankle foot orthosis with a hinged knee joint and straps to further augment the stabilizing characteristics of the brace may be helpful. These types of braces are not typically tolerated in the more active patient, owing to the marked mechanical restrictions they impose. The aesthetics of KAFOs also limits their use, as does their inability to be worn under garments. KAFOs may also make transitioning into and out of a car or seat more problematic.

In both RA and OA, other sources of pain need to be appreciated and explored. Simply assuming that the patient's pain complaints are directly a result of their underlying RA or OA prevents the physician from many times addressing easily managed yet debilitating issues. Nonarticular pain generators can arise from bursa, tendons, as well as muscle and their associated fascial attachments. Bursitis, tendinopathies, and myofascial (muscular) pain syndromes are common sources of pain in patients with underlying RA as well as OA.

The normal function of a bursa is to serve as an interface between muscle and the underlying bone. When viewed by ultrasound, bursas are typically no more than a potential space, many times barely visible. In normal function, they serve to allow for the smooth movement of muscle over areas of bony prominence. Bursitis, an inflammation of bursa, can result from overuse, inflammation, or infection. Patients with RA have an increased incidence of inflammatory mediated bursitis, particularly during episodic flares of their disease. The end result, regardless of the etiology, is swelling of the bursa. This results in alteration of the bursa's normal function, causing pain with activity. The pain leads to decreased activity, which can result in joint stiffness as well as soft tissue stiffness, further causing debility and increasing immobility. As one can see, something as simple as a bursitis can have far-reaching effects upon patient quality of life. As such, promptly identifying and treating the bursitis is imperative to maintaining the activity level of the patient with RA or OA. The first line of treatment of noninfectious bursitis typically uses antiinflammatory modalities. Ice can be very helpful for managing the pain and inflammation of bursitis. Topical NSAIDs can potentially be effective in the management of bursitis for more superficially located bursas, such as the subdeltoid bursa or olecranon, as opposed to a more deeply situated bursa like the trochanteric bursa. Topical NSAIDs also decrease the risk for renal and GI toxicity, which need to be considered in patients on DMARDs to treat their RA, as well as in the typically older OA patient population. Medial and lateral epicondylitis may also respond to both ice and topical NSAIDs. A short course of oral antiinflammatory agents may be helpful, but as noted previously, caution should be exercised, given the side effect profile of oral NSAIDs.

Trochanteric bursitis is typically considered to be the etiology of almost all lateral thigh pain. However, it in fact is not a common source of lateral hip pain. More common causes are tendinopathies involving the gluteus medius, minimus, or tensa fascia lata (TFL) and the iliotibial band (ITB). All of these are common sources of lateral hip pain. In these scenarios patients will note lateral hip pain, worsened with walking and side lying. They may also complain of referral pain that radiates to the level of the knee, especially with ITB syndrome. In addition to these considerations, other possible differentials, including hip OA, referred pain from the lumbar spine, sacro iliac (SI) joint referral pain, and a chronic L5 level radiculopathy, exist and need to be considered. While an injection of corticosteroid with a local anesthetic at the level of the trochanteric bursa can be helpful in ruling out a true trochanteric bursitis, it is of limited utility, as a negative response does not really help one eliminate many of the more common causes of lateral hip pain. In addition, frequent injections should be avoided to decrease the risk of rupture of the gluteus medius tendon, which can result in profound debility and dysfunction. The key to establishing the correct diagnosis lies in the performance of a complete neuromusculoskeletal exam.

Physical therapy can be helpful in the management of bursitis and epicondylitis. Range of motion exercises should be encouraged to avoid issues of joint and associated soft tissue stiffness. Modalities such as ultrasound can be helpful as a source of deep heating to increase soft tissue elasticity and compliance aiding in range of motion activities. In addition, the heat may afford some degree of pain modulation, though in true inflammatory processes heating would be relatively contraindicated and ice would be the modality of choice. Steroid phonophoresis or iontophoresis can be used as a way to drive topical steroids to the site of inflammation. This allows for more focal application of antiinflammatory medication, typically corticosteroids, limiting the potential for systemic side effects. Chronic tendinopathies can be managed with moist heat and stretching exercises, with progression to strengthening exercises with the ultimate inclusion of eccentric loading type exercises to strengthen the myotendinous junction. A supervised exercise program under the guidance of a physical therapist can be extremely beneficial for this patient population.

Myofascial pain or localized muscular derived pain syndromes are an underappreciated source of pain. Not uncommonly they are seen in patients with underlying OA or rheumatologic disorders. Many times patients are frustrated by the time they arrive at the doorstep of a physician with interest in musculoskeletal medicine. The etiology of myofascial pain syndrome, a chronic soft tissue muscle pain syndrome, has yet to be fully elucidated. The hallmark feature, a myofascial trigger point, is theorized to be an area of sensitized nociceptors within muscle. Myofascial pain syndrome can develop after acute trauma or after exposure to long-term repetitive activities. The major question regarding myofascial trigger point or myofascial pain is why the majority of patients who perform repetitive activities or who have sustained musculoskeletal trauma do not develop myofascial trigger points. What factors predispose the approximate 10% of individuals who are involved in trauma such as motor vehicle accidents (MVAs) to progress into chronic muscle pain? Various electrophysiologic studies seem to indicate that an abnormal increase in acetylcholine contributes to endplate hyperexcitability, which causes localized areas of increased muscle tension—hence the taut band. This increase in local muscle tension is theorized to increase the local metabolic demands on the muscle, creating a relative ischemic state, which may well explain patients' complaints of deep aching cramping type pain in the involved musculature. The relative ischemic state of the muscle is theorized to result in an increased release of nociceptive neuropeptides, setting the stage for the development of trigger points and subsequent myofascial pain syndrome.

Various conditions can be associated with myofascial pain syndrome or may exacerbate the condition. Poor sleep, stress, or superimposed painful conditions such as radiculopathy, neuropathy, RA, or OA may exacerbate the problem. As such, attention should focus on trying to elucidate the underlying drivers and associated issues that may be exacerbating the myofascial pain syndrome. Sleep apnea with frequent awakening and poor sleep is a common contributor in the older age overweight population.

Once the diagnosis and underlying contributors to the myofascial pain syndrome have been identified, the first-line interventions typically include a combination of stretching of the involved muscles with the application of ice or heat—whichever is better tolerated. Long-term use of modalities should be avoided to prevent patients from becoming dependent upon physical therapy to manage their pain complaints. Myofascial pain is a chronic pain syndrome; as such the focus needs to be on developing management strategies that the patient can do on their own. Progression to a global conditioning program emphasizing aerobic conditioning and light strength training is key in the management of chronic muscle pain complaints. Strengthening of postural muscles may be helpful as well. Relaxation techniques can be used as adjunct therapy in the management of myofascial pain. Acupuncture and massage can be helpful for managing the trigger points, as the application of strong pressure over the trigger point may cause hyper stimulation analgesia. The same theory applies to the rationale for trigger point injections with local anesthetic or dry needling. In more refractory patients, the broad class of neuromodulators may be helpful.

Medication choices should take into account the potential for myofascial pain to progress to chronic pain. As such, medications with a low risk for renal, GI, or hepatotoxicity are preferred. Medications with abuse potential should be avoided.

KEY POINTS

1. The presence of auto antibodies in RA is a marker of disease severity.
2. There are no true diagnostic criteria for RA.
3. A combination of aerobic conditioning and light strength training can be helpful in the management of RA patients and their associated pain.
4. The pathogenesis of OA is a combination of wear and tear and inflammation.
5. The primary pathology of OA is at the level of the articular cartilage.
6. The primary initial pathology of RA is at the level of the synovium.

BIBLIOGRAPHY

1. Flodin P, Martinsen S, Altawil R, et al. Intrinsic brain connectivity in chronic pain: a resting-state fMRI study in patients with rheumatoid arthritis. *Front Hum Neurosci.* 2016;10:107.
2. Smolen JS, Aletaha D, McInnes IB. Rheumatoid arthritis. *Lancet.* 2016;388(10055):2023-2038.
3. Aletaha D, Neogi T, Silman A, et al. Rheumatoid arthritis classification criteria: an American College of Rheumatology/European League against rheumatism collaborative initiative. *Ann Rheum Dis.* 2010;69:1580-1588.
4. Callahan LF, Pincus T. Education, self-care and outcomes of rheumatics: further challenges to the "biomedical model" paradigm. *Arthritis Care Res.* 1997;10:283-288.
5. McInnes IB, Schett G. The pathogenesis of rheumatoid arthritis. *N Engl J Med.* 2011;365:2205-2219.
6. Gonzalez A, Icen M, Kremers HM, et al. Mortality trends in rheumatoid arthritis: the role of rheumatoid factor. *J Rheumatol.* 2008;35:1009-1014.
7. Mavers M, Ruderman EM, Perlman H. Intracellular signal pathways: potential for therapies. *Curr Rheumatol Rep.* 2009;11:378-385.

8. Choi HK, Hernan MA, Seeger JD, Robins JM, Wolfe F. Methotrexate and mortality in patients with rheumatoid arthritis: a prospective study. *Lancet*. 2002;359:1173-1177.

9. Smolen JS, Breedveld FC, Schiff MH, et al. A simplified disease activity index for rheumatoid arthritis for use in clinical practice. *Rheumatology*. 2003;42:244-257.

10. Smolen JS, Aletaha D, Keystone E. Superior efficacy of combination therapy for rheumatoid arthritis: fact or fiction? *Arthritis Rheum*. 2005;52:2975-2983.

11. Filardo G, Kon E, Longo UG, et al. Non-surgical treatments for the management of early osteoarthritis. *Knee Surg Sports Traumatol Arthrosc*. 2016;24:1775-1785.

12. Bennell KL, Buchbinder R, Hinman RS. Physical therapies in the management of osteoarthritis: current state of the evidence. *Curr Opin Rheumatol*. 2015;27(3):304-311.

13. Hunter DJ. Viscosupplementation for osteoarthritis of the knee. *N Engl J Med*. 2015;372(11):1040-1047.

14. Mushtaq S, Choudhary R, Scanzello CR. Non-surgical treatment of osteoarthritis-related pain in the elderly. *Curr Rev Musculoskelet Med*. 2011;4(3):113-122.

15. Fransen M, McConnell S, Harmer AR, et al. Exercise for osteoarthritis of the knee. *Cochrane Database Syst Rev*. 2015;(1):CD004376.

16. Filardo G, Kon E, Roffi A, et al. Platelet rich plasma intra-articular knee injections show no superiority versus viscosupplementation: a randomized control trial. *Am J Sports Med*. 2015;43(7):1575-1582.

17. Law TY, Nguyen C, Frank RM, Rosas S, McCormick F. Current concepts on the use of corticosteroid injections for knee osteoarthritis. *Phys Sportsmed*. 2015;43(3):269-273.

CHAPTER 29

NEUROPATHIC PAIN: BACKGROUND

David Walk and Anisha Bhangav

1. **What is neuropathic pain?**

   Pain has been defined as "an unpleasant sensory and emotional experience associated with actual or potential tissue damage, or described in terms of such damage." Neuropathic pain is defined as "pain arising as a direct consequence of a lesion or disease of the somatosensory system." Thus neuropathic pain can be thought of as an unpleasant sensory and emotional experience associated with damage to innervated tissues but due to dysfunction of the peripheral or central nervous system. Descriptors (burning, stabbing) will often indicate tissue damage when in fact there is none.

2. **What are the neuroanatomic pathways involved in pain?**

   Physiologic pain transmission begins with nociceptors, which are peripheral axons whose terminals transduce real or potential tissue injury. Cutaneous nociceptors, for example, are small myelinated or unmyelinated axons equipped with surface receptors that transduce real or potential skin injury into neuronal discharges, thus initiating a cascade of information to the brain regarding the nature, location, and severity of the threat. Cutaneous nociceptors are classified according to their fiber type (A-delta or C) and the type of tissue injury to which they respond; thus, for example, there are A-mechanical heat (AMH), a-mechanical (AM), C-mechanical, heat (CMH), C-mechanical, heat, chemical (CMHC), and so forth.

   Nociceptors are present in numerous tissues, including skin, joints, connective tissue, and viscera, in order to signal a variety of external as well as internal threats to the organism. Afferent information is coded in nociceptive discharges; for example, the intensity of skin heating might be proportional to the firing rate of the axon. Nociceptive somatic primary afferent neurons synapse in the dorsal horn of the spinal cord with secondary afferent neurons that cross the spinal cord and form the corticospinal tract, which courses rostrally and forms synapses with thalamic cells. These in turn project to several cortical regions critical to the experience of pain.

   Recall that pain is "an unpleasant sensory and emotional experience." This definition reflects the nature of pain, which is to alert and motivate the organism to change its condition for the purpose of protection. Cortical projections in the physiology of pain reflect this as well. Projections to primary somatosensory cortex enable localization of pain, projections to limbic areas such as insular cortex and amygdala enable attribution of negative valence (unpleasantness), and projections to premotor frontal cortex enable a response to the inciting noxious stimulus, such as withdrawal and avoidance. Numerous other cortical regions are involved in pain projections as well. Thus the neuroanatomy of pain enables us to attend, localize, and react promptly in response to external threats.

   In addition to these afferent pathways, descending modulation of pain plays a critical role in pain perception. Cells in the periacqueductal gray matter (PAG) and rostroventral medulla (RVM) project to the dorsal horn of the spinal cord, where they modulate the afferent signals from primary nociceptors. This descending modulation influences the intensity of the afferent signal from dorsal horn neurons. Physiologic influences on descending modulation can result in substantial differences in pain perception from identical peripheral nociceptive stimuli.

   Finally, other pathways that interact with or synapse with cells in the primary somatosensory system can influence their response to nociceptive input. These include sympathetic efferents and activated glia, both of which can influence nociceptive traffic via their interactions with cells of the primary nociceptive pathway.

3. What are the postulated mechanisms for pathology in these pathways that lead to neuropathic pain?

Experimental evidence exists for multiple mechanisms of neuropathic pain, and different mechanisms may be relevant in different neuropathic pain conditions. These mechanisms can include peripheral sensitization, central sensitization, deafferentation pain, and alterations in descending pain modulation.

- Peripheral nerve disease may result in spontaneous discharges and, as a result, paresthesias or sharp, shooting pains, via several mechanisms. For example, reduced metabolic capacity may result in difficulty maintaining the sodium-potassium pump, leading to spontaneous depolarization. Injured axons can also develop a pacemaker capability, also resulting in spontaneous depolarizations in the absence of external stimuli. Frequent peripheral stimulation or depolarization can result in phosphorylation of peripheral receptors, increasing their sensitivity, increased receptor translation and hence receptor density, increased sensitivity to catecholamines, and activation of "silent nociceptors" that are only active in pathological states.
- Increased firing of primary afferent neurons may result in sensitization of dorsal horn neurons via several mechanisms. These include removal of magnesium-mediated blockade of *N*-methyl-D-aspartate (NMDA) receptors, increased calcium and sodium channel expression, and phenotypic switch, a postulated mechanism in which dorsal horn neurons develop de novo ability to respond to nociceptive input. There is also evidence that glial activation in the spinal cord can sensitize dorsal horn neurons. As a result of these plastic changes in afferent neurons, a given stimulus, such as skin warming to a non-noxious degree, can result in an inappropriately high firing frequency, which will in turn be interpreted as indicating the presence of a noxious stimulus.
- Deafferentation pain is a postulated mechanism of neuropathic pain in the setting of loss of afferent input to thalamus or cortex. It has been demonstrated that in the absence of afferent input, thalamic neurons can develop spontaneous depolarizations. In addition there is some evidence that deafferentation via amputation may lead to alterations in cortical representation of the limb that is associated with the sensation of phantom limb pain (PLP). Thus there are several potential mechanisms of pain due to loss of afferent input, but it is a well-recognized phenomenon in the setting of thalamic or cortical sensory stroke, spinal cord injury, severe ganglionopathy, or amputation.
- Finally, several experimental paradigms have demonstrated alterations in conditioned pain modulation, or descending modulation of pain, in recognized neuropathic pain states as well as other chronic pain states such as fibromyalgia. The degree to which descending modulatory pathways contribute to neuropathic pain states is not well understood, but there is good evidence that pharmacologic manipulation of this pathway (principally norepinephrine reuptake inhibition) can alleviate neuropathic pain.

4. What are the most common neuropathic pain conditions?

The most common peripheral neuropathic pain conditions are distal symmetric painful polyneuropathy, postherpetic neuralgia (PHN), posttraumatic neuralgia (PTN), and trigeminal neuralgia. Neuropathic pain can also follow central nervous system insults, most commonly poststroke pain and spinal cord injury pain; the latter can occur in the context of myelopathy due to trauma, as well as multiple sclerosis (MS) and other inflammatory myelopathies. Finally, complex regional pain syndrome (CRPS) and phantom pain are unique states that arguably have neuropathic components.

Overviews of the most common neuropathic pain states are provided below (see Questions 8 to 24). Their diagnosis and management are described in greater detail in subsequent chapters.

5. What clinical features suggest that a pain is neuropathic?

The following clinical features are most helpful in supporting a suspicion that a given pain state is neuropathic:

- Perhaps most notably, neuropathic pain is usually associated with signs and symptoms of sensory loss, although that sensory loss may be modest or restricted to small fiber (thermal and sharp perception) modalities. A diagnosis of neuropathic pain should be questioned if there are neither signs nor symptoms of sensory loss.
- The presence of spontaneous paresthesias, spontaneous cutaneous burning pain, allodynia, or hyperalgesia strongly supports the conclusion that pain is neuropathic.
- The aforementioned are often referred to as *negative* (sensory loss) and *positive* (spontaneous or stimulus-evoked abnormal sensations) sensory symptoms and signs.

- Neuropathic pain is often worst at night and at rest. Pain that is worst with weight bearing (e.g., foot pain when walking that is relieved with rest) is less likely to be neuropathic, although neuropathic pain at rest may be worse after being on one's feet a great deal than after a sedentary day.
- Most neuropathic pain states present in an anatomic distribution that is consistent with their etiology. Thus, for example, PHN pain should be dermatomal, posttraumatic neuropathy pain should be in the cutaneous territory of the affected nerve, and central poststroke pain should be in a hemibody distribution. A notable exception to this rule is a sensory ganglionopathy, which is non-length-dependent, often asymmetric, and does not necessarily present in a definable dermatomal pattern.

Several discriminative tools have been designed and validated to identify symptoms of neuropathic pain. The presence of paresthesias, sharp, shooting pain, a spontaneous cutaneous burning sensation, allodynia, or hyperalgesia with symptoms of sensory loss correlates with a high likelihood that pain is neuropathic.

6. **How does one examine a person with suspected neuropathic pain?**
The examination of a person in chronic pain should begin with an appropriate general physical examination of the affected area. Thus a musculoskeletal examination (visual inspection and palpation of the joints, range of motion testing, and firm palpation of tendons and fasciae for recognized musculoskeletal conditions, such as extensor tendinitis or plantar fasciitis) is important. Next, examination of the skin and soft tissues for trophic changes, color changes, evidence of vascular insufficiency, and edema is important, especially if CRPS is suspected. It is important not to neglect these fundamental aspects of the general physical examination.

A comprehensive neuromuscular examination, including sensory, motor, and reflex testing, is important if neuropathic pain is suspected. The goal is, in part, as it is in evaluating other neurological problems: Is there evidence of a neurological deficit, and if so, what is the localization?

The sensory examination should explicitly include the following:
- *Large fiber modalities:* Typically light touch and vibration; position sense testing is unlikely to be revealing unless vibration perception is substantially impaired.
- *Small fiber modalities:* Typically perception of pinprick and temperature. Only one of these may be sufficient, and testing of pinprick perception is generally better at identifying the margins of the symptomatic area.

Particular attention should be paid to the presence of sensory disturbances other than sensory loss alone. These can include:
- *Allodynia:* Light stroking of the skin with cotton or a fingertip might demonstrate allodynia (a painful perception in response to a non-noxious stimulus). This is particularly prevalent and severe, for example, in PHN, and can be present in PTNs and painful small fiber neuropathy.
- *Hyperalgesia:* Testing with a pin may evoke excessive pain, and often a person with hyperalgesia will withdraw promptly as one approaches with the pin to guard the region, or will refuse pinprick testing. Sometimes, in distal symmetric painful polyneuropathy, the distal zone of sensory loss abuts a zone of hyperalgesia, which in turn yields to normal sensation as one moves proximally.
- *Other dysesthesias:* At times people with neuropathic pain report other abnormal and unpleasant responses to external stimuli, or a delayed or lingering perception after the stimulus is removed. Because they are inconsistent with expectations of normal physiologic responses, patients themselves sometimes discount such sensations, but they can be indicators of a neuropathic process.
- *Profound sensory loss:* When this occurs in a painful area, consider the possibility of a deafferentation pain. The clinical context should be informative in this regard.

In the case of a possible posttraumatic neuropathy, explore the course of the nerve for the presence of a Tinel's sign.

7. **What confirmatory tests are helpful in confirming the presence of a neuropathic pain condition?**
Pain is a clinical diagnosis, but in the following conditions testing can be useful in confirming the presence of a lesion of the somatosensory system and thus more clearly establish the case for a neuropathic pain diagnosis:
- *Painful distal symmetric polyneuropathy:* While typically a distinct clinical syndrome, in some cases the clinical presentation is less compelling and diagnostic confirmation of the presence of a neuropathy is helpful.

- Nerve conduction studies (NCS) can only demonstrate the presence of a large fiber neuropathy, which, in isolation, is often not painful; however, insofar as both large and small fibers are commonly affected in painful distal symmetric polyneuropathy, NCS are a good initial examination.
- NCS are, essentially by definition, normal in a pure small fiber neuropathy. The most commonly utilized confirmatory test for the presence of pathology in small myelinated and unmyelinated fibers is skin biopsy for epidermal nerve fiber (ENF) density measurement. There is a generally good correlation between a reduction in ENF density and other clinical indicators of neuropathy. Reduction in ENF density, in combination with clinical evidence of either punctate or thermal sensory loss, has been included as a criterion in a proposed "gold standard" for the diagnosis of small fiber neuropathy. A 3-mm punch biopsy is used and several laboratories are available for processing and reporting results.
- Tests of *sudomotor* function are also sometimes used to confirm small fiber neuropathy, as denervation of cutaneous sweat glands is common in small fiber neuropathy. Such tests include quantitative sudomotor axon reflex test (QSART) and thermoregulatory sweat test (TST).
- In patients with diabetes or other conditions in which a mild subclinical neuropathy is common, ENF density or tests of sudomotor function are likely to be abnormal in most patients, and therefore are less useful in demonstrating a cause for pain.

- *Posttraumatic neuropathy and other focal, painful neuropathies:* If there is clinical uncertainty regarding the presence of a nerve lesion, NCS can be useful if they are available for the nerve in question. In many cases, however, there is not an established NCS for the nerve in question. In such cases a skin biopsy for ENF density can be useful. If normal values are not established for the body region of interest, bilateral biopsies can be performed and a substantial side-to-side asymmetry in ENF density can be taken as supportive evidence of a nerve lesion.
- *Central pain states:* In poststroke pain and neuropathic pain from myelopathy or spinal cord injury, imaging has almost always been performed in the acute phase of the injury.

  Quantitative sensory testing (QST) can be a useful adjunct to the neurological examination in postulated neuropathic pain states. QST is used to quantify sensory and pain thresholds to thermal or vibratory stimuli. While the term is usually applied to testing performed with specialized equipment, in its broader sense it can refer to any quantitation of sensory thresholds. QST provides supportive evidence of a somatosensory deficit and can also demonstrate allodynia, hyperalgesia, and hyperpathia, which are all clinical features of neuropathic pain; however, it does not localize the deficit or provide pathologic or neurophysiologic confirmation of a lesion in the somatosensory system.

8. How does distal symmetric painful polyneuropathy present clinically?
   Distal symmetric painful polyneuropathy presents with paresthesias or burning in the feet in a symmetric distribution. Because it is length-dependent, the symptoms usually begin in the toes and progress proximally. Foot pain beginning in the instep, heels, or ankles is less likely to be neuropathic. Symptoms are commonly most severe at rest and in the evening. Although pain is often more severe after an active day, it is not generally precipitated by weight bearing, and pain that immediately develops upon standing or walking and improves promptly with sitting down is most likely to be mechanical foot pain rather than neuropathy pain. As noted previously, sensory loss is usually present, and many patients are aware of this. In almost all cases this is an indolently progressive disorder, with pain and sensory deficits progressing proximally very slowly over a matter of years, and often stabilizing with little detectable worsening within a few years of onset.

9. What are the etiologies of distal symmetric painful polyneuropathy?
   - Diabetes is the most commonly established cause. While it is not clear why pain severity varies among people with diabetic neuropathy, evidence of some genetic factors is emerging.
   - There is also evidence that prediabetes (impaired glucose tolerance or impaired fasting glucose) is prevalent among nondiabetic people with distal symmetric painful polyneuropathy, often in the context of the metabolic syndrome, or a combination of glucose dysmetabolism, hypertension, hyperlipidemia, and obesity. For this reason, a 2-hour oral glucose tolerance test and fasting lipid panel are commonly performed in nondiabetic people presenting with painful polyneuropathy. In such cases one can only say that there is an association between the metabolic syndrome or prediabetes and neuropathy, but given the fact that these are modifiable risk factors for vascular events, it is important to consider the development of unexplained painful polyneuropathy as an opportunity to test for these conditions.

- *Infections:* Most commonly, chronic hepatitis C and HIV.
- *Neurotoxins:* Alcohol is perhaps the most common neurotoxin to cause a painful polyneuropathy. The other major class is medications. Principal among these are antiretroviral drugs and several cancer treatments, including oxaliplatin, cis-platinum, and taxanes.
- *Inflammatory disorders:* Most notably Sjogren's syndrome, which can cause either a non-length-dependent ganglionopathy or a distal symmetric sensory polyneuropathy.
- The precise cause of distal symmetric painful polyneuropathy is often undiscovered despite appropriate investigations.

10. **How is small fiber neuropathy different from painful distal symmetric polyneuropathy?**
    Small fiber neuropathy is a term reserved for the circumstance in which distal symmetric painful polyneuropathy is largely restricted to small myelinated and unmyelinated axons. It is often the presenting form of painful polyneuropathy, with involvement of large myelinated axons developing later. Clinically it presents with painful paresthesias and reduced sharp perception distally, as described previously. Because by definition large myelinated axons are normal, NCS, vibration perception, reflexes, and strength are normal in small fiber neuropathy. The clinical diagnosis of small fiber neuropathy can be supported by a demonstrated reduction in cutaneous axons via a skin biopsy. While neurophysiologic tests of small somatic fibers are not available, several tests of sudomotor function can be utilized to support the clinical diagnosis.

11. **What is erythromelalgia?**
    Erythromelalgia is a very specific syndrome of severe burning pain in both feet that is reproducibly precipitated by skin warming, alleviated by cooling, and associated with striking erythema and swelling. All of these features should be present for the diagnosis to be made with confidence, as many patients with painful distal symmetric polyneuropathy will note some changes in the severity of their pain with skin warming or cooling but do not demonstrate the dramatic erythema, warmth, and temperature sensitivity seen in this condition.

    Erythromelalgia has been described in the presence of hematologic malignancies and chronic inflammatory states, and therefore a careful investigation for both is important. In these circumstances, exquisite responsiveness to treatment with aspirin or nonsteroidal antiinflammatory medications has been reported. When it does not respond to these simple measures, erythromelalgia is usually treated with medications used for distal symmetric painful sensory polyneuropathy, but can be refractory to treatment.

    Erythromelalgia also occurs in a familial form, which has been shown to be due to a mutation in the SCN9A gene encoding for a sodium channel in nociceptors. The causative mutation results in a lowered firing threshold in affected neurons, essentially resulting in a neuropathic pain state with thermal allodynia and hyperalgesia, whereby skin warming into the normally innocuous range is perceived as painful. Familial erythromelalgia is allelic to paroxysmal extreme pain disorder, which presents with episodic facial or rectal pain.

12. **What are the evidence-based treatments of painful distal symmetric polyneuropathy and small fiber neuropathy?**
    Nearly all evidence-based treatments are based upon studies performed in people with diabetic neuropathy. There is a strong evidence base for the efficacy of tricyclic agents (principally amitriptyline) pregabalin, gabapentin, and SNRIs (principally duloxetine). Some evidence also exists for efficacy of opioids in neuropathic pain, but these are not considered first-line therapies for neuropathic pain states. Many other agents have been investigated with equivocal evidence to support their use.

    Among topical agents, only one, 0.1% clonidine gel, has been shown to be beneficial among patients with paraclinical evidence of some preserved small fiber function.

    For unclear reasons, HIV infection and chemotherapy are two etiologies of painful neuropathy that tend to be particularly refractory to treatment. A 30-minute application of high-potency (8%) capsaicin has demonstrated statistically meaningful benefit for neuropathic pain from HIV, but is not FDA approved for this indication.

13. **What is the natural history of postherpetic neuralgia?**
    PHN is, by definition, a persistent pain state and commonly does not resolve spontaneously. Since neuropathic pain is a common but transient feature of zoster, PHN cannot be diagnosed unless pain persists well beyond healing of the acute zoster lesions. Typically therefore it is defined as pain that

persists more than 3 or 6 months after resolution of zoster. Even then, PHN can improve slowly thereafter, but it is often persistent for years or indefinitely and can be a refractory neuropathic pain. In addition to the spontaneous burning and paresthesias common to many neuropathic pain states, PHN is characteristically associated with prominent allodynia and hyperalgesia, which can often be the most disabling aspects of the condition.

14. What are the evidence-based treatments of postherpetic neuralgia?
There is a strong evidence base for treatment of PHN with tricyclics, pregabalin, and gabapentin. Unlike distal symmetric polyneuropathy, two topical agents have demonstrated benefit in this condition: Lidoderm patches (lidocaine in an adhesive patch), and high-potency (8%) capsaicin, which is applied once by a medical provider and may provide several months' improvement in PHN pain.

15. What is posttraumatic neuralgia, and how is it diagnosed?
PTN is characterized by posttraumatic sensory loss, pain, and allodynia or hyperalgesia in the cutaneous distribution of a single peripheral nerve. PTN can develop after trauma or iatrogenic injury, and is a recognized complication of surgical procedures, including herniorraphy, mastectomy, and thoracotomy. Mechanisms likely include spontaneous depolarizations from a nerve stump with secondary central sensitization and, in some cases, deafferentation pain.

Like painful distal sensory polyneuropathy, geographically restricted PTN can sometimes be treated with topical as well as systemic pharmacotherapy. In addition, interventional pain management modalities can be of diagnostic and therapeutic utility in PTN.

16. What are the causes of trigeminal neuralgia?
In many cases, evidence of demyelination presumably due to chronic irritation from an adjacent vascular structure can be demonstrated in trigeminal neuralgia (TGN). TGN can also develop in multiple sclerosis. In this context the condition is a consequence of loss of central myelin affecting fascicles of the trigeminal nerve within the pons.

17. What are the evidence-based treatments of trigeminal neuralgia?
Trigeminal neuralgia responds most consistently to treatment with carbamazepine, the only pharmacologic agent with a strong evidence base in this context. Oxcarbazepine has also been demonstrated to be beneficial in TGN. For patients with pain refractory to medical therapy, surgical therapies have been shown to be beneficial.

18. What are the most common central pain syndromes? What are the evidence-based treatments of central pain syndromes?
The most common central pain syndromes are poststroke pain, spinal cord injury pain, and myelopathic pain due to MS. Central pain syndromes typically develop in a delayed fashion—that is, several months after the inciting clinical event. Poststroke pain, unsurprisingly, usually occurs after a stroke affecting somatosensory pathways (thalamus or, less commonly, parietal cortex). Spinal cord injury pain can have two components: an "at-level" radicular pain and a "below-level" central pain state referable to interruption or dysfunction of ascending somatosensory pathways.

Central pain syndromes are often refractory to typical treatments for peripheral neuropathic pain. Amitriptyline, pregabalin, and lamotrigine have been demonstrated to be beneficial in poststroke pain, and pregabalin has been demonstrated to be beneficial in spinal cord injury pain.

19. What is complex regional pain syndrome?
CRPS is a clinical disorder characterized by spontaneous or stimulus-induced pain that is out of proportion to the provoking event and is accompanied by autonomic, sensory, and motor disturbances. There are two types: CRPS 1 and CRPS 2. By definition, CRPS 1 is not associated with previous nerve injury, and represents the current terminology for the condition previously referred to as reflex sympathetic dystrophy. CRPS 2 is associated with previous nerve injury and represents the current terminology for the condition previously referred to as causalgia.

20. Is complex regional pain syndrome a neuropathic pain state?
Proposed mechanisms of CRPS include neurogenic inflammation, altered blood flow due to efferent sympathetic activity, cortical reorganization, and autoimmunity. Although the precise mechanism or group of mechanisms is unknown, CRPS shares some clinical and pathologic features with neuropathic pain states. In particular, people with CRPS demonstrate exquisite allodynia and hyperalgesia, and skin biopsy in CRPS demonstrates reduced ENF density. That said, CRPS is a very

distinct clinical entity and the trophic changes, temperature changes, and severity of cutaneous sensitivity and guarding make it clearly different from other neuropathic pain states.

21. **How is complex regional pain syndrome diagnosed?**
The diagnosis of CRPS is made clinically. The Budapest diagnostic criteria for CRPS require the following:
- Continuous pain which is disproportionate to an inciting event
- Symptoms in at least three of four domains (sensory, vasomotor, sudomotor/edema, and motor/trophic). Specific aspects of each domain are described in the criteria.
- Signs in at least two of four domains (sensory, vasomotor, sudomotor/edema, and motor/trophic). Specific aspects of each domain are described in the criteria.
- No other diagnosis that better explains the signs and symptoms.
  Although there is no specific diagnostic test for CRPS, in certain circumstances, investigations such as QST, autonomic testing, x-rays, bone scintigraphy, and Doppler flow studies can be performed to interrogate for findings that have been described in people with CRPS.

22. **How is complex regional pain syndrome treated?**
There is a limited evidence base for effective treatment of CRPS, in part because its response to interventions is limited. A principal goal of treatment is functional restoration, as CRPS is associated with striking loss of function of the affected limb because of severe hyperalgesia. Therefore the foundation of CRPS management is a graded multimodal therapy program designed to overcome a fear-avoidance cycle of disuse and commonly led by occupational or physical therapists familiar with the relevant techniques. Several behavioral interventions have been designed to supplement this. Finally, pharmacologic and interventional therapies are used to reduce edema, sympathetic tone, or bone loss, and to alleviate pain so as to allow rehabilitative interventions to proceed.
Because of the typical need for multimodal therapy, CRPS is often managed in a multidimensional pain management setting.

23. **What is phantom limb pain?**
PLP is chronic, severe pain perceived to be located in amputated body regions. People with PLP may also report feeling movement of the amputated body part or other phantom limb sensations such as paresthesias or temperature changes.

24. **Is phantom limb pain a neuropathic pain state?**
Evidence exists that cortical reorganization as well as peripheral and central sensitization may contribute to PLP. Should these prove to be correct, PLP would fit the criteria established by the definition of neuropathic pain; furthermore, as PLP is pain referable to tissues that do not exist, it can only be either referred pain or neuropathic pain.

25. **Does neuropathic pain require multidisciplinary pain management?**
Many people with neuropathic pain can be treated successfully by a primary care provider or neurologist familiar with the diagnostic and management principles relevant to their condition. That said, neuropathic pain states are often difficult to treat for the following reasons:
- Many established treatments are of limited efficacy.
- Many established pharmacologic interventions have limiting adverse effects. This is not surprising, as medications designed to impact neurotransmission or neuromodulatory systems are inherently more likely to cause undesirable centrally mediated symptoms such as difficulty concentrating, nausea, and weight gain.
- Much like people with other causes of chronic pain, people with neuropathic pain often have musculoskeletal, psychological, and medical comorbidities that are best managed by a multidisciplinary team. These can include the following:
  - Musculoskeletal: Neuropathic pain often results in guarding, disuse, or unconscious excessive muscle contraction that leads to secondary musculoskeletal and myofascial pain. Physical therapists with expertise in treating people in pain are skilled in diagnosing and managing these comorbidities.
  - Behavioral: Pain and distress can be alleviated or exacerbated by a person's psychological traits and state. Mental health professionals with experience in pain management can be instrumental in making an initial assessment, providing counseling when indicated, and implementing behavioral interventions, such as cognitive-behavioral therapy and relaxation techniques that can alleviate pain, distress, and pain-related disability.

• Medical and pharmacological: Anxiety, sleep disturbances, and alterations in physical functioning related to pain impact medical comorbidities and general health. Medications for pain have the potential for adverse effects and drug-drug interactions that require monitoring.

Awareness of the following principles increases the likelihood of satisfactory outcomes in management of neuropathic pain:

• Identify the patient's goals and concerns at the outset of care. Obtaining medical care is a complex process and therefore does not occur without motivation. Find out what is motivating the patient; typically it is not pain *per se* but distress due to pain, questions about their diagnosis or prognosis, or concerns about disability or loss of life roles. Knowing the patient's goals and concerns enables the provider to focus their efforts appropriately. As an example, in people with painful distal symmetric polyneuropathy, an explanation of the possible causes and prognosis of their condition is often more important to the patient than achieving pain relief.

• Make an accurate and precise diagnosis. Utilizing the principles enumerated previously, determine as accurately as possible whether the pain is neuropathic and, if it is, what syndrome is represented. In the author's experience imprecise or inaccurate diagnoses, such as use of the term "neuropathy" as a catch-all for sensory symptoms, or "CRPS" as a catch-all for unexplained severe limb pain, are common and lead to inappropriate diagnostic and therapeutic interventions.

• Establish realistic goals of therapy early. Often people expect complete pain relief when in fact alleviation of distress and disability are more realistic and, in fact, more important goals. In such cases it is prudent to discuss this early in the management process.

KEY POINTS

1. Neuropathic pain is a distinct category of chronic pain due to dysfunction of the somatosensory system, in contradistinction to pain as an appropriate indicator of injury to innervated tissues.
2. Postulated mechanisms of neuropathic pain include spontaneous depolarizations of dysfunctional nociceptors, peripheral sensitization, central sensitization, deafferentation, and alterations in descending pain modulation. In addition to primary alterations in nociceptive and pain modulatory pathways, activation of glia and sympathetic efferents can contribute to neuropathic pain.
3. Neuropathic pain is diagnosed on the basis of the presence of characteristic positive and negative neuropathic sensory symptoms and signs in an appropriate neuroanatomic distribution. When clinically indicated, the diagnosis can be supported by physiologic or anatomic studies of the nervous system such as NCS, ENF density determination, and imaging.
4. Common neuropathic pain states include distal symmetric painful polyneuropathy, PHN, PTN, trigeminal neuralgia, and central pain states in the context of stroke or myelopathy. CRPS and PLP are other distinct chronic pain conditions with neuropathic features.
5. Depending upon the condition in question, neuropathic pain states can be treated with several forms of interventions, including topical pharmacotherapy, systemic pharmacotherapy, interventional, and surgical treatments.
6. Neuropathic pain is often accompanied by musculoskeletal, myofascial, and behavioral comorbidities that are substantial contributors to the patient's distress and disability. Assessment and treatment of these by an appropriate multidisciplinary team increases the likelihood of a good outcome.
7. Understanding the patient's goals of care and concerns, making an accurate and precise diagnosis, and establishing realistic goals of therapy are critical keys to success in management of neuropathic pain.

BIBLIOGRAPHY

1. Costigan M, Scholz J, Woolf CJ. Neuropathic pain: a maladaptive response of the nervous system to damage. *Annu Rev Neurosci.* 2009;32:1-32.
2. Bennett MI, Attal N, Backonja MM, et al. Using screening tools to identify neuropathic pain. *Pain.* 2007;127:199-203.
3. Treede RD, Jensen TS, Campbell JN, et al. Neuropathic pain: redefinition and a grading system for clinical and research purposes. *Neurology.* 2008;70:1630-1635.
4. Chan AC, Wilder-Smith AC. Small fiber neuropathy: getting bigger! *Muscle Nerve.* 2016;53:671-682.
5. International Association for the Study of Pain. Classification of chronic pain. In: Merskey H, Bogduk N, eds. *IASP Task Force on Taxonomy.* 2nd ed. Seattle: IASP Press; 1994:209-214. http://iasp-pain.org/Taxonomy?navItemNumber=576.

CHAPTER 30

NEUROPATHIC PAIN: SPECIFIC SYNDROMES AND TREATMENT

Katherin Peperzak and Brett R. Stacey

1. **What is neuropathic pain?**

   Neuropathic pain is "pain caused by a lesion or disease of the somatosensory nervous system." A lesion refers to an abnormality that is evidenced by diagnostic tests (e.g., imaging, neurophysiologic studies, biopsies) or a known trauma to the nervous system. The term "disease" refers to lesions from a known underlying cause such as diabetes mellitus, stroke, vasculitis, and so on. Neuropathic pain can be due to aberrant somatosensory processing in either the peripheral or central nervous system (CNS). Of note, neuropathic pain is a clinical descriptor and not a diagnosis.[5]

2. **List some other definitions I should know.**

   Neuropathy is a disturbance of function of pathologic change in a nerve. If it is present in one nerve, it is called "mononeuropathy." If neuropathy is present in several nerves, it is called "mononeuropathy multiplex," whereas if it is diffuse and bilateral, it is often called "polyneuropathy." Neuritis is a special case of neuropathy when nerves are affected by inflammation. Neuralgia is used to refer to any pain in the distribution of a nerve or nerves.[5]

3. **How common is neuropathic pain, and who gets it?**

   Epidemiologic studies estimate a prevalence of 7% to 9.8% of the adult population may experience neuropathic pain, and up to 20% of patients with chronic pain may have neuropathic components.

4. **How does neuropathic pain affect quality of life?**

   Neuropathic pain impacts mood, sleep, function, and overall health. The higher a patient rates their neuropathic pain on a scale of 0 to 10, the higher the negative impact of the pain on all of these domains. Negative mood associated with neuropathic pain includes both anxiety and depression. Similarly, higher pain scores are associated with more direct and indirect medical expenditures and more use of medications.

5. **Describe some conditions that sound similar to neuropathic pain.**

   Fibromyalgia is a pain disorder characterized by widespread musculoskeletal pain and heightened pain response to pressure, often accompanied by fatigue, mood, and cognitive disturbance. Although patients may describe some symptoms including numbness, tingling, and paresthesia-like sensations, technically the International Association for the Study of Pain criteria for neuropathic pain is not met, as there is no demonstrable disease state or demonstrable lesion. Similarly, patients with complex regional pain syndrome (CRPS) type 1 may complain of neuropathic-like symptoms, including burning pain or allodynia, but there is no lesion, as opposed to CRPS type 2, which does include a component of specific nerve injury. Still many do not consider CRPS type 2 an entirely neuropathic syndrome.

6. **What are common descriptors of the pain that a patient might give you when describing their possible neuropathic pain?**

   Patients may describe their pain as burning, tingling, electric-like, or shooting, and often report that the pain is unfamiliar or unlike typical pain experienced before. Many terms used to describe neuropathic pain are consistent with a dysesthesia, which is defined as an abnormal pain complaint. Patients may also describe unpleasant numbness or a painful itch sensation.

7. **What history may a patient with neuropathic pain report?**

   People with neuropathic pain may report a history of disease, toxin exposure, or injury that can cause nerve damage and therefore neuropathic pain. Examples include a history of diabetes (possible diabetic peripheral neuropathy [DPN]), human immunodeficiency virus (HIV) infection with treatment (HIV associated neuropathy), treatment with chemotherapy, orthopedic or spine surgery with persistent pain after the surgery, or other injury associated with loss of motor or sensory function. Additionally, patients with neuropathic pain may already have a history of another neuropathic pain problem.

8. **What are common physical exam findings in patients with neuropathic pain?**
   Exam may reveal allodynia (pain created by a normally nonpainful stimulus such as a light brush or touch), hypoalgesia or hyperalgesia (relatively decreased or increased perception of a noxious stimulus, respectively), hypoesthesia or hyperesthesia (relatively decreased or increased perception of a non-noxious stimulus, respectively), or hyperpathia (exaggerated pain response). There may be focal neurologic deficits including weakness, reflex changes, or motor weakness. In an extremity there may be autonomic changes such as swelling and vasomotor instability (observed as color changes, livedo reticularis, and temperature changes). Trophic changes may also be seen including alterations of the skin, subcutaneous tissues, hair, or nails.

9. **What is central neuropathic pain?**
   Central neuropathic pain is pain caused by a lesion of the CNS—typically the brain or spinal cord. Examples are pain following stroke, pain associated with disease of the CNS such as multiple sclerosis or Parkinson's disease, plexus avulsion, or pain associated with spinal cord injury (SCI). The pain may develop concurrent with the initial injury or over time. While the injury that starts the process is in the CNS, peripheral input may modify the pain, either making it worse or better.

10. **What is peripheral neuropathic pain?**
    In peripheral neuropathic pain, the initiating lesion is located outside of the CNS—in the periphery. A classic example is painful peripheral diabetic neuropathy, in which there is confirmed damage to the peripheral nerves in the hands and feet. While the initiating problem is in the periphery, peripheral neuropathic pain is often accompanied by changes in CNS function and physiology that may be more important than peripheral changes in maintaining the ongoing pain. An interesting example is phantom limb pain, in which the initial injury (amputation of a body part) is clearly outside the CNS, but the main pathology for ongoing pain is often in cortical and subcortical structures in the brain.

11. **What is the difference between central and peripheral neuropathic pain?**
    While central neuropathic starts with a process in the CNS, the peripheral nervous system can impact and modify the pain, as patients may have allodynia and hyperalgesia and note that some types of touch or stimulus of the body can lessen pain. Similarly, while damage to the nervous system outside of the CNS is required for peripheral neuropathic pain, central sensitization and changes in CNS pain processing are often the primary reasons for the ongoing pain. In general, central neuropathic pain states appear to be more difficult to treat, and there are fewer treatments established as effective for them. Additionally, patients with central neuropathic pain may have more profound neurological deficits accompanying their pain complaints. See Table 30.1 for examples.

12. **What are some assessment and screening tools available specifically for neuropathic pain?**
    Aside from determining a numeric pain score for severity of pain, there are many validated neuropathic pain assessment tools used to aid in diagnosis and assess response to treatment, including the Neuropathic Pain Questionnaire (NPQ), PainDetect, the Neuropathic Pain Symptom Inventory (NPSI), IDpain, DN4, the Leeds Assessment of Neuropathic Pain, and Signs-LANSS. History and physical exam are of course imperative to diagnosis.

13. **Describe some diagnostic tools that may aid in diagnosis.**
    Electrodiagnostic studies like electromyogram (EMG) and nerve conduction studies can sometimes be helpful in confirming existence of a neurologic lesion. Some patients may dislike these tests, as they require many tiny needle electrodes to be placed, often in painful areas. Thermography, quantitative sensory testing (QST), and quantitative sudomotor axon reflex testing (QSART) may be useful in confirming autonomic dysregulation. Skin biopsy is used to assess intraepidermal nerve fiber density (IENFD) and determine severity of axon loss in patients with possible small-fiber sensory neuropathy. Functional magnetic resonance imaging (fMRI) has been useful in research regarding central pain mechanisms, but it is unclear what, if any, role this modality may have in diagnosis or routine clinical care.

14. **Are any labs useful?**
    Judicious laboratory testing will be dependent on suspected etiology and risk factors. Labs to consider if a disease state is suspected include complete blood count, comprehensive metabolic panel, liver function tests, fasting blood glucose, hemoglobin A1C, thyroid stimulating hormone, and

Table 30.1. Common Neuropathic Pain Syndromes

CENTRAL NEUROPATHIC PAIN STATES	PERIPHERAL NEUROPATHIC PAIN STATES	MIXED NEUROPATHIC STATES
Compressive myelopathy (spinal stenosis)	Painful diabetic peripheral neuropathy	Postherpetic neuralgia
Poststroke pain	HIV-associated neuropathy	Complex regional pain syndrome type 2
Posttraumatic spinal cord injury	Radiculopathy	—
HIV myelopathy	Entrapment neuropathies (e.g., carpal tunnel)	—
Postischemic myelopathy	Nerve injury after trauma	—
Syringomyelia	Pressure or nerve infiltration injury (e.g., tumor growth)	—
Phantom limb pain	Trigeminal neuralgia	—
Pain related to multiple sclerosis	Chemotherapy-associated peripheral neuropathy	—

serum vitamin B12 level. Vitamin D level (deficiency is associated with painful peripheral neuropathy) and erythrocyte sedimentation rate (elevated in various autoimmune, infectious, and other system conditions) may also be useful. If a specific cause of neuropathy remains elusive, more extensive testing based upon the history and physical examination such as HIV, Lyme antibody, rapid plasma reagin (RPR), antinuclear antibody, or paraneoplastic syndrome testing should be considered.

15. What is small fiber peripheral neuropathy?

Small fiber peripheral neuropathy (SFPN) is a type of peripheral neuropathy due to damage of small, unmyelinated C fibers and thinly myelinated A-delta fibers that innervate the skin or autonomic system. It can present with paresthesias, dysesthesias, pain, or numbness. Other symptoms include changes in skin color and temperature, sweating, or the presence of edema. Most commonly symptoms and signs are length-dependent, starting in the distal portion of longer nerves. There are many causes of small fiber neuropathy from diabetes (the most common) to nutritional deficiencies and infectious causes such as Lyme disease, many of which will be described later. Because large fibers are spared, routine electrodiagnostic studies do not confirm the presence of SFPN.

16. Tell me more about diabetic peripheral neuropathy

DPN most commonly presents as a distal, symmetric polyneuropathy. Typically feet are predominantly effected (stocking distribution) and involvement of the hands comes later (stocking glove distribution). Duration and severity of hyperglycemia are major risk factors, as well as dyslipidemia, hypertension, and smoking. A small fraction of those with DPN will develop painful DPN, and of those approximately half may have spontaneous resolution in 12 months. There are some acute painful DPN syndromes associated with rapid glycemic control or in the setting of intentional or unintentional weight loss. These are potentially reversible or may have spontaneous resolution. In general, optimal glucose control is key to treatment, though tricyclic antidepressants (TCAs), serotonin reuptake inhibitors (SNRIs), and anticonvulsants all may be effective[1].

17. Tell me about human immunodeficiency virus–associated neuropathy.

HIV infection itself is associated with multiple neuropathic syndromes (30% to 67% of patients), including axonal as well as acute and chronic demyelinating neuropathies, with distal, symmetric polyneuropathy being most common. Between 30% and 67% of HIV patients will develop a neuropathy. CD4 count and HIV viral load were previously thought to be risk factors, but recent studies do not substantiate this claim. Treatment with neurotoxic drugs such as didanosine, stavudine, and zalcitabine was previously associated with neuropathy, causing them to fall out of favor.[6]

18. **How about chemotherapy-induced peripheral neuropathies?**
Chemotherapy drugs are known to most commonly cause a sensory neuropathy in a "stocking and glove" distribution known as chemotherapy-induced peripheral neuropathy (CIDP). This effect is dose dependent and cumulative. Cisplatin, oxaliplatin, paclitaxel (can also be associated with a motor neuropathy), vincristine, and thalidomide have all been implicated in chronic neurotoxicity. Neuropathy may improve over time after therapy is stopped, though it may continue to worsen for several months before improvement. Oxaliplatin and paclitaxel may also cause acute neurotoxicity syndromes, which typically improve several days after each dose but may recur with repeated dosing. Studies on antiepileptics and antidepressants for treatment have shown underwhelming efficacy despite utility in other forms of neuropathy, causing a shift toward studying chemoprotectant agents like amifostine or nimodipine.

19. **What are some less common peripheral neuropathies?**
There are *many* other peripheral neuropathies. Hypothyroidism can cause a sensory polyneuropathy as well as mononeuropathy due to entrapment (most commonly carpal tunnel syndrome). Uremia and chronic renal failure are associated with a sensory polyneuropathy. Amyloidosis is associated with pain, small-fiber dysfunction (e.g., loss of pain and thermal senses), and autonomic neuropathy. Meanwhile, patients with the rare lipid storage disorder Fabry's disease can develop painful polyneuropathy with continuous, burning dysesthesias of the distal extremities. Exposure to toxins like arsenic and cyanide may also lead to polyneuropathies.

20. **Are there any other peripheral neuropathies?**
Yes—there are many. More examples include hereditary sensory neuropathy type I (a rare autosomal dominant disorder), painful polyneuropathy associated with Guillan-Barre syndrome (an acute myelinopathy), or chronic inflammatory demyelinating polyneuropathy (a chronic myelinopathy), as well as neuropathies related to porphyria and autoimmune disorders. Sensorimotor neuropathies may present as part of a paraneoplastic syndrome with various carcinomas, with small cell carcinoma being most common. "Idiopathic neuropathy" should also be mentioned.

21. **True or false: surgery can lead to persistent neuropathic pain.**
True. Surgery causes either direct nerve injury through severing during surgery or stretch during retraction. In some patients scar tissue formation may also cause nerve compression. Inguinal hernia repair may lead to persistent groin pain due to inguinal and/or iliohypogastric neuralgia and/or genitofemoral neuralgia. Spine surgery may lead to "failed back syndrome" or "postlaminectomy pain syndrome," which is a well-described phenomenon, particularly after laminectomy, that may involve neuropathic components or nerve injury. Orthopedic surgeries can also lead to various peripheral neuralgias, depending on location and in some instances CRPS, type 2.

22. **How is trauma to nerves classified?**
Laceration, stretch, compression, or drug toxicity can all cause trauma to a nerve. Seddon's classification grades the severity of a nerve injury. Neurapraxia (class I) describes temporary interruption of conduction spontaneously recovering in days to weeks, whereas axonotmesis (class II) involves the loss of continuity of an axon and myelin, while the epineurium and perineurium framework are preserved. Surgical intervention is sometimes needed. Lastly, neurotmesis (class III) involves total disruption of the nerve fiber, and surgical intervention is required. Sunderland's classification is similar, with first degree and second degree referring to neurapraxia and axonotmesis, respectively, and third through fifth degree being further divisions of neurotmesis.

23. **What is a neuroma?**
Neuroma represents abnormal growth of neural tissue that can be from nerves, the myelin sheath, or other nervous structure. The growth usually is localized and benign; less commonly it is malignant. Neuromas may form at the end of a cut nerve, along the course of a regenerated nerve or as result of disease, compression, or disease. Regardless of location, neuromas pathologically appear similar to regenerating small nerve fibers and are prone to generating spontaneous discharges both at the area of the neuroma and at the dorsal root ganglion. These aberrant discharges may be caused by mechanical stimulation or by changes in the local environment such as ischemia or electrolyte disturbances, and may be associated with pain.

24. **What is a plexopathy?**
Plexopathy refers to a disorder of a network of nerves causing pain, weakness, and sensory deficits. This may be due to trauma to an area (such as with an avulsion injury), mass effect (such as from metastatic cancer), or entrapment (such as with the brachial plexus in thoracic outlet syndrome). Plexopathies include brachial plexopathy affecting areas innervated by C5 to T1, lumbar plexopathy affecting areas innervated by L1 to L4, and sacral plexopathy affecting areas innervated by L5 to S3. Any plexopathy would be expected to provoke neuropathic symptoms in the correlating distribution. Magnetic resonance imaging (MRI) and/or electromyography/nerve conduction study (EMG/NCS) may be helpful in diagnosis.

25. **Explain radiculopathy.**
Radiculopathy refers to an injury at a nerve root that can cause pain, weakness, or numbness along the entire course of the nerve. This is often due to compression of the nerve root as it exits the neural foramen of the spine. This may be secondary to degenerative disc disease, herniated disc, osteoarthritis, calcification of ligaments, or spondylolisthesis, among other causes. Less commonly, radiculopathy may be caused by diabetes, neoplastic lesions, or infectious processes. On exam, aside from thorough sensory and motor exam, Spurling's test and straight-leg testing are often used to identify cervical or lumbar radiculopathy, respectively. Deep tendon reflexes of the corresponding nerve root may also be diminished. As in plexopathies, MRI and/or EMG/NCS may be useful.

26. **Erythromelalgia sounds interesting. What is it?**
Erythromelalgia is a "zebra" diagnosis occurring in 1 : 100,000 people that also happens to the first chronic neuropathic pain disorder associated with a discovered ion channel mutation, specifically in the Na_v 1.7 channel. A subset of erythromelalgia has this mutation. Erythromelalgia can be familial (hereditary, more likely associated with the Na_v 1.7 mutation) or spontaneous. It is primarily a vascular peripheral pain disorder in which peripheral blood vessels (typically in the lower extremities or hands) periodically spasm, causing skin redness and severe burning pain via small sensory fibers. Attacks can be precipitated by heat exertion (even mild), pressure, dependent position, or stress. Differential diagnosis includes polycythemia and SFPN.

27. **That's a lot of information about peripheral neuropathy. Tell me more about central neuropathic pain.**
As mentioned earlier, deafferentation pain (including phantom pain, plexus avulsion, and SCI) is a type of central neuropathic pain. Research shows that "central sensitization" has a prominent role in deafferentation syndromes. Central sensitization is a complex process involving functional and structural changes in the CNS pathways involved in nociception. This is an area of continued research, but one mechanism involves the interaction of excitatory amino acids like glutamate with the *N*-methyl-D-aspartate receptor (NMDA), producing sensitization of the nociceptive neurons in the dorsal horn of the spinal cord. Central neuropathic pain may also involve changes in cortical pain processing that may be seen with positron emission tomography (PET) scans or functional MRI scanning.

28. **What is postherpetic neuralgia?**
Postherpetic neuralgia (PHN) is considered a deafferentation pain. It is defined by prolonged pain following acute herpes zoster (HZ) infection that persists beyond crusting of lesions and disappearance of the rash. Following resolution of systemic varicella infection (which usually occurs in childhood), the virus remains dormant in the dorsal root ganglia. Later, HZ produces diffuse inflammation of peripheral nerves, dorsal root ganglion, and in some cases, the spinal cord. Long after the acute infection resolves, the pathology reveals chronic inflammatory changes in the periphery, neuronal loss in the dorsal root ganglion, and a reduction of both axons and myelin in affected nerves.

29. **What is the epidemiology of postherpetic neuralgia?**
The incidence of HZ is approximately 1.3 to 4.8 cases per 1000 person-years, with a higher incidence in the elderly and immunocompromised. Overall, 10% of those with acute HZ will go on to experience pain for more than 1 month, with an increasing frequency with advancing age and severity of both the rash and acute zoster pain. In one survey, the prevalence of pain 1 year after the eruption was 4.2% in patients 20 years old and younger, and 47% in those older than 70. With advent of the varicella vaccine, future studies will likely show a reduction in incidence of PHN, and at least one large trial has determined that repeat vaccination during late adulthood reduces the incidence of PHN.

30. **What are important clinical features of postherpetic neuralgia?**
HZ erupts in the thoracic dermatomes in more than 50% of patients. The trigeminal distribution (usually V1) is next most common. Lumbar and cervical zosters each occur in 10% to 20% of patients. PHN pain is in the same dermatomal location as the original HZ rash. The pain of PHN is described as a combination of deep aching, superficial burning, and paroxysmal pain. Itch is often reported. Allodynia or hyperpathia is common but variable; in some patients, the sensitivity to touch is the most distressing component. About 10% of patients with HZ infection experience pain without the concomitant presence of skin lesions. PHN can also occur in the ear following Ramsay-Hunt syndrome, in which varicella spreads from the geniculate ganglion.

31. **What is an appropriate management strategy for acute zoster?**
Studies of antiviral treatment, such as famcyclovir and valacyclovir, have shown that early treatment shortens the time of pain associated with the acute attack, in essence reducing the incidence of PHN. Antivirals are recommended for those over the age 50 or for anyone with a more complicated or extensive initial presentation such as facial involvement, severe rash, poorly controlled pain, or those who are immunocompromised. Corticosteroids such as prednisone and early sympathetic nerve block can have valuable analgesic effects during acute zoster. Epidural administration of local anesthetic and steroid may reduce both the severity of HZ pain and chance of developing PHN. The use of low-dose amitriptyline during acute zoster may reduce PHN according to some studies. Once PHN develops, pain can be aggressively managed with a combination of systemic analgesics, using the same general approach as for other types of neuropathic pain, as well as topical agents like a lidocaine patch.

32. **What is central poststroke pain?**
Central poststroke pain (CPSP), also known as thalamic pain, results from injury to the thalamus or parietal lobe by ischemic or hemorrhagic lesions. The pain is usually dysesthetic with continuous burning, and may be associated with uncomfortable paresthesias. Allodynia is common, and some patients experience dramatic hyperpathia, with diffuse radiation of pain and continued pain for a prolonged period after a stimulus is removed from the skin. The pain can present in the entire hemibody or be localized to a small region. Occasional patients have a so-called cheiro-oral distribution (perioral region and ipsilateral hand). CPSP typically occurs months to years after injury.

33. **True or false. Chronic central pain is common in patients with multiple sclerosis.**
This is partially true. Chronic pain occurs in 23% to 80% of patients with multiple sclerosis. Central pain is the most common and is most common in those with disease of long duration. Pain is often described as continuous burning and may be associated with other dysesthesias or lancinating pains that fluctuate in intensity spontaneously or in response to activity, stress, or change in weather. Typically pain is in the distal legs or feet, but may present in a dermatomal distribution or in another region of the trunk or an extremity. The pain may come and go.

34. **Describe the central pain caused by spinal cord injury.**
Damage to the spinal cord from trauma or demyelinating lesions is known to cause central pain. In fact, 10% to 49% of patients may develop chronic pain following acute SCI. There is significant variation in clinical presentation of central pain caused by SCI. Patients may have spontaneous or evoked dysesthesias with or without associated paresthesias, described as tingling, numbness, or squeezing. Painful areas may be small or large, unilateral or bilateral, and stable or fluctuating in size and location. Flexor or extensor spasms, which may be spontaneous or precipitated by movement or distention of the bladder or bowel, can contribute significantly to pain. The pain may be at level of the lesion (also known as transitional zone pain) or "below level," primarily impacting the more distal body. Some patients have secondary musculoskeletal pain including of the trunk, shoulders, or limbs that often has different characteristics and responds to different treatments than the neuropathic SCI pain.

35. **What is known about the mechanisms of phantom limb pain?**
Phantom pain can occur after amputation of any body part, whether it be postsurgical or traumatic limb amputation or following mastectomy or tooth extraction. The specific pathophysiology that causes phantom pain is not known. Some research suggests that "shrinkage" of the somatosensory cortical representation of an amputated limb correlates with the development of pain. Other research suggests phantom pain is a somatosensory "memory" that involves complex interactions of neural

networks in the brain. We do know that phantom pain is rare in congenital amputees or children who lose a limb prior to age 6, suggesting some degree of CNS maturation is required to develop pain. Changes in cortical pain processing accompany phantom limb pain and can be seen with PET or functional MRI scanning.

36. **Does every patient with an amputation get phantom pain?**
Surveys have reported incidence of phantom pain from 25% to 98% in amputees. Some epidemiologic studies suggest about half of patients with phantom pain will continue to have pain for at least 1 to 2 years, while others indicate a large majority will experience resolution of pain within one year. The experience of pain in the limb prior to amputation may predispose to the development of phantom pain. Other suggested predisposing factors include older age, proximal amputations, upper limb lesions, sudden amputations, and preexisting psychological disturbances. Most patients develop phantom pain and sensations soon after nerve injury and amputation, but symptoms may develop at any time.

37. **How is phantom pain different from phantom sensation?**
Phantom pain is one element among many phantom sensations. Pain is considered an exteroceptive sensation, a description that has also been applied to the perception of touch, temperature, pressure, and itch, among others. Kinesthetic sensation involves the perception of posture, length, as well as willed and spontaneous movements. Some other kinesthetic phantom sensations include unusual postures, foreshortening of a limb ("telescoping"), or distortion of size of body parts (usually reduction in proximal regions and expansion of distal regions). All of these sensations tend to be most vivid immediately after amputation and gradually fade in intensity.

38. **How is phantom pain different from stump pain?**
Phantom pain is generated by the CNS, whereas stump pain (also known as residual limb pain) originates from the peripheral nervous system, presumably related to an ill-fitting prosthetic, scar tissue formation, skin or tissue breakdown, ischemia, or development of a neuroma at the end of a severed nerve. Patients describe stump pain as aching, squeezing, throbbing, and stabbing pain localized to the distal stump. Stump pain may not present for several months after amputation. A patient may suffer from both phantom limb pain and stump pain. Patients with severe stump pain may be more likely to have symptomatic phantom limb pain.

39. **What nonpharmacologic and interventional treatments should be considered in neuropathic pain?**
In general, treatment of neuropathic pain should include a combination of pharmacological and nonpharmacological strategies. See Table 30.2 for a general approach to treatment. Physical therapy with emphasis on balance and gait training is particularly important in distal, symmetric neuropathies, as well as radiculopathies. Graded motor imagery and mirror therapy take advantage of neuroplasticity and may be useful in those with phantom limb pain, poststroke pain, or CRPS, as patients learn to "move" or "unclench" phantom limbs out of painful positions and change perception of their affected extremity. Transcutaneous electrical stimulation (TENS) may also be applied to painful areas as stimulation of peripheral C-beta sensory fibers has been shown to suppress nociceptive processing by A-delta fibers.

40. **Describe some specific exercise techniques that may be useful.**
Yoga and Tai Chi, an Eastern art that involves slow and deliberate relaxation and balance techniques, are becoming increasingly popular in the treatment of neuropathic pain. Yoga has been studied specifically in multiple sclerosis and has shown benefit in fatigue level and other MS symptoms. Studies on Tai Chi in peripheral neuropathy have shown improvement in balance, sensation, and overall health compared to walking alone or low-impact weight training.

41. **What medications are available for treatment of neuropathic pain?**
Antiepileptics, antidepressants, and opioids have all demonstrated efficacy in treatment of neuropathic pain. Various professional societies and academic groups have published recommendations for different types of neuropathic disorders based on the literature. For example, the American Academy of Neurology recommends pregabalin as first-line treatment for DPN, with duloxetine, tricyclic antidepressants, and gabapentin being second-line agents, and opioids third. Unfortunately, data suggest that half of patients will only obtain partial relief. In practice, drug rotations and trialing of additional agents (rational polypharmacy) is very common to obtain satisfactory pain relief[2].

Table 30.2. Ten-Step Approach to Treatment of Neuropathic Pain

1. Establish diagnosis and cause of neuropathic pain.

2. When possible, treat underlying cause or refer to appropriate specialist (e.g., primary care physician for diabetes management, surgeon for carpal tunnel release).

3. Identify comorbidities and medication interactions that may affect choice of treatment (e.g., renal impairment may require reduced dosing of gabapentin).

4. Initiate therapy with one or more of the following:
   - TCA (nortryptiline, amitryptiline, desipramine)
   - Antiepileptic (gabapentin, pregabalin, carbamazepine)
   - Serotonin reuptake inhibitors (duloxetine, venlafaxine)
   - Topical agents such as lidocaine or capsaicin gels or patches
   - Opioid analgesics (tramadol, methadone tapentadol, oxycodone, morphine, etc., in select patients with acute onset or cancer-related neuropathies)

5. Consider interventional approaches such as epidural steroid injections or peripheral nerve blocks with local anesthetic and/or steroid depending on source.

6. Consider appropriate nonpharmacologic strategies:
   - Physical and occupational therapy
   - Transcutaneous electrical stimulation unit
   - Yoga, Tai Chi, and other exercise for balance and gait training
   - Specialized therapies such as mirror therapy in phantom limb pain
   - Pain psychology approaches: cognitive behavioral therapy, mindfulness, acceptance

7. Evaluate effectiveness of treatment after adequate dosage and duration of medication trial reached.

8. If ineffective, consider rotation to alternative first-line medications or addition of medications of different mechanism ("rational polypharmacy").

9. Consider non-first-line therapies or agents under investigations such as mexelitine or memantine.

10. If quality of life and function remain inadequate or medications are poorly tolerated, evaluate for more invasive treatment options, including spinal cord stimulation and intrathecal drug delivery.

42. **What are the US Food and Drug Administration approved medications for the treatment of neuropathic pain?**
Pregabalin, gabapentin, gastroretentive gabapentin, gabapentin enacarbil, the 8% topical capsaicin patch, and the 5% lidocaine patch are U.S. Food and Drug Administration (FDA) approved for PHN. Duloxetine, pregabalin, and the opioid tapentadol are FDA approved for painful DPN. Pregabalin is FDA approved for neuropathic pain associated with SCI. Carbamazepine is FDA approved for trigeminal neuralgia. Many other medications such as TCAs are not FDA approved but are commonly suggested in guidelines and used in clinical practice.

43. **Name some of the antiepileptics commonly used for neuropathic pain.**
A multitude of antiepileptic drugs exist that are useful in treatment of neuropathic pain. They work by various mechanisms including effects on sodium or calcium conduction, increase in gamma-aminobutyric acid (GABA) levels, reduction in glutamate levels, or other unknown mechanisms. Gabapentin is an alpha-2 delta calcium channel ligand and has been shown to significantly reduce pain in DPN and PHN, and has a favorable side-effect profile compared to first-generation anticonvulsants. There are two longer acting forms of gabapentin, once daily gastroretentive gabapentin and a twice daily prodrug, pregabalin. Pregabalin is similar to gabapentin by binding at the same site on voltage-dependent calcium channels, and both drugs have similar side effects of dizziness and sedation and require dose adjustments in renal insufficiency. Controlled trials reveal carbamazepine to be effective in trigeminal neuralgia and DPN, but not in PHN or central pain.

Oxcarbazepine and sodium valproate also have benefit in DPN. Topiramate, levetiracetam, phenytoin, lamotrigine, and the newer antiepileptic lacosamide, among others, have all been considered in treatment, though they have limited data supporting their efficacy. Eventual choice in antiepileptic should be based on side effect profile and trial and error.

44. **Which antidepressants are most useful in neuropathic pain?**
Tricyclic antidepressants (e.g., amitriptyline, nortriptyline, desipramine, imipramine) are known to have analgesic benefit independent of antidepressant effect, likely through inhibition of reuptake of norepinephrine and serotonin at the spinal dorsal horn. It is thought that lower doses than what is required for treatment of depression are sufficient for pain benefit, and they continue to be first-line treatment for DPN and PHN. Concern for cardiac toxicity and anticholinergic side effects such as orthostatic hypotension, urinary retention, and dry mouth tend to be limiting, though nortriptyline may be the best tolerated. Selective norepinephrine and SNRIs such as duloxetine and venlafaxine may be even better tolerated, but may take several weeks to become effective. For SNRIs, the dose that treats neuropathic pain is similar to the antidepressant dose. Duloxetine has shown sustained efficacy in painful DPN and has some suggestive evidence in HIV-associated neuropathy and CIDP, but has not been formally studied in other neuropathies. Meanwhile, venlafaxine has also some efficacy in DPN, but not in PHN.

45. **Local anesthetics should help too, right?**
Studies have established the 5% lidocaine patch (Lidoderm) to be effective in patients with PHN. Some patients with PHN and other neuropathic pain may obtain relief from the cutaneous anesthesia provided by the eutectic mixture of lidocaine and prilocaine (EMLA) or 5% or 10% lidocaine gel or cream. Typically this is applied in a thin layer several times daily. Temporary nerve blocks with local anesthetic to both peripheral nerves and sympathetic nerves may also be beneficial in some patients. Intravenous lidocaine in a dose of 3 to 5 mg/kg can reduce neuropathic pain short term and in some cases there may be a more prolonged response.

46. **Speaking of blocking sodium channels, can mexiletine be used in neuropathic pain?**
Yes. Mexiletine, an oral analogue of intravenous lidocaine, has shown some modest benefit in chronic neuropathic pain, but it still considered a second- or third-line treatment option. It is a class IB antiarrhythmic used in life-threatening ventricular arrhythmias; it should be used with caution in patients with preexisting conduction defects and is specifically contraindicated in second- and third-degree atrioventricular block.

47. **True or false: Opioids are a first-line treatment for neuropathic pain.**
False. The adverse and complex psychosocial effects of opioids and existence of other more targeted therapies makes the role of opioids unclear. Some double-blind, randomized, controlled trials of opioids have shown efficacy for treatment of neuropathic pain. If opioid therapy is deemed appropriate, there are multimechanism mu-opioid agonists that may be especially worth considering. Tramadol inhibits serotonin and norepinephrine reuptake and has proven useful in DPN and polyneuropathy. Similarly, tapentadol also inhibits norepinephrine reuptake. Studies have shown benefit from the extended-release formulation in diabetic painful neuropathy. Methadone is well known for its NMDA antagonism and has been shown to be beneficial at a 10- to 20-mg total daily dose in various types of neuropathy.

48. **Ketamine seems to be en vogue. Are *N*-methyl-D-aspartate receptor antagonists useful?**
Patients who do not respond to the treatments discussed previously could consider ketamine (intranasal formulation), memantine, or dextromethorphan. Despite having the usual indications of anesthesia, treatment of Alzheimer's disease, or cough suppression, respectively, each of these drugs causes some degree of NMDA receptor antagonism. Ketamine IV has also been studied in CRPS and phantom limb pain, with inconsistent results. Based on current meta-analysis, no definitive conclusion on the efficacy of NMDA receptor antagonists in chronic neuropathic pain can be made. Given the NMDA receptor's role in spontaneous pain, allodynia, and hyperalgesia, it remains an area of research.[7]

49. **What is ziconotide?**
In short, it is a synthetic form of sea snail toxin. The toxin is known to cause selective blockade of the N-type voltage-gated calcium channel, leading to the inhibition of release of glutamate,

calcitonin gene-related peptide, and substance P in the brain and spinal cord. The drug is delivered through an intrathecal infusion pump, and thus is only considered in those who have failed therapy with oral medications. Originally ziconitide was only studied in cancer pain, but there have been some studies and case reports on its utility in neuropathic pain. It has been known to induce psychosis, as well as cause other central side effects such as sedation and mental clouding.

50. **Is capsaicin still being used?**
Yes. Capsaicin is a naturally occurring compound that selectively depletes peptide neurotransmitters (such as substance P) from small-diameter primary afferent neurons and is toxic to the TRPV1 receptors on small axons responsible for thermal pain. Capsaicin cream has been used in PHN and in neuropathy due to HIV. A typical trial could include application to the affected area 3 to 4 times daily for 4 weeks, after which some patients may have a significant response. Due to the pain and logistics involved in typical dosing, a high-concentration (8%) capsaicin patch was approved for treatment by the FDA in 2009 that only requires application for 1 hour every 3 months, with relief lasting days to months.

51. **My patient tells me they use marijuana for neuropathic pain. Is this legit?**
It could be. As of April 2016, 24 states and the District of Columbia have enacted laws to allow medical marijuana for a variety of indications, generally including chronic or severe pain. A clinical review on cannabinoids and marijuana in pain recently published in *JAMA* points to 6 trials (396 patients) in neuropathic pain and 12 trials (1600 patients) on multiple sclerosis, of which several high-quality studies had positive results suggesting efficacy. The American Academy of Neurology has also indicated support of certain oral cannabis products for spasticity and central pain associated with multiple sclerosis. Given inconsistency between marijuana products and delivery methods, it is difficult to make specific recommendations. (Hill KP. Medical marijuana for treatment of chronic pain and other medical and psychiatric problems: a clinical review. *JAMA* 2015;313(24):2474–2483).

52. **My patient is interested in over-the-counter supplements. Which ones might be helpful?**
Although treatment with antiepileptics and antidepressants has good results, these medications may also cause side effects prompting patients to explore other options. Some supplements that have had promising results with neuropathic pain include alpha-lipoic acid, n-acetyl-cysteine, L-carnitine, selenium, and vitamin C. Vitamin C is currently being extensively studied in both the treatment of and prevention of diabetic neuropathy and other peripheral neuropathies. Patients with known vitamin deficiencies should be treated accordingly, with repletion of B vitamins (particularly B1, B6, and B12), vitamin E, or niacin.

53. **Is there a role for procedural interventions in neuropathic pain?**
Yes. Procedures are particularly appropriate when trials of oral medications have failed to provide adequate relief or medications cause undesirable or intolerable side effects. Peripheral nerve blocks, neuraxial nerve blocks, sympathetic blocks, implanted spinal cord stimulators, and implanted intrathecal catheters may all have a role. Unfortunately, literature supporting interventional procedures for neuropathic pain in particular is limited. Given the lack of quality data and consensus, no strong recommendations can be made, but there is sufficient evidence to support consideration of some specific procedures for selected neuropathic pain states.

54. **When are peripheral nerve blocks useful?**
In patients with focal peripheral neuropathic pain, diagnostic nerve blocks may be used to determine if a particular nerve is involved in a patient's symptoms. The response to injection can help determine candidacy for therapeutic blocks (with steroids or a series of injections), neuroablative techniques, or surgical therapy. Currently, there are no clear standard recommendations for injectate (medication and volume) or treatment pathways. However, some studies do show perineural steroids as being useful in treatment in neuropathic pain secondary to trauma or compression, presumably due to the antiinflammatory effect and immunosuppression action on injured nerves.

On a related subject, limited data suggest that using regional anesthesia in patients with preamputation limb pain *may* help prevent phantom limb pain. There is not a clear role for this treatment after development of chronic phantom pain.

55. **Name some indications for epidural steroid injections in neuropathic pain.**
Epidural steroid injections (ESIs) may be useful in treatment of radicular pain as well as pain related to acute HZ or PHN. Some studies have shown a favorable response in patients with prolonged PHN

to a series of epidural injections with local anesthetic and steroid. The most common indication for ESIs is radicular pain[3].

56. How useful are epidural injections for radicular pain?

This could be the subject of a 50-page chapter with varying conclusions, but in general epidural injections, particularly with local anesthetic and steroids, are useful. A recent review of randomized-controlled trials concluded a modest effect size lasting less than 3 months most often when using a transforaminal approach (>70%), as compared with caudal (60%) and interlaminar (50%) techniques. Further response to injection for a radicular pain, particularly due to herniated disc, is more likely to be positive than when procedures are performed for spinal stenosis or axial back pain. In select patients, strategic use of epidurals should be considered.

57. True or false: Epidural injections may prevent postherpetic neuralgia.

They might. Multiple randomized-controlled trials have shown at least some modest reduction in pain and allodynia, with a single epidural injection of local anesthetic and steroid soon after onset of HZ, but prevalence of chronic pain 6 months later was not significantly reduced. However, results of another randomized controlled study suggest that repetitive epidural injections of local anesthetic and steroid may prevent PHN, similar to previous observational or cohort studies. It is also possible that repetitive paravertebral blocks with local anesthetic and steroids may have a role, as one study revealed significantly reduced pain with acute injection, as well as reduced incidence of postherpetic neuralgia 3, 6, and 12 months posttherapy[4].

58. When should sympathetic blocks be considered for treatment of neuropathic pain?

Sympathetic blocks such as the classic stellate ganglion block and lumbar sympathetic block (depending on affected region) should be considered when CRPS or sympathetic involvement in pain is suspected. CRPS, types 1 and 2, may have significant sympathetic involvement. Aside from typical neuropathic pain description and allodynia, vasomotor instability, swelling, hair and nail changes, and temperature changes can indicate sympathetic system dysfunction. Traditionally sympathetic blocks have had both diagnostic and therapeutic roles in management of sympathetically maintained pain, despite the fact that there is weak evidence to support its role in diagnosis.

59. Describe some more invasive techniques used in treatment such as spinal cord stimulation.

Spinal cord stimulation (SCS) includes percutaneous placement of electric leads or surgical placement of a "paddle" lead in the posterior epidural space. The leads are secured in place and tunneled under the skin to a pulse generator implanted subcutaneously. The device sends electric impulses to the spinal cord with multiple possible pain relieving mechanisms, including alterations in wide dynamic range neuron function, facilitation of inhibition, changes in multiple neurotransmitters, and dorsal column activation to alter nociceptive processing at the spinal cord and brain. The devices are programmable with many parameters under patient control. A temporary preimplantation trial of SCS is typically performed prior to permanent system implantation. The technology is rapidly evolving with new waveforms and programming, hardware improvements, and new indications. SCS has evidence for efficacy in radicular pain, postlaminectomy pain syndrome, peripheral neuropathy, and CRPS. In postlaminectomy pain syndrome, SCS appears to be more efficacious than either reoperation or traditional medical management.

60. What about intrathecal drug delivery?

Intrathecal pumps may be used to deliver medication directly to the intrathecal space with immediate access to the spinal cord and via the cerebrospinal circulation to the brain. Typically opioids or a combination of opioids and local anesthetic are placed in a programmable reservoir located in the lower abdominal wall, where it connects to a catheter anchored in the intrathecal space. Baclofen is sometimes used for spasticity, clonidine can be used as an adjunct, and ziconotide is a nonopioid option. This method of delivery is much more efficient than the oral route, allowing for approximately 1/300th of the amount of morphine to be given and reducing associated side effects. It has been used in multiple types of pain complaints, including postlaminectomy pain syndrome, multiple sclerosis, and CRPS, as well as nonneuropathic conditions like cancer or chronic pancreatitis. Long-term pain reduction is often modest.

61. Anything *more* invasive than that? What about dorsal root entry zone lesioning and deep brain stimulation?

   Dorsal root entry zone (DREZ) lesioning involves a neurosurgeon exposing the spinal canal via a laminectomy and inserting a small probe under a microscope to destroy dorsal horn cells of the spinal cord via radiofrequency ablation. The procedure has had promising results in treatment of brachial or sacral plexus avulsion and SCI, but has not been found to be useful in phantom limb pain. Risks include unintentional injury to the spinal cord, which could cause long-term weakness or sensation changes. Deep brain stimulation (DBS) has been used in epilepsy, Tourette syndrome, and psychiatric disorders, as well as chronic pain. It involves placement of electrodes to the ventral posterior lateral and medial thalamic nuclei, or the periventricular grey matter. Long-term results have been mixed, though may be effective for neuropathic pain and phantom limb pain in well-selected patients.

62. Woah. I'm not ready to send my patient to a surgeon yet. Or should I?

   It is important to treat the underlying cause if there is specific target for treatment. Obviously, DREZ lesioning and DBS are drastic measures, but surgeons may have a role earlier on as well in specific neuropathic syndromes. Carpal tunnel release is a straightforward example of how surgery may be indicated in a specific entrapment peripheral neuropathy (median nerve). Similarly, spinal surgery may become indicated in severe central stenosis or radiculopathy due to significant neural foraminal stenosis, particularly if a neurologic deficit appears. Spine surgery should be very carefully considered if the patient's only indication is pain, as results are variable.

63. Are there any new treatment options in the pipeline?

   Transcranial magnetic stimulation (TMS) is an intriguing option that utilizes a magnetic field to alter brain activity, as a noninvasive alternative to surgical DBS. TMS was approved by the FDA in 2008 for treatment of major depression and is now being explored for use in chronic, intractable pain. It has become clear that repetitive TMS (rTMS) may be required for meaningful treatment, though the optimal number and interval between sessions is unclear, as is the duration of effect on neuroplasticity.

Acknowledgments

Thank you to Drs. Russell K. Portenoy, MD; Ricardo Cruciani, MD, PhD; and Charles Argoff for providing the basis on which this chapter was developed, as authors of "Neuropathic Pain" in the prior edition of *Pain Secrets*.

KEY POINTS

1. Neuropathic pain is a clinical descriptor of pain caused by a lesion or disease of the somatosensory nervous system.
2. Both peripheral and CNS mechanisms may be responsible for neuropathic pain conditions.
3. Identifying as specifically as possible the etiology of the neuropathic pain syndrome may lead to more effective treatment.
4. Numerous therapies, including pharmacologic, interventional, and physiatric, are available for the treatment of neuropathic pain.

REFERENCES

1. Dworkin RH, O'Connor AB, Audette J, et al. Recommendations for the pharmacologic management of neuropathic pain: an overview and literature update. *Mayo Clin Proc*. 2010;85(3 suppl):S2-S14.
2. Backonja M. Neuropathic pain therapy: from bench to bedside. *Semin Neurol*. 2012;32:264-268.
3. Cohen SP, Bicket MC, Jamison D, Wilkinson I, Rathmell JP. Epidural steroids: a comprehensive, evidence-based review. *Reg Anesth Pain Med*. 2013;38:175-200.
4. Ji G, Niu J, Shi Y, et al. The effectiveness of repetitive paravertebral injections with local anesthetics and steroids for the prevention of postherpetic neuralgia in patients with acute herpes zoster. *Anesth Analg*. 2009;109:1651-1655.
5. International Association for the Study of Pain (IASP). Taxonomy. http://www.iasp-pain.org/Taxonomy. Updated on 22 May 2012. Accessed 4 March 2017.
6. Bhatia N, Chow F. Neurologic complications in treated HIV-1 infection. *Curr Neurol Neurosci Rep*. 2016;16:62.
7. Collins S, Sigtermans MJ, Dahan A, Zuurmond WW, Perez RS. NMDA receptor antagonists for the treatment of neuropathic pain. *Pain Med*. 2010;11(11):1726-1742.

CHAPTER 31

DEPRESSION AND ANXIETY IN CHRONIC PAIN

Sarah Narayan, Alycia Reppel and Andrew Dubin

INTRODUCTION

In recent years, the biopsychosocial nature of chronic pain has become more widely recognized, and efforts to understand the complex interactions between physiologic and psychosocial aspects of chronic pain have increased. In particular, depression and anxiety have been noted to be present in many people with chronic pain; in some cases, these psychologic illnesses are present prior to the onset of pain, and in others, they develop following the onset of pain. Depression is the most common comorbid psychologic diagnosis associated with chronic pain, but anxiety is also common and can contribute to fixation on symptoms.

1. **What is the DSM-5? What are differences between the DSM-5 and the DSM-4 as they pertain to chronic pain?**

   The *Diagnostic and Statistical Manual of Mental Disorders*, Fifth Edition (DSM-5) is the 2013 update to the American Psychiatric Association's classification and diagnostic tool. DSM-5 classifications are used to determine psychiatric diagnoses, treatment recommendations, and payment in the United States. There are many differences between the DSM-4 and the DSM-5. The DSM-5 does not employ a multiaxial system as the DSM-4 did, and instead is divided into three sections. Section I is the introductory section. Section II is diagnostic criteria and codes, and Section III is emerging measures and models.

   Some changes pertain to the field of pain medicine, specifically those changes having to do with somatoform disorders, which are now called somatic symptom and related disorders. Patients that present with chronic pain can now be diagnosed with somatic symptom disorder with predominant pain, psychological factors that affect other medical conditions, or with an adjustment disorder. "Psychological factors affecting other medical conditions" is a new diagnosis. These changes are based in large part on a movement away from an emphasis on medically unexplained symptoms, to a focus on the way patients present and interpret their somatic symptoms, rather than solely the symptoms themselves.

   Mental disorders such as major depressive disorder and anxiety disorders may initially present with primarily somatic symptoms (e.g., pain). These disorders may fully account for the symptoms, or they may be concurrent with symptoms that have an identifiable organic etiology. Patients may suffer from major depressive disorder, dysthymia, or an anxiety disorder prior to the development of chronic pain. In others, these psychiatric illnesses arise as a consequence of chronic pain. In this case, a diagnosis of "depressive disorder due to another medical condition" or "anxiety disorder due to another medical condition" may be made.

   The somatic symptom disorders and related disorders have multiple contributing factors: genetic and biological vulnerability, early traumatic experiences, presence of learned behaviors, and social and cultural norms that devalue and stigmatize psychological suffering versus physical suffering. This group of disorders is characterized by the prominent focus on somatic concerns and the tendency to initially present mainly in medical rather than mental health care settings. Psychological factors affecting other conditions is a common entity in the world of chronic pain; the presence of one or more clinically significant psychological or behavioral factors that adversely affect a medical condition by increasing the risk for suffering, death, or disability is necessary for this diagnosis. Although an individual may not have official psychiatric diagnoses, psychological factors can hamper their ability to recover appropriately from a period of acute pain as well as encourage their transition to a chronic pain state.

2. What are the DSM-5 diagnostic criteria for major depressive disorder?

A. Five (or more) of the following symptoms have been present during the same 2-week period and represent a change from previous functioning; at least one of the symptoms is either (1) depressed mood or (2) loss of interest or pleasure.

1. Depressed mood most of the day, nearly every day, as indicated by either subjective report (e.g., feels sad, empty, hopeless) or observation made by others (e.g., appears tearful)
2. Markedly diminished interest or pleasure in all, or almost all, activities most of the day, nearly every day (as indicated by either subjective account or observation)
3. Significant weight loss when not dieting or weight gain (e.g., a change of more than 5% of body weight in a month), or decrease or increase in appetite nearly every day
4. Insomnia or hypersomnia nearly every day
5. Psychomotor agitation or retardation nearly every day (observable by others, not merely subjective feelings of restlessness or being slowed down)
6. Fatigue or loss of energy nearly every day
7. Feelings of worthlessness or excessive or inappropriate guilt (which may be delusional) nearly every day (not merely self-reproach or guilt about being sick)
8. Diminished ability to think or concentrate, or indecisiveness, nearly every day (either by subjective account or as observed by others)
9. Recurrent thoughts of death (not just fear of dying), recurrent suicidal ideation without a specific plan, or a suicide attempt or a specific plan for committing suicide

B. The symptoms cause clinically significant distress or impairment in social, occupational, or other important areas of functioning.

C. The episode is not attributable to the physiological effects of a substance or to another medical condition.

D. The occurrence of the major depressive episode is not better explained by schizoaffective disorder, schizophrenia, schizophreniform disorder, delusional disorder, or other specified and unspecified schizophrenia spectrum and other psychotic disorders.

E. There has never been a manic episode or a hypomanic episode.

3. What are the DSM-5 diagnostic criteria for depressive disorder due to another medical condition?

A. A prominent and persistent period of depressed mood or markedly diminished interest or pleasure in all, or almost all, activities that predominates in the clinical picture.

B. There is evidence from the history, physical examination, or laboratory findings that the disturbance is the direct pathophysiological consequence of another medical condition.

C. The disturbance is not better explained by another mental disorder (e.g., adjustment disorder, with depressed mood, in which the stressor is a serious medical condition).

D. The disturbance does not occur exclusively during the course of a delirium. The disturbance causes clinically significant distress or impairment in social, occupational, or other important areas of functioning.

4. What are the DSM-5 diagnostic criteria for somatic symptom disorder?

A. One or more somatic symptoms that are distressing or result in significant disruption of daily life

B. Excessive thoughts, feelings, or behaviors related to the somatic symptoms or associated health concerns as manifested by at least one of the following:

1. Disproportionate and persistent thoughts about the seriousness of one's symptoms
2. Persistently high level of anxiety about health or symptoms
3. Excessive time and energy devoted to these symptoms or health concerns

C. Although any one somatic symptom may not be continuously present, the state of being symptomatic is persistent (typically more than 6 months).

If the somatic symptoms predominantly involve pain, the specifier "with predominant pain" is added. Severity (mild, moderate, or severe) is also specified. If the symptoms are severe and there is marked impairment with duration more than 6 months, the specifier "persistent" is added.

There are multiple associated features that may be present in conjunction with somatic symptom disorder. There may be increased attention focused on somatic symptoms, attribution of normal bodily sensations to physical illness (sometimes with catastrophizing), worry about illness, and fear that any physical activity may damage the body. The individual may repeatedly check their body for abnormalities, seek medical help and reassurance repeatedly, and avoid physical activity. Somatic symptom disorder is associated with depressive disorders, and therefore there is an increased suicide risk. It is unclear whether somatic symptom disorder has an independent association with suicide risk.

Somatic symptom disorder is likely more prevalent in females versus males. It is more common in those with lower education level and lower socioeconomic status, those who are unemployed, as well as those individuals who have experienced a recent traumatic life event and/or have a past history of sexual abuse. The individuals often have concurrent medial and/or psychiatric diagnoses. The personality trait of neuroticism is associated with greater number of somatic symptoms. The disorder is associated with marked impairment of health status.

5. What are the DSM-5 diagnostic criteria for psychological factors affecting other conditions?
   A. A medical symptom or condition (other than a mental disorder) is present.
   B. Psychological or behavioral factors adversely affect the medical condition in one of the following ways:
      1. The factors have influenced the course of the medical condition as shown by a close temporal association between the psychological factors and the development or exacerbation of, or delayed recovery from, the medical condition.
      2. The factors interfere with the treatment of the medical condition (e.g., poor adherence).
      3. The factors constitute additional well-established health risks for the individual.
      4. The factors influence the underlying pathophysiology, precipitating or exacerbating symptoms or necessitating medical attention.
   C. The psychological and behavioral factors in criterion B are not better explained by another mental disorder (e.g., panic disorder, major depressive disorder, posttraumatic stress disorder). Severity (mild, moderate, severe, or extreme) is specified.
      Psychological or behavioral factors include psychological distress, patterns of interpersonal interaction, coping styles, and maladaptive health behaviors. The affected medical conditions include ones with a clear pathophysiology, but also include functional syndromes such as migraine and fibromyalgia, and medical symptoms such as fatigue and chronic pain.

6. What are the DSM-5 diagnostic criteria for generalized anxiety disorder?
   A. Excessive anxiety and worry (apprehensive expectation), occurring more days than not for at least 6 months, about a number of events or activities (such as work or school performance).
   B. The individual finds it difficult to control the worry.
   C. The anxiety and worry are associated with three (or more) of the following six symptoms (with at least some symptoms having been present for more days than not for the past 6 months):
      1. Restlessness or feeling keyed up or on edge
      2. Being easily fatigued
      3. Difficulty concentrating or mind going blank
      4. Irritability
      5. Muscle tension
      6. Sleep disturbance (difficulty falling or staying asleep, or restless, unsatisfying sleep)
   D. The anxiety, worry, or physical symptoms cause clinically significant distress or impairment in social, occupational, or other important areas of functioning.
   E. The disturbance is not attributable to the physiological effects of a substance (e.g., a drug of abuse, a medication) or another medical condition (e.g., hyperthyroidism).
   F. The disturbance is not better explained by another mental disorder.

7. What are the DSM-5 diagnostic criteria for anxiety disorder due to another medical condition?
   A. Panic attacks or anxiety is predominant in the clinical picture.
   B. There is evidence from the history, physical examination, or laboratory findings that the disturbance is the direct pathophysiological consequence of another medical condition.
   C. The disturbance is not better explained by another mental disorder.
   D. The disturbance does not occur exclusively during the course of a delirium.
   E. The disturbance causes clinically significant distress or impairment in social, occupational, or other important areas of functioning.

8. What is the prevalence of depression in the setting of chronic pain?
   The prevalence of depression in people with chronic pain ranges from 31% to 100% across sources. The variability between studies is likely due to a number of factors, including varying time duration

used for the definition of chronic, varying definitions of depression, and differing checklists and questionnaires.

The prevalence of depression in chronic pain patients does seem to be consistently higher than the prevalence in the general population. A large survey performed in Michigan found that the prevalence of chronic pain due to any cause was 21.9%, and approximately 35% of the participants with chronic pain had comorbid depression.

In one large epidemiologic study, the prevalence of depression in individuals with chronic pain conditions was 11.3% versus 5.3% in those without. The data suggested that there are approximately twice as many pain disorders with a higher prevalence in women versus men. Also, women suffer from both depression and chronic pain conditions at approximately twice the prevalence of men.

9. What is the prevalence of anxiety in the setting of chronic pain?
The exact prevalence of anxiety disorder in chronic pain is unclear, due to a lack of studies specifically looking at this. However, it is widely recognized that it is not uncommon for patients with chronic pain to be anxious and worried. When patients with chronic pain do carry a diagnosis of anxiety disorder, it is rarely the only psychiatric diagnosis; often there is a comorbid depression or dysthymia diagnosis. It is important to note that often the anxiety can be diminished or even eradicated when treatment is directed at the mood disorder.

In patients with chronic pain, it is important not to overlook a potential diagnosis of panic disorder, as this may present with complaints of chronic headache, chronic abdominal pain, and/or chronic chest pain. Panic disorder is more common in females than in men, and usually the onset is before the fourth decade of life. Often these patients have a fear of an undiagnosed life-threatening medical illness, and therefore they often first present in the medicine setting.

10. What is the relationship between anxiety and depression and chronic pain?
A cause and effect relationship between chronic pain and depression and anxiety may be present. However, the exact relationship has yet to be defined and continues to be a topic of debate among clinicians and researchers. One 4-year longitudinal study in the Netherlands found that there appears to be a synchrony of change in anxiety, depression, and pain over time. However, even after their anxiety and depression are in remission, subjects reported higher pain ratings. It was concluded that even a history of depression and anxiety puts individuals at higher risk for chronic pain.

There seems to be an association between chronic pain and depression in different ethnic groups. However, reporting varies across ethnic groups and there are differences in health seeking behavior across groups, and this makes gathering data difficult. There are also differences due to cultural barriers regarding expression of concern about mood and pain, coping strategies, and language barriers. These aspects need to be taken into account and addressed when managing chronic pain and depression in minorities.

It has been found that the association between obesity and back pain is stronger in people who have an emotional disorder. This association is still present after accounting for the prevalence of emotional disorders in those who are obese. Obesity, depression, and anxiety are all recognized as inflammatory states and higher levels of proinflammatory cytokines that have been shown to have a relationship with the progression to chronic pain. Therefore, one hypothesis regarding this relationship is that people with an emotional disorder may be sensitized to experience pain, and this may be magnified by the presence of the inflammatory state associated with increased adipose tissue. This suggests that weight loss counseling may be especially important for those patients who are obese and have comorbid depression and/or anxiety.

Depression and anxiety are more common in patients with chronic headaches than episodic headaches, and have a significant impact on quality of life in patients with both episodic headaches and chronic headaches. Depression and anxiety have a significant impact on employment status, earnings, career success, and these patients feel less understood in general, according to one Austrian study. Persisting anxiety in the early phase of acute neck pain and depression at baseline have been found to be risk factors for poor self-reported recovery and may contribute to the transition from acute to chronic neck pain. Therefore, these factors should be addressed early in the course of the illness.

A more recent theory regarding the relationship between mood disorders and chronic pain is that emotions lie at the interface between physical and psychological processes. Therefore, it has been hypothesized that emotional processing deficits play a role in the development of chronic low back pain (CLBP). The results of one study exploring whether patients with chronic low back pain process their emotions differently compared to asymptomatic individuals suggests that dysfunctional emotional processing is indeed associated with chronic low back pain. However, a causal relationship has yet to be established. One hypothesized model is the fear-anxiety-avoidance model, which proposes that pain-related anxiety and anxiety sensitivity are important factors in the development and maintenance of chronic musculoskeletal pain.

Attempts have been made to identify syndromes that might unify the presence of multiple comorbidities, including anxiety, mood disorders, and chronic pain. For example, one such proposed syndrome is called anxiety-laxity-pain-immune-mood (ALPIM) syndrome. A study found significant relationships between a cluster of comorbidities that includes a core anxiety disorder, joint laxity, chronic pain syndromes, immune disorders, and mood disorders. It is therefore postulated that there may be a genetic predisposition for development of ALPIM.

Researchers have attempted to elucidate the biological basis of the relationship between chronic pain and psychological disorders. One study using a rat model of neuropathic pain shows that chronic neuropathic pain leads to affective behavioral dysfunctions related to classical anxiety and depression symptoms. These changes are accompanied by a noradrenergic impairment similar to that described for depressive disorders. A theory regarding the neurobiological basis of anxiety and chronic pain proposes that anxiety is mediated through presynaptic long-term potentiation in the anterior cingulate cortex, which is a key region for pain perception, and that postsynaptic long-term potentiation plays a role in the behavioral sensitization to chronic pain.

11. How is depression diagnosed in the setting of chronic pain?

Diagnosing depression in the setting of chronic pain is challenging due to the presence of symptom overlap. Because of this, it has been suggested that questionnaires such as the Beck Depression Inventory may have less utility in the setting of chronic pain. One method that has been proposed to improve ease and specificity of diagnosis is to separately analyze somatic and cognitive-emotional symptoms. However, the association between these separate categories and variables such as chronic pain intensity and disability has yet to be elucidated.

It is important to note that a depressed mood does not always equate to a diagnosis of major depression; however, it is also important to realize that the presence of chronic pain does not exclude one from a diagnosis of major depression. Often, patients with symptoms of depression will attribute all of those symptoms to their chronic pain. A good number of chronic pain patients will endorse anhedonia, the inability to enjoy activities or experience pleasure, even when they are not experiencing pain or an increase in pain during the activities. In the same vein, poor sleep and poor concentration are also often attributed to pain when they are not direct physiologic effects of pain, and therefore they should be considered symptoms of depression.

Regardless of the presence or absence of a specific psychiatric diagnosis, a differential diagnosis including bipolar disorder, dysthymic disorder, and substance-induced mood disorder should be considered. A psychiatric or psychology practitioner with a focus in pain should be involved in order to provide the most comprehensive chronic pain care.

12. What is the stress and coping model?

Initially presented by Lazarus, the stress and coping model explains a possible network of relationships between psychological processes and pain. The basis of this model is the belief that coping starts with appraisals of a stressful situation. In chronic pain, appraisal involves characterizing the threats that the pain poses and identifying coping strategies that address the threats. These appraisals reflect the person's beliefs about their condition. These beliefs can be associated with positive or negative coping. The belief that one can control one's own pain is associated with better adaptation to pain than belief that one cannot control one's own pain. The belief that one can recover from pain is also positively associated with coping ability.

Patients often have intense emotional reactions to cognitive appraisal, and in turn cognition can influence these emotions. Most of these emotional reactions can be characterized as anxiety, depression, or anger. These emotions may lead to maladaptive coping strategies, which may lead to increased and/or prolonged pain. Therefore, many treatment strategies have focused on interrupting this self-perpetuating cycle.

13. What is pain catastrophizing?

Pain catastrophizing is a negatively distorted perception of pain as awful, horrible, and unbearable. It is strongly associated with depression and pain. Functional magnetic resonance imaging (fMRI) has shown that pain catastrophizing is independently associated with increased activity in areas related to anticipation of pain, attention to pain, and emotional aspects of pain and motor control.

A study exploring the relationship among catastrophizing, depression, and chronic pain found that elements of catastrophizing, particularly magnification and helplessness, partially mediate the relationship between pain intensity and depressed mood in older adult patients with chronic pain. It also found that these elements completely mediate the relationship between pain intensity and depressed mood in patients 80 years and older. This supports a cognitive-behavioral mediation model and has implications for the treatment of persistent pain in older individuals, especially the "oldest old" who can especially benefit from efforts to reduce catastrophizing.

Catastrophizing is associated with poorer outcomes. One Scandinavian study exploring the relationship among social anxiety, catastrophizing, and return-to-work self-efficacy in chronic pain patients found that social anxiety and pain catastrophizing correlated positively with each other and negatively with the perceived ability to communicate pain-related needs. Social anxiety was found to be a significant predictor of an individual's ability to communicate pain-related needs to the work environment. Pain severity was not found to be associated with the individual's confidence in communicating pain-related needs. It was concluded that anxiety and fears relating to pain-related social situations at work may have a significant impact on the return-to-work process and rehabilitation in chronic pain.

14. How does depression in the setting of chronic pain impact medical costs?

Patients with major depressive disorder (MDD) and comorbid disabling chronic pain have higher medical service costs when compared to patients with depression and nondisabling chronic pain, major depressive disorder alone, and disabling chronic pain alone, and patients with neither depression nor chronic pain. It appears that the cost increase is additive rather than multiplicative.

15. What is the relationship between chronic pain and suicide?

Chronic pain is associated with a higher risk for suicidal thoughts and suicide across all age groups. The relationship between pain and suicidal thoughts and behaviors is complex.

A recent meta-analysis concluded that:

- Individuals with physical pain were more likely to show a lifetime death wish, both current and lifetime suicidal ideation, suicide plans, and suicide attempts, and to die by suicide.
- There is high between-studies heterogeneity due to differences in pain characteristics, type of pain, intensity, and duration, as well as differences in methods of evaluation of pain, assessed suicide outcomes, study designs, control samples, age of population, geographic location of population, number of physical disorders, and the presence of comorbid psychiatric disorders.
- Due to this heterogeneity, further investigation is needed regarding specific pain conditions and suicidality, as well as chronic versus acute pain, and risk factors for suicide in chronic pain patients.

What are the treatment strategies for chronic pain with co-morbid depression and/or anxiety?

Mindfulness-based stress reduction (MBSR) is a structured training program that aims to provide adaptive coping, focused attention, and cognitive restructuring skills to distressed populations. These programs have been shown to have positive outcomes in patients with chronic pain, especially chronic back pain. It has been suggested that an abbreviated 4-week MBSR program (as opposed to the traditional 8-week program) may be an effective complementary intervention for back pain patients. However, there appears to be a dose-response relationship among pain, depression, anxiety, and MBSR; therefore, a course that is at least 8 weeks provides a more solid foundation and likely leads to more enduring positive cognitive and emotional changes. On fMRI, patients who have gone through both abbreviated and full MBSR courses show increased frontal lobe hemodynamic activity, which is thought to be associated with gains in awareness of their emotional state.

Intensity of pain correlates with intensity of psychological symptoms, including depression, anxiety, and worry. Active pain coping strategies such as striving to function in spite of pain and distracting oneself from pain are adaptive strategies. Passive strategies that involve withdrawal or relinquishing control are maladaptive strategies that are related to greater pain and depression.

Cognitive-behavioral methods (CBT) of pain treatment in the domains of pain experience, cognitive coping, and appraisal are effective in reducing pain. Multifaceted cognitive behavioral treatment regimens need further study—more specifically, they need to be compared to placebo. Recently, web-based CBT has been proposed as a potentially cost- and time-effective treatment strategy. It is important to take into account comorbidities when developing the CBT plan. For example, it has been shown that children with chronic pain and anxiety are more likely to initiate and complete CBT than those that have chronic pain without anxiety, but still have poorer outcomes. One proposed strategy to address this is to identify these individuals with anxiety prior to CBT and initiate tailored behavioral interventions.

Managing expectations prior to an event that may be uncomfortable or painful (giving information regarding procedural and objective aspects as well as information about the specific sensations that the patient may experience during the event) may alter patients' cognitive appraisal of an event, which may result in shorter subjective pain duration and intensity. Combining the provision of this preparatory information with information/training regarding coping skills and reduction of stress and anxiety reactions appears to be more effective than providing preparatory information alone.

Stress-inoculation training is a CBT intervention that has three phases. It takes into account the multidimensional nature of differences between individuals' reactions to pain and provides multiple options for coping skills. There is an educational phase, a rehearsal phase, and an application phase. The effectiveness of this method is unclear.

Yoga has been shown to be an effective complementary component of comprehensive chronic pain management programs, especially for individuals with anxiety, depression, and chronic low back pain.

KEY POINTS

1. The DSM-5 employs a format that differs from the DSM-4. Chronic pain patients may fall under the "somatic symptom disorders and related disorders" diagnostic category.
2. The relationship between depression, anxiety, and chronic pain is unclear. Depression and anxiety are more prevalent in the chronic pain population than in the population without chronic pain.
3. Making the official diagnosis of depression in the setting of chronic pain is complicated by symptom overlap. An official diagnosis need not be made before involving a psychiatry and/or psychology practitioner in the patient's care.
4. Chronic pain is associated with a higher risk for suicidal thoughts and suicide across all age groups.
5. The relationship between psychological processes, emotions, and pain is complex. Pain catastrophizing is a negatively distorted perception of pain as awful, horrible, and unbearable. It is strongly associated with depression and pain.

BIBLIOGRAPHY

1. American Psychiatric Association. *Diagnostic and Statistical Manual of Mental Disorders: DSM-5.* 5th ed. Washington, DC: American Psychiatric Association; 2013.
2. Miller L, Cano A. Comorbid chronic pain and depression: who is at risk? *J Pain.* 2009;10:616-627.
3. Nicholl BI, Smith DJ, Cullen B, et al. Ethnic differences in the association between depression and chronic pain: cross sectional results from UK Biobank. *BMC Fam Pract.* 2015;16:128.
4. Chou L, Brady SR, Urquhart DM, et al. The association between obesity and low back pain and disability is affected by mood disorders: a population-based cross-sectional study of men. *Medicine (Baltimore).* 2016;95(15):e3367.
5. Zebenholzer K, Lechner A, Broessner G, et al. Impact of depression and anxiety on burden and management of episodic and chronic headaches—a cross-sectional multicentre study in eight Austrian headache centres. *J Headache Pain.* 2016;17:15.
6. Knaster P, Estlander AM, Karlsson H, Kaprio J, Kalso E. Diagnosing depression in chronic pain patients: DSM-IV major depressive disorder vs. Beck depression inventory (BDI). *PLoS ONE.* 2016;11(3):e0151982.
7. Wirth B, Humphreys BK, Peterson C. Importance of psychological factors for the recovery from a first episode of acute non-specific neck pain—a Longitudinal Observational Study. *Chiropr Man Therap.* 2016;24:9.
8. Arnow BA, Blasey CM, Lee J, et al. Relationships among depression, chronic pain, chronic disabling pain, and medical costs. *Psychiatr Serv.* 2009;60(3):344-350.
9. Braden BB, Pipe TB, Smith R, et al. Brain and behavior changes associated with an abbreviated 4-week mindfulness-based stress reduction course in back pain patients. *Brain Behav.* 2016;6(3):e00443.
10. Gorczyca R, Filip R, Walczak E. Psychological aspects of pain. *Ann Agric Environ Med.* 2013;1:23-27.
11. Esteves JE, Wheatley L, Mayall C, Abbey H. Emotional processing and its relationship to chronic low back pain: results from a case-control study. *Man Ther.* 2013;18(6):541-546.
12. Munce SE, Stewart DE. Gender differences in depression and chronic pain conditions in a national epidemiologic survey. *Psychosomatics.* 2007;48(5):394-399.

13. van Tilburg MA, Spence NJ, Whitehead WE, Bangdiwala S, Goldston DB. Chronic pain in adolescents is associated with suicidal thoughts and behaviors. *J Pain.* 2011;12(10):1032-1039.
14. Calati R, Laglaoui Bakhiyi C, Artero S, Ilgen M, Courtet P. The impact of physical pain on suicidal thoughts and behaviors: meta-analyses. *J Psychiatr Res.* 2015;71:16-32.
15. Alba-Delgado C, Llorca-Torralba M, Horrillo I, et al. Chronic pain leads to concomitant noradrenergic impairment and mood disorders. *Biol Psychiatry.* 2013;73(1):54-62.
16. Howe CQ, Robinson JP, Sullivan MD. Psychiatric and psychological perspectives on chronic pain. *Phys Med Rehabil Clin N Am.* 2015;26(2):283-300.
17. Zhuo M. Neural mechanisms underlying anxiety—chronic pain interactions. *Trends Neurosci.* 2016;39(3):136-145.
18. Coplan J, Singh D, Gopinath S, Mathew SJ, Bulbena A. A novel anxiety and affective spectrum disorder of mind and body—the ALPIM (anxiety-laxity-pain-immune-mood) syndrome: a preliminary report. *J Neuropsychiatry Clin Neurosci.* 2015;27(2):93-103.
19. Thomtén J, Boersma K, Flink I, Tillfors M. Social anxiety, pain catastrophizing and return-to-work self-efficacy in chronic pain: a cross-sectional study. *Scand J Pain.* 2016;11:98-103.
20. Carleton RN, Abrams MP, Asmundson GJ, Antony MM, McCabe RE. Pain-related anxiety and anxiety sensitivity across anxiety and depressive disorders. *J Anxiety Disord.* 2009;23(6):791-798.
21. Gerrits MM, van Marwijk HW, van Oppen P, van der Horst H, Penninx BW. Longitudinal association between pain, and depression and anxiety over four years. *J Psychosom Res.* 2015;78(1):64-70.
22. Cunningham NR, Jagpal A, Tran ST, et al. Anxiety adversely impacts response to cognitive behavioral therapy in children with chronic pain. *J Pediatr.* 2016;17(1):227-233.
23. Macea DD, Gajos K, Daglia Calil YA, Fregni F. The efficacy of web-based cognitive behavioral interventions for chronic pain: a systematic review and meta-analysis. *J Pain.* 2010;11(10):917-929.
24. Tekur P, Nagarathna R, Chametcha S, Hankey A, Nagendra HR. A comprehensive yoga programs improves pain, anxiety and depression in chronic low back pain patients more than exercise: an RCT. *Complement Ther Med.* 2012;20(3):107-118.

CHAPTER 32

PERSONALITY DISORDERS IN CHRONIC PAIN

Michael R. Clark and Michael A. Bushey

1. **What is a personality disorder?**
   The *Diagnostic and Statistical Manual of Mental Disorders,* Fifth Edition (DSM-5), defines a personality disorder as "an enduring pattern of inner experience and behavior that deviates markedly from the expectations of the individual's culture, is pervasive and inflexible, has an onset in adolescence or early adulthood, is stable over time, and leads to distress or impairment."

2. **Are there types of personality disorders?**
   The DSM-5 recognizes 10 distinct personality disorders, which are arranged into clusters. Cluster A personalities are the "odd" types, including paranoid (suspicious), schizoid (detached), and schizotypal (eccentric). Cluster B personality disorders are considered "dramatic" types and include antisocial (disregard for others), narcissistic (self-important), borderline (emotionally unstable), and histrionic (attention-seeking). Cluster C personality disorders are "anxious" types and include dependent (submissive and clingy), avoidant (feels inadequate), and obsessive-compulsive (perfectionistic). The DSM also recognizes personality change due to a medical condition or unspecified/other specified personality disorder to include patients with significant personality dysfunction that do not meet specific criteria for other diagnoses. Due to considerable shortcomings with interrater reliability, and with patients often meeting criteria for more than one personality disorder, the DSM-5 introduces a second system that defines personality dysfunction based on traits rather than categorical diagnoses.

3. **Do certain personality disorders predispose patients to chronic pain?**
   While chronic pain strikes patients of all personality types, patients meeting criteria for Cluster C personality disorders are especially at risk. These patients tend to be high in harm avoidance and lower in self-directedness, which have been shown to be overrepresented in patients with chronic pain. These traits predispose a person to engaging in fear-avoidance behaviors, which have been implicated in the initiation of chronic pain-related disability. These patients tend to be highly anxious, which can also promote avoidance of negative experiences, leading to underutilization of rehabilitation therapies, muscle atrophy, and global deconditioning.

4. **Are personalities influenced by chronic pain?**
   Personality trait pathology, especially in the domains of anxiety, self-efficacy, and somatization, has been demonstrated to improve with treatment of chronic pain. As the patient's symptoms improve, the vulnerability of their trait composition is less likely to be provoked. Conversely, the emergence of chronic pain can lead to the development of maladaptive reactions that are manifestations of personality trait vulnerabilities under stress in patients that did not previously exhibit them.

5. **Are certain personality disorders predisposed to developing problematic substance use?**
   Patients with Cluster B types are particularly vulnerable to the positively reinforcing effects produced by taking medications that provide immediate positive psychoactive effects (euphoria). This is especially true of opiates and benzodiazepines. These patients do not tolerate the strong negative emotions produced by pain, and therefore, they are primed for the negative reinforcement of pain relief. As a result, even when the negative consequences of substance abuse begin to mount, these patients have difficulty discontinuing their use because of powerful reinforcements already established.

6. **If a patient is "difficult," does that mean that they have a personality disorder?**
   Difficult patients generally fall into three categories: demanding, noncompliant, and high-utilizing. In each case, the difficulty may be related to an underlying personality disorder or may be from

another secondary cause. In each case, a personality disorder should be considered just one possibility in the differential diagnoses.

7. How do you treat the difficult patient?

Patient Type	Characteristics	Treatment Goal	Therapeutic Tactic
Demanding	Doesn't take "no" for an answer	Turn patient from a client into a patient	Set expectations (role induction), and follow through with consequences
Noncompliant	Is unable or unwilling to comply with treatment	Understand why they either "can't" or "won't" comply	Address the root cause, which can be anything from untreated depression (can't) to drug diversion (won't)
High-utilizing	High distress, unexplained symptoms, many previous treatment failures	Recognize and validate distress	Identify and treat the cause of the underlying distress

8. Do patients with personality disorder have altered pain sensitivity?
This relationship has most frequently been studied in patients with borderline personality disorder. Early studies conducted in mental health settings suggested that patients with borderline personality disorder have an insensitivity to pain. However, more recent studies of patients in the primary care setting suggest that patients scoring high on borderline personality scales tend to have higher sensitivity to pain and exhibit greater levels of pain catastrophizing. One recent study suggests that this discrepancy may be linked to self-injurious behaviors, with patients who have engaged in such behavior reporting lower levels of acute pain in a cold pressor task compared with borderline personality disorder patients who had not engaged in such self-injurious behavior.

9. How prevalent are personality disorders in chronic pain patients?
A recent review of eight prevalence studies suggests that the prevalence of borderline personality disorder in patients presenting to pain clinics is approximately 30%, which is significantly higher than the estimated 2% to 6% reported for the general population.

10. Are the goals of treatment different for pain patients with borderline personality disorder?
The goals of treatment for borderline personality disorder parallel the goals of treating chronic pain. In both cases, patients are working toward improving their function and developing skills to help tolerate discomfort. The goals of therapy are based upon changing behavior in the face of intense and distressing emotional states. Dialectical behavior therapy is the most widely recognized treatment for borderline personality disorder. This treatment is based on validating strong emotions and negative experiences, while helping the patient choose healthier behaviors despite these feelings.

11. Is there a role for medication in treating borderline personality disorder?
Because of the high prevalence of comorbid mood disorders in patients with borderline personality disorder, treatment of underlying mood disorders with appropriate antidepressants or mood stabilizers can provide significant benefit. Medications can help dampen their profound emotional reactivity, diminish their impulsive behaviors, and allow these patients sufficient relief from distress to engage in meaningful psychotherapy.

12. What is the prognosis of borderline personality disorder?
While personality or character is thought to consolidate in early adulthood as a result of life experience, personality disorders are independent paradigms based on personality trait extremes that incorporate numerous maladaptive behavioral responses. However, a 10-year follow-up study demonstrated that 88% of patients with borderline personality disorder entered remission, at which time they no longer meet criteria for the disorder.

13. **Is there a "right way" to interact with patients who have borderline personality disorder?**

Patients with borderline personality disorder are sensitive to the emotional attention paid to them by others, especially health care workers. Utilizing praise to positively reinforce even small progress while ignoring maladaptive behaviors is the most useful technique. Confrontation should be reserved for the most inappropriate actions. In these circumstances, emphasis should be placed on the potential immediate benefits to be gained or negative outcomes to be avoided if the patient engages in alternative behaviors.

14. **What practices should be avoided in treating patients with borderline personality disorder?**

Patients with borderline personality disorder are more likely than controls to report the use of prescription opiates. Prescribing opiates and benzodiazepines provide unique challenges in patients with borderline personality disorder. These medications provide an opportunity to escape, rather than cope with, unpleasant sensations. These medications produce robust positive reinforcement that is difficult to extinguish. As a result, poor coping strategies are rewarded. Scolding such patients should also be avoided, as this provides attention to negative behaviors, and may actually result in their reinforcement.

15. **How prevalent are suicide attempts and completion in patients with borderline personality disorder?**

An important consideration when managing patients with borderline personality disorders is their elevated rates of suicide attempts and completion of suicide. Suicide attempt rates are as high as 70% in this group, with 5% to 10% having completed suicides. Patients presenting to treatment for pain who have comorbid borderline personality disorder should be prescribed potentially lethal medications with caution given the potential for any prescribed medication to be taken intentionally with the intent to commit self-harm or suicide. In general, it is important to screen for suicidality in high-risk patients and to prescribe smaller quantities of medications more frequently than the usual monthly or even 90-day supply.

16. **Are there specific guidelines for treating patients with borderline personality disorder?**

Role induction is crucial in the treatment of patients with personality disorders. There should be very clear instructions regarding the appropriate ways to utilize the clinic and expectations regarding appointment adherence and following recommended prescriptions for treatment. Consequences for not following the rules should be made clear and reinforced. Despite the difficulty that these patients may have with meeting agreed upon goals, it is important that the clinician not lower expectations of the patient, as this will lead to worsening function and outcomes.

17. **When is it OK to call it quits with a difficult patient?**

As outlined previously, expectations for treatment should be clearly delineated. Generally, it is preferred that the practitioner not give up on the patient unless explicitly fired by the patient, which may be the result of the clinician not giving in to the patient's demands. It should be made clear that the patient is rejecting the clinician's help, and that the door would remain open, should the patient be willing in the future to adhere to treatment recommendations and act as a patient instead of a consumer.

KEY POINTS

1. Personality disorders do not cause chronic pain, but will affect the way that a particular patient presents and responds to treatment.
2. 30% of patients presenting to pain clinics meet criteria for borderline personality disorder.
3. Borderline personality disorder and chronic pain have similar treatment goals: working toward improving function and developing skills to help tolerate discomfort.
4. Patients with Cluster C personality disorders are highly susceptible to developing pain avoidant behaviors.
5. Patients with borderline personality disorder are vulnerable to the immediate rewards provided by opiates and benzodiazepines, which increases the risk of abuse.

BIBLIOGRAPHY

1. American Psychiatric Association. *Diagnostic and Statistical Manual of Mental Disorders.* 5th ed. Arlington, VA: American Psychiatric Publishing; 2013.
2. Carpenter RW, Trull TJ. The pain paradox: borderline personality disorder features, self-harm history, and the experience of pain. *Personal Disord.* 2015;6(2):141-151.
3. Clark M. The madwoman in the attic: pain and borderline personality disorder. *PainWeek.* 2014;2(Q3):22-29.
4. Frankenburg FR, Fitzmaurice GM, Zanarini MC. The use of prescription opioid medication by patients with borderline personality disorder and axis II comparison subjects: a 10-year follow-up study. *J Clin Psychiatry.* 2014;75(4):357-361.
5. Links PS, Ross J, Gunderson JG. Promoting good psychiatric management for patients with borderline personality disorder. *J Clin Psychol.* 2015;71(8):753-763.
6. Wasan AD, Sullivan MD, Clark MR. Psychiatric illness, depression, anxiety, and somatoform pain syndromes. In: Fishman SM, Ballantyne JC, Rathmell JP, eds. *Bonica's Management of Pain.* 4th ed. Baltimore, MD: Lippincott Williams & Wilkins; 2009.

CHAPTER 33

SUBSTANCE ABUSE IN CHRONIC PAIN

Eric Gruenthal and Julie G. Pilitsis

1. How is chronic pain management defined in this chapter?
Here we define chronic pain as pain that lasts for at least 90 days. Chronic pain management is defined as the use of medications or interventions with a goal of alleviating pain. The focus of this chapter is the use of opioids for chronic pain management and the possible consequence of addiction.

2. What is addiction?
The 2013 *Diagnostic and Statistical Manual of Mental Disorders*, Fifth Edition (DSM-5), defines addiction (substance use disorder) as a multifaceted disorder including behavioral, cognitive, and physiological symptoms. Characteristics are as follows:
1. Taking the substance in larger amounts or over a longer period than was originally intended
2. A persistent desire to cut down or regulate substance use and multiple unsuccessful efforts to decrease or discontinue use
3. Spending a great deal of time obtaining the substance, using the substance, or recovering from its effects
4. Craving manifested by an intense desire or urge for the drug
5. A failure to fulfill major role obligations at work, school, or home
6. Persistent or recurrent social or interpersonal problems caused or exacerbated by the effects of the substance
7. Important social, occupational, or recreational activities may be given up
8. Recurrent substance use in situations in which it is physically hazardous
9. Continued use despite knowledge of having a persistent or recurrent physical or psychological problem
10. Tolerance signaled by requiring a markedly increased dose of the substance to achieve the desired effect
11. Withdrawal when blood or tissue concentrations of a substance decline
    Mild substance use disorder is defined as two to three of these symptoms, moderate as four to five symptoms, and severe as six or more symptoms.

3. List the five main characteristics of addiction.
The "ABCDE" as provided by the American Society of Addiction Medicine as follows:
A. Inability to **A**bstain
B. Impaired **B**ehavioral control
C. **C**raving
D. **D**iminished recognition of problems with one's behaviors and relationships
E. Dysfunctional **E**motional response

4. What is physical dependence?
Physical dependence results from repeated use of a substance. The body becomes used to a substance, and withdrawal symptoms may occur when the substance is decreased, stopped, or an antagonist is used.

5. What are the symptoms of opioid intoxication?
Opioid intoxication is characterized by behavioral manifestations such as memory impairment, sleepiness, euphoria, confusion, delirium, and apathy, and by physical manifestations including lack of coordination, nausea, vomiting, pupillary constriction, slurred speech, bradycardia, and respiratory distress.

6. What are the symptoms of opioid withdrawal?

Opioid withdrawal is characterized by behavioral manifestations such as restlessness, anxiety, insomnia, and low energy, and physical manifestations such as muscle aches, nausea or vomiting, tearing, runny nose, sweating, pupillary dilation, and persistent yawning.

7. What is opioid tolerance, and how does it relate to addiction?

In the context of treating pain with opioids, tolerance is the need for higher doses in order to relieve pain. Patients using opioids for the treatment of pain may exhibit tolerance without addiction.

8. When is it appropriate to prescribe opioids for chronic pain management?

Two broad classes of chronic pain are typically defined: cancer-related pain and non-cancer-related pain. There is general agreement that for cancer-related pain, opioids may be an appropriate option.

For non-cancer-related chronic pain, however, patients often show little change in their reported pain scores during the course of long-term treatment. In fact, there is some evidence that opioids may do more harm than good and may diminish efforts to exercise to regain function and reduce pain. This is especially true for musculoskeletal pain: after an initial round of opioids to enable rehabilitation, guidelines suggest stopping opioid treatment. A multiyear study of postmenopausal patients with chronic pain showed that those who received opioids were less likely to experience improvement in their pain than those who did not. Similarly, opioids are contraindicated for headaches, which may actually worsen with treatment. However, if normal activity is not a realistic goal, such as in the elderly, or when other forms of pain management have failed, opioids may be a good choice for chronic pain management.

9. Is addiction common, and are patients vulnerable to dependence on opioid analgesics used for chronic pain syndromes?

The relationship between increased prescribing rates of opioids for chronic pain and opioid addiction is well known. In a recent meta-analysis, Vowles et al. in 2015 found that misuse (defined as underuse, overuse, erratic or disorganized use, and use with alcohol or illegal substances) occurs in nearly 25% of patients and addiction occurs in approximately 10% of patients treated with opioids for chronic pain. In addition, the sharing and stealing of prescriptions is a common practice that has contributed to the opioid addiction epidemic.

10. What are the risk factors for addiction to opioid treatment for pain management?

Risk factors include:

- Genetic and environmental factors including sexual abuse
- Family and personal history of addiction
- Psychiatric conditions like anxiety and impulse control disorders
- Age between 16 and 45

Using opioid risk screening tools that assess for these and other factors can help physicians identify patients who are at increased risk. See websites at the end of this chapter for such resources.

11. How has the landscape changed for physician liability with respect to addiction and pain management in the last 6 years?

The public health and political environment for physicians regarding addiction, opioids, and pain management has changed substantially since the last edition of this book. By 2012 drug overdose was the leading cause of injury deaths (more than car accidents) of individuals between 25 and 64 years old in the United States, and nearly 500,000 emergency room visits each year were related to opioids, an almost doubling of the number reported in the early 2000s. In 2014, both the US Department of Health and Human Services and the Centers for Disease Control designated deaths resulting from prescription opioids as an epidemic.

According to national surveys, physicians are largely blamed by the general public for the diversion and inappropriate use of opioids due to the excessive and prolonged treatment with these drugs for chronic pain management.

As a reaction, many states are enacting new laws to regulate prescribing habits of physicians. In March 2016 the federal government issued the first national guidelines on this topic. In those guidelines, while it is recognized that surgeons are often the first prescribers of opioids to reduce pain during initial recovery, it is postulated that the primary care physician typically manages the patient's opioid use. Awareness of the changing landscape of pain management is critical for maintaining the best practices possible and for minimizing the risk of litigation.

12. **What are the newest guidelines for physicians to minimize the risk of addiction to opioids in chronic pain management?**
    According to the Centers for Disease Control (CDC) Opioid-Prescribing Guidelines (March 2016):
    - Nonpharmacologic and nonopioid therapy are preferred for chronic pain.
    - Establish treatment goals with patients before starting opioid therapy.
    - When starting therapy, use immediate-release opioids instead of extended-release.
    - Initiate treatment with the lowest effective dose and avoid greater than 90 mg morphine equivalent per day.
    - Reevaluate for benefits and harms within 1 to 4 weeks of starting or escalating therapy.
    - Consider offering naloxone for high-risk patients such as those with history of overdose, history of substance use disorder, doses greater than 50 mg morphine equivalent per day, or concurrent benzodiazepine use, which should be avoided.
    - Use a state prescription drug monitoring program (PDMP).
    - Use urine drug screening at initiation and at least annually.

13. **What are the newest formulations of opioids that are designed to mitigate addiction?**
    There are new opioid formulations aimed at reducing the risk of addiction. Since the rapid "rush" that amplifies the risk of addiction is associated with intranasal, inhaled, or intravenous routes of opioid use, new formulations that deter crushing can be helpful. In addition, some formulations include a substance that is irritating if inhaled, injected, or chewed. Other formulations now include an antagonist such as naloxone, which is deactivated only if the medication is swallowed. These formulations help reduce but do not completely mitigate the risk of addiction.

14. **What are some of the newer, nonopioid options for the outpatient management of chronic pain?**
    Since the general lack of benefit of long-term treatment with opioids for chronic pain and the risk of addiction have been documented, the new CDC guidelines state that the nonopioid interventions of exercise therapy, weight loss, cognitive behavioral therapy, interventions to improve sleep, nonsteroidal antiinflammatory drugs (NSAIDs) for low back pain, neuromodulation, and antidepressants for neuropathic pain are preferred for chronic pain not related to cancer or end-of-life care.

15. **What is the utility of written medication agreements in patients suspected of opioid abuse?**
    When opioids are the treatment of choice, a pain management contract that sets out the parameters of treatment may be useful. In general, these contracts include agreements that prescriptions cannot be refilled early (even if lost or stolen) and that refills will require a physical exam, or at least an office visit. The contracts specify that any medications prescribed by other physicians must be reported to the opioid-prescribing physician. Agreements to undergo random urine drug screening and not to share or sell medications should be considered.

16. **What actions on the part of the patient should alert you to the possibility of "drug-seeking" behavior?**
    Drug-seeking behaviors include complaints of abnormally high levels of pain, reoccurring headaches, back or dental pain, requests for narcotics by name, and early requests for refills or for replacements of lost medications. Other suspicious behaviors include the hesitancy to produce past medical records, making a direct request for drugs without a concomitant request for evaluation of the problem causing the pain, and seeking appointments with multiple practitioners.

17. **What should be done if addiction is suspected?**
    If addiction is suspected, use of long-acting opioids and the other new formulations mentioned previously, which are more difficult to abuse, may be a better option. Reducing the number of pills prescribed or shortening the interval between refills and involving family members in the safekeeping and distribution of pills may be advisable. Requiring random urine screens and pill counts can unveil an ongoing addiction.
    Realize that chemical and some psychological dependence on opioids is almost unavoidable when long-term opioid therapy is used, and withdrawal-associated symptoms will be an outcome of cessation or decreases in dosage. Your patients may need assistance through drug counseling or other resources when transitioning off their medication.

18. How can a practitioner actively prevent drug diversion?

It is important to document all of your findings and your individualized treatment plan for each patient, including any suspicion of addiction and diversion. Your best defense against diversion of the drugs you prescribe is to limit the duration of treatment and intervals between refills. Other tools that can help include the use of:
- State PDMPs, which can be checked prior to prescribing
- If used, prescription pads that are not easily copied
- Writing out the dose and number of refills, including "zero" if no refills are allowed

19. How common are practitioner sanctions from regulating bodies?

Due to concerns regarding prescription drug abuse, the Drug Enforcement Agency (DEA) doubled its Tactical Diversion Squads from 37 in March 2011 to 66 in March 2014. State-based medical review and licensure boards and prosecutors are scrutinizing physicians at an increasing rate for the prescription of controlled substances. The federal U.S. Department of Justice lists 28 registrant actions for physicians and nurse practitioners in 2015. In 15 cases, the DEA certificate was revoked. In an additional seven cases, the reapplication for a DEA certificate was denied after an action short of revocation had been taken.

WEBSITES

To learn more about signs and risks of addiction to opioids associated with pain management and the physician sanctions for diversion, visit:

Actions Against Pain Physicians: www.aapsonline.org

American Academy of Pain Management: www.aapainmanage.org

American Academy of Pain Medicine: www.painmed.org

American Pain Society: www.americanpainsociety.org

American Society of Addiction Medicine: www.asam.org

PROP I Physicians for Responsible Opioid Prescribing: www.supportprop.org

In addition, the following website offers information about legal drug disposal as well as physician sanctions: www.deadiversion.usdoj.gov.

KEY POINTS

1. The US Department of Health and Human Services and the Centers for Disease Control designated the deaths resulting from prescription opioids as an epidemic, and physicians are being held accountable by government and the public.
2. Best estimates are that misuse occurs in nearly 25% of patients and addiction occurs in around 10% of patients treated with opioids for chronic pain.
3. Long-term opioid treatment is not first-line treatment of chronic pain.

BIBLIOGRAPHY

1. Alam A, Juurlink DN. The prescription opioid epidemic: an overview for anesthesiologists. *Can J Anaesth.* 2016;63(1):61-68.
2. American Psychiatric Association. *Diagnostic and Statistical Manual of Mental Disorders (DSM-5).* 5th ed. Washington, DC: American Psychiatric Association; 2013.
3. Ballantyne JC. Opioid therapy in chronic pain. *Phys Med Rehabil Clin N Am.* 2015;26(2):201-218.
4. Barry CL, Kennedy-Hendricks A, Gollust SE, et al. Understanding Americans' views on opioid pain reliever abuse. *Addiction.* 2016;111(1):85-93.
5. Bruera E, Paice JA. Cancer pain management: safe and effective use of opioids. *Am Soc Clin Oncol Educ Book 2015 Edition.* 2015;e593-e599.
6. Buchman DZ, Ho A, Illes J. You present like a drug addict: patient and clinician perspectives on trust and trustworthiness in chronic pain management. *Pain Med.* 2016;17(8):1394-1406.
7. Cheatle MD. Facing the challenge of pain management and opioid misuse, abuse and opioid-related fatalities. *Expert Rev Clin Pharmacol.* 2016;9(6):751-754.
8. Cheatle MD. Prescription opioid misuse, abuse, morbidity, and mortality: balancing effective pain management and safety. *Pain Med.* 2015;16(suppl 1):S3-S8.
9. Conrardy M, Lank P, Cameron KA, et al. Emergency department patient perspectives on the risk of addiction to prescription opioids. *Pain Med.* 2015;17(1):114-121.

10. Frieden TR, Houry D. Reducing the risks of relief—the CDC opioid-prescribing guideline. *N Engl J Med.* 2016;374(16):1501-1504.

11. Gould HJ, Paul D. Critical appraisal of extended-release hydrocodone for chronic pain: patient considerations. *Ther Clin Risk Manag.* 2015;11:1635-1640.

12. Kanner R. Addiction and pain management. In: Dubin A, Pilitsis J, Argoff CE, Mcleane G, eds. *Pain Management Secrets.* 3rd ed. Philadelphia: Mosby/Elsevier; 2009:1-9.

13. Hoffman J. Patients in pain, and a doctor who must limit drugs. New York Times. March 16, 2016.

14. Lasser KE, Shanahan C, Parker V, et al. A multicomponent intervention to improve primary care provider adherence to chronic opioid therapy guidelines and reduce opioid misuse: a cluster randomized controlled trial protocol. *J Subst Abuse Treat.* 2016;60:101-109.

15. Leonardi C, Vellucci R, Mammucari M, Fanelli G. Opioid risk addiction in the management of chronic pain in primary care: the addition risk questionnaire. *Eur Rev Med Pharmacol Sci.* 2015;24:4898-4905.

16. Sacco LN. Drug enforcement in the United States: history, policy and trends. October 2, 2014. Congressional Research Service Report; www.crs.gov. Accessed 15 July 2016.

17. Vowles KE, McEntee ML, Julness PS, et al. Rates of opioid misuse, abuse, and addiction in chronic pain: a systematic review and data synthesis. *Pain.* 2015;156(4):569-576.

PAIN IN CHILDREN

Renee C.B. Manworren

CHAPTER 34

1. **What types of pain do children experience?**
   Like adults, children experience acute pain from injury, illness, and invasive medical procedures. Neonates experience 1 to 10+ painful procedures per day during their first week of hospitalization. Children receive 49 doses of 14 vaccines by their 6th birthday; and over 6 million children per year have surgery. Children also experience recurrent, persistent, and chronic pain. Unlike the pain from disease or trauma, the pain itself, rather than the underlying disease, becomes the problem. Chronic pain of childhood is associated with a mean loss of 3.43 quality-adjusted life years. Prevalence estimates of chronic pain in children range from 11% to 38%. The most common pains are headaches (10% to 30% of children and the reason for 1%–2% of pediatric visits), stomachaches (7% to 25% and the reason for 2% to 4% of pediatric visits), and musculoskeletal pain (over 50% of children). Functional pain syndromes are a less common, complex, loosely defined group of pediatric chronic conditions characterized by pain, suffering, and disability with unclear disease etiology or biomechanical cause. It is important for parents and children to understand that there is no single source of tissue damage that causes the child's recurrent, persistent, chronic, or functional pain syndrome (Fig. 34.1).

2. **How do children's pain experiences differ from those adults?**
   There is evidence that children experience pain differently than adults. Normative quantitative sensory testing (QST) values demonstrate that younger children (<8 years of age) are less sensitive to thermal and mechanical stimuli and more sensitive to pain stimuli than older children (>9-year-olds). Reference values for QST differ for children as compared to adults. Research also demonstrates that noxious stimuli experienced during the vulnerable neonatal period of neuronal plasticity may trigger unpredicted long-term epigenomic changes that affect the brain, neurodevelopment, and pain reactivity into adulthood. Very preterm infants exposed to repeated neonatal procedural pain and stress may have alterations in their brain microstructure and function, stress systems, neurodevelopment, and stress-sensitive behaviors. However, despite different engagement of brain regions during functional brain imaging, there is no evidence for greater prevalence of pain syndromes for children born prematurely and exposed to early repeated painful events when compared with children and adults born healthy at full term.

3. **What is plasticity?**
   Plasticity refers to the capacity to respond differently or change in response to tissue damage. Neuroplasticity due to early or repeated exposure to pain may result in a maladaptive reorganization of the peripheral and central nervous system. Noxious stimuli including inflammation may cause elevated nociceptive input and elicit a neuroplastic response causing physical changes to individual neurons, how neurons communicate with each other, and the cortical and whole-brain level (remapping). Children's perceptions of pain depend on complex neuronal interactions that include both ascending pain transmission and descending pain modulation and suppression. Children are more vulnerable to pain given their frequent exposures, variable developmental and cognitive ability to evaluate the meaning of the pain experienced, and lack of autonomy to seek pain prevention interventions and treatments.

4. **What myths have complicated our management of children's pain?**
   Research indicates knowledge regarding children's pain has improved and the myths, like "infants have immature nervous systems and do not feel pain," have been dispelled. However, attitudes regarding children's pain have not changed. For example, despite documented knowledge that developmentally appropriate children over 3 to 4 years of age can accurately report pain intensity,

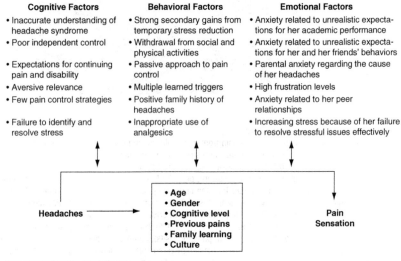

Factors Involved in Pain of 10-Year-Old Girl with Recurrent Headaches

Cognitive Factors	Behavioral Factors	Emotional Factors
• Inaccurate understanding of headache syndrome	• Strong secondary gains from temporary stress reduction	• Anxiety related to unrealistic expectations for her academic performance
• Poor independent control	• Withdrawal from social and physical activities	• Anxiety related to unrealistic expectations for her and her friends' behaviors
• Expectations for continuing pain and disability	• Passive approach to pain control	• Parental anxiety regarding the cause of her headaches
• Aversive relevance	• Multiple learned triggers	• High frustration levels
• Few pain control strategies	• Positive family history of headaches	• Anxiety related to her peer relationships
• Failure to identify and resolve stress	• Inappropriate use of analgesics	• Increasing stress because of her failure to resolve stressful issues effectively

Headaches →
- Age
- Gender
- Cognitive level
- Previous pains
- Family learning
- Culture

Pain Sensation

Treatment Recommendations:

1. Assist child in identifying and resolving stressful situations.
2. Teach child to cope more effectively with routine frustrations.
3. Teach parents and child about pain systems, recurrent pain syndromes, and true vs. learned headache triggers.
4. Reduce secondary gains associated with child's pain by providing consistent and nonmaladaptive responses to her pain complaints.
5. Teach child nonpharmacologic methods of pain control, such as muscle relaxation through biofeedback and nonstressful exercise.

Figure 34.1. Factors involved in pain of 10-year-old girl with recurrent headaches.

health care providers and parents are more likely to believe and attend to behaviors when children's behaviors are inconsistent with children's self-reports of pain. Children's reports of pain are not believed. Adverse effects of pain are discounted, and the adverse effects of pain treatments are overestimated. Thus inappropriate attitudes and concerns regarding the underrecognition and undertreatment of children's pain perpetuate the underrecognition and undertreatment of children's pain.

Children are typically regarded as resilient, but children can become significantly disabled by recurrent, persistent, and chronic pain. When the protective behaviors appropriate for acute disease or trauma pain persist, it can lead to progressive loss of function. Children and parents need to understand that when significant disability is present, the pain diagnosis and disability must both be addressed. Parents require assistance understanding that the treatment of chronic pain is different from that of pain due to disease or trauma. Opioids are rarely used to treat children's recurrent, persistent, and chronic pain, and gradual return to activity is encouraged despite pain. Chronic pain affects the entire family, and the emotional suffering, impaired physical function, decreased independence, and uncertain prognosis must be addressed as a family. Children and parents of children with chronic pain require more specialized therapy to return to school and physical and social activities.

5. How do you assess infants' pain experiences?

Valid and reliable pain assessment tools for infants and preverbal children are actually indirect measures of pain (Table 34.1). Because these tools rely on observed behaviors and physiologic measures, they do not measure pain intensity but rather quantify responses to pain-related distress. Scores from these tools are influenced by contextual factors, such as gestational age and physiologic stability. Therefore pain assessment tools for infants and preverbal children are most

Table 34.1. Tools for Assessing Pain of Infants and Preverbal Children

TOOL (ACRONYM) AND REFERENCE (YEAR)	AGE RANGE	TYPE OF PAIN	PARAMETERS
Children's and Infants' Postoperative Pain Scale (CHIPPS) *Bringuier et al. (2009); Buttner and Finke (2000)*	Birth to 5 years	Acute, postop	Scored from 0 to 10: • Cry • Facial • Leg posture motor/restlessness • Trunk poster
COMFORT Behavior Scale *de Jong et al. (2010); van Dijk et al. (2000, 2005)*	Neonates to 3 years	Acute, intensive care postop	Used to assess distress, sedation, and pain. Scored from 8 to 40: • Alertness • Blood pressure • Calmness • Facial tension • Heart rate • Muscle tone • Physical movement • Respiratory distress Also valid without physiologic parameters (COMFORT B).
Crying, Requires oxygen, Increased vital signs, Expression, and Sleeplessness (CRIES) *Ahn and Jun (2007); Krechel and Bildner (1995)*	Neonates	Acute, intensive care procedural, post-op	Scored from 0 to 10: • Crying • Requires oxygen—oxygenation • Increased vital signs, Expression • Sleeplessness
Distress Scale for Ventilated Newborn Infants (DSVNI) *Sparshott (1996)*	Ventilated, neonates and infants	Acute, intensive care procedural	Sum of four physiologic parameters: • Blood pressure • Heart rate • Oxygen saturation • Temperature differential And three behavioral parameters: • Body movements • Facial expressions
Faces, Legs, Activity, Cry, and Consolability Observational Tool (FLACC) *Ahn and Jun (2007); Manworren and Hynan (2003); Merkel et al. (1997); Voepel-Lewis et al. (2002, 2010); Willis et al. (2003)*	0–3 years, Up to 7 years in post-anesthesia care unit	Acute, procedural, postop, disease-related	Scored from 0 to 10: • Faces • Legs • Activity • Cry • Consolability
Neonatal Infant Pain Scale (NIPS) *Lawrence et al. (1993)*	Preterm and term infants		Scored 0 to 7: • Breathing pattern • Crying • Facial expression • Movement of arms and/or legs • State of arousal

Continued on following page

Table 34.1. Tools for Assessing Pain of Infants and Preverbal Children *(Continued)*

TOOL (ACRONYM) AND REFERENCE (YEAR)	AGE RANGE	TYPE OF PAIN	PARAMETERS
Neonatal Pain, Agitation, and Sedation Scale (N-PASS) *Hummel et al. (2008); Hummel et al. (2010)*	Premature neonates 23–40 weeks gestation	Procedural and postop during mechanical ventilation neonatal intensive care unit	Used to assess sedation and pain. Scored from −2 to +2 for each parameter: • Behavior • Cry • Extremity tone • Facial expression • Vital signs in the context of gestational age.
Premature Infant Pain Profile (PIPP) and Premature Infant Pain Profile—Revised (PIPP-R) *Ahn and Jun (2007); Gibbins et al. (PIPP-R, 2014); Stevens et al. (1996); Stevens et al. (2010)*	Premature and term neonates	Procedural and postop in neonatal intensive care unit	Scored from 0 to 21: • Brow bulge • Eye squeeze • Heart rate • Nasolabial furrow • Oxygen saturation in the context of gestational age and behavioral state.

reliable for procedural pain, rather than ongoing chronic pain assessments. These validated behavioral pain assessment tools should always be considered as proxy pain measures to be interpreted based on expected or potential tissue damage.

As children gain control over their ability to express themselves verbally and control their behaviors, behavioral tools become inappropriate for assessing their pain. Toddlers can report the presence and location of pain, adopting words learned to express pain and pain location from their parents and caregivers. As children develop more complex verbal skills and cognitive understanding, they also develop a more diverse pain vocabulary.

6. How do you assess children's pain experiences?
Self-report is the gold standard for assessing children's pain. By 3 to 4 years of age, children can differentiate pain intensity with pictorial adaptations of the numeric rating scale (NRS) and visual analogue scale (VAS; Table 34.2). Most children over 7 to 8 years of age can understand rank order and rank pain severity on a scale of 0 to 10 or 0 to 5, with the 0 anchor representing "no pain" and 5 or 10 representing the "worst possible pain." Therefore, like adults, most school-age children can use the NRS and VAS to report and quantify their pain intensity. Children 6 to 16 years of age, however, report a preference for using the faces scale to the NRS. No single pain intensity scale is valid, reliable, and appropriate for all pediatric age groups or types of pain.

Pain intensity is the most common component of pain assessed with children and adults, but a more comprehensive pain assessment is often necessary. Pediatric self-report tools of pain quality, pattern, triggers, aggravating, and alleviating factors, and how pain interferes with everyday life has been developed and validated for children and adolescents with acute and chronic pain. Few self-report multidimensional pain assessment tools have been developed and validated for assessing children with chronic pain (Table 34.3). The Patient-Reported Outcomes Measurement Information System (PROMIS) comprises valid, person-centered measures for (1) assessing symptoms and functions across chronic health conditions, (2) enhancing communication between health care providers and patients, and (3) evaluating and monitoring physical, social, and emotional health. PROMIS self-report measures are available for children 8 to 17 years of age, and parent-proxy measures are available for children 5 to 17 years of age. Pain interference, emotional distress, fatigue, physical activity, physical function, strength impact, physical stress experiences, psychological stress experiences, family relationships, peer relationships, global health, and life satisfaction are all PROMIS measures appropriate for obtaining a more comprehensive assessment of children with chronic pain.

Table 34.2. Valid and Reliable Pictorial Adaptations of the Numeric Rating Scale and Visual Analogue Scale for Assessing Children's Pain

TOOL (ACRONYM) AND REFERENCE (YEAR)	AGE RANGE	TYPE OF PAIN	COMMENTS
Faces Pain Scale—Revised (FPS-R) Bieri et al. (1990); Hicks et al. (2001)	4–12 years	Acute, disease-related, postop, procedural	Highly feasible. Neutral anchors. Recommended by PediIMMPACT.
Oucher Beyer and Aradine (1986)	3+	Acute, disease-related, postop, procedural	Available with photographs of different races/ethnicities to facilitate cultural competency.
Wong–Baker FACES Pain Scale (WBPRS) Wong and Baker (1988)	3+	Acute, disease-related, postop, procedural	Validated with 0 to 5 and 0 to 10 anchors. Anchor faces are smiling and crying, which may confuse measurement of intensity and affect.

Table 34.3. Valid and Reliable Multidimensional Pediatric Self-Report Pain Assessment Tools for Chronic Pain

TOOL (ACRONYM) AND REFERENCE (YEAR)	AGE RANGE	TYPE OF PAIN	COMMENTS
Adolescent Pediatric Pain Tool (APPT) Jacob et al. (2014); Savedra et al. (1989)	8+	Acute, chronic, disease-related, postop, procedural	Validated to assess pain intensity, pattern or timing, location, and quality. Available in English and Spanish.
Bath Adolescent Pain Questionnaire (BAPQ) Eccleston et al. (2005)	11–18	Chronic	Validated to assess the impact of chronic pain.
Pediatric Pain Assessment Tool (PPAT) Abu-Saad et al. (1990)	5+	Acute, chronic, disease-related, postop	Validated to assess pain intensity and quality of pain by circling words in the sensory, affective, evaluative, and temporal domains of pain.
Pediatric Pain Questionnaire (PPQ) Varni and Thompson (1985)	5+	Chronic, disease-related	Validated to assess pain intensity, location, sensory, evaluative, and affective qualities of pain. Available in seven languages.

7. **How do you assess pain experiences of children with intellectual disabilities?**
   Children with intellectual disabilities are the most burdened by pain due to their need for frequent medical procedures and their inability to communicate pain with the simple self-report tools. A hierarchy of pain assessment techniques has been recommended. The first step on this hierarchy is to still attempt to obtain a self-report of pain whenever possible. The second step on the hierarchy is to use a pain assessment tool that has been validated for use with children with intellectual disabilities (Table 34.4). These pain assessment tools are also indirect measures of pain. These observational pain assessment tools are not validated to quantify pain intensity, but instead quantify the intensity of pain-related distress and pain reactivity. Despite being validated pain assessment tools, these behavioral tools are proxy measures of pain that must be interpreted based on actual or

Table 34.4. Tools for Assessing Pain of Nonverbal Pediatric Patients With Intellectual Disabilities

TOOL (ACRONYM) AND REFERENCE (YEAR)	AGE RANGE	TYPE OF PAIN	PARAMETERS
Revised Faces, Legs, Activity, Cry, and Consolability Observational Tool (rFLACC) *Malviya et al. (2006); Voepel-Lewis et al. (2002, 2003, 2005)*	4–19 years with mild to severe intellectual disabilities	Acute, postop	Observations and scoring are similar to the FLACC with descriptions to parameters to characterize behaviors of children in pain who also have intellectual disabilities. Allows the addition of individual patient's pain behaviors.
Individualized Numeric Rating Scale (INRS) *Solodiuk and Curley (2003); Solodiuk et al. (2010)*	6–18 years with severe intellectual disabilities in acute care settings	Postop	Personalized assessment tool to assess pain in nonverbal children with intellectual disability based on the parent's knowledge of the child. Parents describe and then rank order their child's usual and pain indicators and behaviors.
Noncommunicating Children's Pain Checklist (Acute care NCCPC) *Breau (2003); Breau et al. (2000, 2001, 2002, 2004); Breau and Camfield (2011); Burkitt et al. (2011); Lotan et al. (2009)*	3–18 years with intellectual disabilities in hospital, rehab, home or residential settings	Chronic, postop	Caregivers of children with severe cognitive impairments recorded their observations of their children. The NCCPC-PV (postoperative version) has eight parameters scored 0–3 each (vocal, social, facial, activity, body/limbs, physiologic).

potential tissue damage and expected or previously experienced pain from similar procedures and conditions. These tools should be interpreted by a parent or caregiver familiar with the child's verbalizations and behaviors. Proxy report and concern regarding pain is the third step of the pain assessment hierarchy. The fourth and final step is to attempt an analgesic trial.

8. **How do you assess pain experiences of children with autism spectrum disorders?**
   As previously mentioned, health care providers and parents are more likely to believe and attend to children's behaviors when they are consistent with expected pain-related behaviors. Children with autism spectrum disorders (ASD) do not consistently demonstrate socially expected interactions and nonverbal behaviors that facilitate interpersonal communication. However, most individuals with ASD are able to describe and locate their pain but require a variety of approaches. Most are able to report pain intensity but prefer not to focus on pain. Language to communicate pain should be simple and familiar. Parent involvement is essential; both to help interpret the child's needs and provide trusted support.

9. **Which pain assessment tools should be incorporated into routine clinical practice?**
   Pain is the most common reason individuals seek health care services, so all patients should be screened for pain at every health care visit. If pain is the focus of the visit, a thorough pain assessment, medical history, and physical examination are necessary to establish clinical diagnosis.

Pain assessment is a critical component for the diagnosis and treatment of children's pain. Always ask a child directly about their pain experience. Obtain objective information about pain pattern, intensity, and quality of children's pain to facilitate diagnosis and treatment plan. A few structured questions and valid and reliable pain assessment tools can be easily incorporated into regular health care visits.

Pain diaries are a way to track children's pain experiences and provide more information for clinical diagnosis and treatment planning. Real-time, electronic, handheld diaries have been developed for children with recurrent and chronic pain. Electronic pain diaries are readily available, but availability should not be confused with quality. Health care professionals must evaluate e-diaries and pain apps for reliability, validity, and efficacy as thoroughly as other pain assessment tools or treatment prior to recommending them for patients.

10. **Is there a basic treatment algorithm to control children's pain?**
There are substantial disparities in pain treatment with undertreatment and inadequate treatment common in children. One significant contributing factor to undertreatment is lack of US Food and Drug Administration (FDA) approval and guidance for prescribing pain medications to children. Another factor is the lack of robust evidence for the effectiveness of nonpharmacologic treatments for children's pain. In spite of these contributing factors, the basic treatment algorithm to control children's pain is similar to that of treating any individual with pain. Begin with a thorough assessment. Evaluate the primary sensory characteristics of pain, including pain location, intensity, duration, timing, pattern, quality, and aggravating and alleviating components. Also assess the extent to which cognitive, behavioral, and emotional factors may influence the pain experience. Obtain a thorough medical history, pain history, and physical examination. Complete any necessary diagnostic tests. Then develop a differential diagnosis and a multimodal treatment plan (include analgesics, cognitive, physical, and behavioral interventions) to address all dimensions of the pain experience. Partner with children and parents to promote adherence to treatment plans by first explaining and addressing potential causes of the pain and any contributing factors. Finally, regularly evaluate treatment plan effectiveness, and revise the plan as needed.

11. **What are the basic guidelines for selecting and administering analgesics to children with pain?**
Selection of analgesics for children with pain should be part of a multimodal treatment plan. Consistent with principles of analgesia, consider the six rights of medication administration: (1) right patient, (2) right drug, (3) right route, (4) right dose, (5) right time, and (6) right way.

First, right patient—is an analgesic even recommended to treat the child's pain? Most minor cuts and abrasions are well tolerated with a parent's kiss and a bandage. Local anesthetics are also available in over-the-counter topical antibiotics. Does the patient have any comorbid conditions that would prevent the use of certain analgesics, such as the contraindication to use acetaminophen with patients with liver failure, or over-the-counter ibuprofen for patients with bleeding disorders? Analgesic agents should be based on each child's circumstances. No analgesic will reliably relieve pain for all children who have a similar medical condition or a similar location, quality, or intensity of pain.

Second, right drug—the choice of analgesics should be based on diagnosis, mechanisms of pain, and the mechanisms of action of the analgesic. Thus nonsteroidal antiinflammatory drugs (NSAIDs) are preferred for inflammatory pain. As previously mentioned, most analgesics are not approved by the FDA for administration to children. However, few are contraindicated for children. Thus treatment of children's pain with analgesics often requires the prescriber to translate knowledge gained from adult use of the drug to determine the drug's actions, dose, duration of analgesia, and adverse effects when used with children. Prescribers are forced to make patient care decisions based on professional experience with the analgesic and off-label dosing guidelines and recommendations.

Third, right route—consider the location of the pain and the pharmacokinetics and dynamics of the analgesic. For example, a topical anesthetic is far more appropriate for the prevention of pain from a needle procedure than a strong opioid would be for treating the pain after the procedure. Also consider the pattern of the pain. For severe pain of sudden onset, the fast action of the parental route may be preferred. However, the intramuscular (IM) route should be avoided whenever possible. The IM route is painful, dangerous, and results in erratic drug absorption. Analgesics administered by the oral route tend to have a longer duration of analgesia and may be less expensive. The oral route is considered the preferred route for analgesic administration. This route, however, may not be appropriate if the child cannot tolerate enteral medications, if the appropriate dose is not available in an oral formulation, if the child cannot swallow pills, or the child may not prefer this route if the liquid analgesic has a particularly nasty taste!

Fourth, right dose—analgesic doses are based on empiric evidence and extrapolation of adult doses to children's sizes. Initial analgesic dose is based on the child's weight up to the normal starting dose for an adult. Health care professionals may use current body weight, adjusted body weight, or ideal body weight to calculate dose—since there is no accepted standard for weight-based dose calculations. The dose for nonopioids, like acetaminophen and NSAIDs, are standardized by age and weight, whereas opioid doses need to be titrated to determine the optimal safe dose to use to relieve each individual child's pain. Predetermined pain intensity scores for different pain treatments or different analgesic doses are inappropriate. There is no research linking analgesic dose to specific pain intensity scores. This practice puts children at risk for oversedation, respiratory depression, and poorly managed pain. Analgesic dosage may vary by route. Consider the relative strength of analgesics given by different routes.

Fifth, right time—analgesics may be given before the painful event to prevent pain, intermittently to quickly treat pain, or infused on a continuous basis to maintain pain relief. Analgesics should be given on a timed schedule consistent with their duration of action for predictable or continuous pain.

Sixth, right way—pain treatment should always be multimodal. Could pain be prevented by avoiding triggers or using preventative medication strategies, such as topical anesthetics for needle procedures? Are patient controlled analgesia (PCA) and epidural analgesics appropriate for child?

12. **Are there special dosing considerations for neonates and infants?**
Yes. The pharmacokinetics and pharmacodynamics among neonates, preterm infants, and full term infants require special attention until 6 to 12 months of age. In general, analgesics are recommended for a shorter course of therapy. Dosing interval (time between doses) may be shorter or longer depending on how the drug is metabolized. Opioids should be dosed at one-fourth to one-third of the recommended weight-based starting dose for children. Subsequent doses must be titrated based on further evaluation of efficacy and monitoring for adverse effects.

13. **Can patient-controlled analgesia be used by children?**
Yes. PCA allows children to administer small intermittent doses of analgesics when needed. PCA is prompt, economical, adjusts for variability in children's analgesic needs, and removes the barrier of assessment judgment and bias. Research indicates children use less opioids when delivered with a PCA device than when intermittent doses are administered by nurses for their pain. PCA has been used in children for more than 30 years and has a high degree of safety. Most children more than 6 years of age can appropriately use PCA. Screen children for their ability to activate the device, provide self-report of pain, understand the need to activate the device before their pain is severe, and report poorly controlled pain despite a PCA. Family members should also be screened to ensure they do not activate the device when the child is asleep, since this overrides the inherent safety of PCA. Continuous infusions or background infusions are not recommended with a PCA for opioid naïve children, although there is some debate among pediatric health care professionals who routinely use PCA to treat children's pain, particularly those who use it with children less than 6 years of age. Due to the risk of excessive sedation and respiratory depression, monitoring is recommended.

14. **Can regional techniques be used for children?**
Regional techniques for the administration of local anesthetics and other analgesics are an integral part of postoperative pain management. For example, a one-shot caudal may prevent the need for outpatient analgesics after hernia repair, local anesthetic catheters may prevent the need for epidural analgesia and facilitate transition home after major postoperative procedures, and Bier blocks may facilitate fracture reduction. The only absolute contraindication to catheter placement is the inability to place the catheter—for example, in children with myelomeningocele. Epidurals or spinal analgesia are recommended for the management of postoperative pain in patients undergoing thoracic, abdominal, hip, and lower extremity procedures. Catheters can be placed caudally and advanced under ultrasound guidance to achieve thoracic level analgesia (e.g., for newborns requiring cardiac surgery). There are no absolute limits for length of time the catheter can remain in the epidural space, but if longer duration is anticipated, the catheter should be tunneled. Catheters should be immediately assessed and removal considered if a child becomes septic (due to risk of

catheter seeding), is at great risk of bleeding (due to risk of epidural hematoma), exhibits a new motor block (potential epidural hematoma), or the catheter is no longer functional or needed. Children who have received regional anesthetic techniques should be monitored for these adverse effects, and these techniques should only be used in settings where health care providers have adequate training in these techniques, have early recognition of adverse effects, and are prepared to rapidly treat adverse effects from regional anesthesia.

15. **How do parents know which pain medications (prescription and over the counter) are safe and effective for children?**
Parents should be advised that most pain medications have not been specifically evaluated and approved for use in children. Unfortunately sharing of prescription analgesics and diversion of opioids has increased to the point of being considered a national epidemic. For children's safety, all over-the-counter (OTC) and prescription medications should be secured and controlled. Analgesics and other medications can be deadly if taken in a manner other than as prescribed or by someone other than who they were prescribed. Therefore analgesics should be kept in locked storage containers or cabinets. The same medications should be disposed of as soon as they are no longer indicated for the reason prescribed. In other words, children and parents should be taught not to share analgesics or store analgesics for future use even if they anticipate needing the medication again for similar pain during the year.

16. **How do parents know which pain complementary and alternative therapies are safe for children?**
Complementary and alternative medications (CAM) and therapies (CAT) are popular and generally considered safe. Despite little evidence of effectiveness, prevalence rates for overall CAM use in children ranges from 10% to almost 90% for lifetime use and slightly less at 8% to almost 50% for current use. Fish oil, garlic, chamomile, and acidophilus are the most commonly used CAM, but their use is rarely reported to children's treating health care providers. Among children seen at a pediatric chronic pain center, CAM users tended to have higher pain intensity and greater functional disability. CAT most frequently used by children with chronic pain are also those most frequently recommended by health care providers, including guided imagery, biofeedback, journaling, yoga, hypnosis, transcutaneous electrical nerve stimulation (TENS), massage, and acupuncture (Table 34.5). Parents should be advised of potentially dangerous CAM use (St. John's wort, ginseng) and the benefit of biobehavioral techniques, which have been associated with adaptive coping skills.

17. **What about marijuana—is it safe to use to treat children's pain?**
No. Cannabis use alters neurodevelopment, with most alterations documented in the frontal lobe. Adolescent initiation of cannabis use has long been known as a significant risk factor for subsequent addiction. With increased legalization of marijuana for medical or recreational use, the number of marijuana poisonings has increased each year. The most common age groups poisoned were ≤5 years and 13 to 19 years. Symptoms included drowsiness/lethargy (43%), tachycardia (31%), agitated/irritable (14%), and confusion (14%). While most clinical effects are minor, ventilatory support has been necessary, and deaths reported.

Table 34.5. Complementary and Alternative Therapies for Children's Pain

COGNITIVE	BEHAVIORAL	PHYSICAL
Information	Behavior modification	Acupuncture
Choices and control	Biofeedback	Massage
Distraction and attention	Exercise	Physiotherapy
Guided imagery	Relaxation therapy	Sensory stimulation
Hypnosis	Yoga	Thermal stimulation
Psychotherapy	Parental response modification	TENS (transcutaneous electrical nerve stimulation)

18. **How are cognitive therapies used to treat pain in pediatric clinical practice?**
Cognitive therapies are an important component of multimodal pain treatment plans when directed at a child's beliefs, expectations, and coping abilities. Cognitive therapies include approaches from basic developmentally appropriate education to more formal psychotherapy. A basic cognitive intervention is providing children with age-appropriate information about pain and teaching them how to use simple strategies to cope with pain and pain-related fear and anxiety. When children receive accurate information about what they may feel, they can improve their understanding, increase their control, lessen their distress, and reduce their pain. Distraction and focused attention, as well as guided imagery, are strategies that health care professionals and parents can coach children to use routinely when children experience pain. Focused attention, also known as hypnosis, is a very active process that can lessen neuronal responses evoked by pain and tissue damage.

19. **What is the role of behavioral therapy in pain management for children?**
Behavioral therapies are directed toward changing either children's behaviors or the behaviors of the adults who respond to their pain. The therapeutic objective is to lessen behaviors that may increase children's pain, distress, and disability, while increasing behaviors that may reduce pain, anxiety, and distress. The objective is to help children reduce their stress, increase their independent pain management, and increase their participation in school and social events to return them to full participation and enjoyment in activities of daily life.

20. **Which children should be referred to pediatric pain management specialists?**
Children with recurrent, persistent, and chronic pain benefit from interdisciplinary teams implementing multimodal pain treatment plans. Unfortunately most major American cities still do not have specialized pediatric pain management teams available to address the needs of this vulnerable population. Board certification in pediatric pain management does not exist, and pediatric pain management specialists are as varied as the patients they treat. Despite the lack of appropriate specialists to accept patient referrals, most pediatric pain management specialty teams at leading children's hospitals will consult with primary care providers to develop a plan to address children's pain and best meet the needs of these children and their families.

KEY POINTS

1. Like adults, children experience acute, persistent, recurrent, and chronic pain, but children are not little adults. Children's pain is more likely to be unrecognized, undertreated, and inadequately relieved.
2. Pain should be assessed with valid, reliable, and developmentally appropriate tools. A high degree of suspicion for pain from actual and potential tissue damage is required.
3. Children's pain is treated with many of the same medications and therapies used to treat pain in adults, but these treatments are rarely approved for use in children because they have not been systematically tested in children.

BIBLIOGRAPHY

1. Basch MC, Chow ET, Logan DE, Schechter NL, Simons LE. Perspectives on the clinical significance of functional pain syndromes in children. *J Pain Res.* 2015;8:675-686. doi:10.2147/JPR.S55586.
2. Blankenburg M, Boekens H, Hechler T, et al. Reference values for quantitative sensory testing in children and adolescents: developmental and gender differences of somatosensory perception. *Pain.* 2010;149(1):76-88.
3. Cao D, Srisuma S, Bronstein AC, Hoyte CO. Characterization of edible marijuana product exposures reported to United States poison centers. *Clin Toxicol.* 2016;15:1-7.
4. Chou R, Gordon DB, de Leon-Casasola OA, et al. Management of postoperative pain: a clinical practice guideline from the American Pain Society, the American Society of Regional Anesthesia and Pain Medicine, and the American Society of Anesthesiologists' Committee on Regional Anesthesia, Executive Committee, and Administrative Council. *J Pain.* 2016;17(2):131-157.
5. Connelly M, Neville K. Comparative prospective evaluation of the responsiveness of single-item pediatric pain-intensity self-report scales and their uniqueness from negative affect in a hospital setting. *J Pain.* 2010;11(12):1451-1460.
6. Courtois E, Droutman S, Magny JF, et al. Epidemiology and neonatal pain management of heelsticks in intensive care units: EPIPPAIN 2, a prospective observational study. *Int J Nurs Stud.* 2016;59:79-88. doi:10.1016/j.ijnurstu.2016.03.014. [Epub 2016 Mar 30].

7. Craig BM, Hartman JD, Owens MA, Brown DS. Prevalence and losses in quality-adjusted life years of child health conditions: a burden of disease analysis. *Matern Child Health J.* 2016;20(4):862-869. doi:10.1007/s10995-015-1874-z.

8. Dell ML, Campo JV. Somatoform disorders in children and adolescents. *Psychiatr Clin North Am.* 2011;34(3):643-660.

9. Ely E, Chen-Lim ML, Carpenter KM 2nd, Wallhauser E, Friedlaender E. Pain assessment of children with autism spectrum disorders. *J Dev Behav Pediatr.* 2016;37(1):53-61. doi:10.1097/DBP.0000000000000240.

10. Fowler-Kerry S, Lander JR. Assessment of sex differences in children's and adolescents' self-reported pain from venipuncture. *J Pediatr Psychol.* 1991;16(6):783-793.

11. Grunau RE. Neonatal pain in very preterm infants: long-term effects on brain, neurodevelopment and pain reactivity. *Rambam Maimonides Med J.* 2013;4(4):e0025. doi:10.5041/RMMJ.10132. eCollection 2013.

12. Hatfield LA. Neonatal pain: what's age got to do with it? *Surg Neurol Int.* 2014;5(suppl 13):S479-S489. doi:10.4103/2152-7806.144630. eCollection 2014.

13. Herr K, Coyne PJ, Manworren RCB, McCaffery M, Merkel S. Pain assessment in the patients unable to self-report: position statement update. *Pain Manag Nurs.* 2011;12(4):230.

14. Italia S, Wolfenstetter SB, Teuner CM. Patterns of complementary and alternative medicine (CAM) use in children: a systematic review. *Eur J Pediatr.* 2014;173(11):1413-1428. doi:10.1007/s00431-014-2300-z.

15. Jacobs E, Stinson J, Duran J, et al. Usability testing of a smartphone for accessing a web-based e-diary for self-monitoring of pain and symptoms in sickle cell disease. *J Pediatr Hematol Oncol.* 2012;34(5):326-335.

16. King S, Chambers C, Huguet A, et al. The epidemiology of chronic pain in children and adolescents revisited: a systematic review. *Pain.* 2011;152:2729-2738.

17. Manworren RC. Pediatric nursing knowledge and attitude survey regarding pain. *Pediatr Nurs.* 2014;40(1):50.

18. Miró J, Castarlenas E, Huguet A. Evidence for the use of a numerical rating scale to assess the intensity of pediatric pain. *Eur J Pain.* 2009;13(10):1089-1095.

19. Noll M, Candotti CT, Rosa BN, Loss JF. Back pain prevalence and associated factors in children and adolescents: an epidemiological population study. *Rev Saude Publica.* 2016;50:pii: S0034-89102016000100219. doi:10.1590/S1518-8787.2016050006175.

20. Northwestern University. PROMIS® (Patient-Reported Outcomes Measurement Information System), National Institutes of Health grant U2C CA186878 01; 2016. http://www.healthmeasures.net/resource-center/about-us.

21. Pagé MG, Katz J, Stinson J, et al. Validation of the numerical rating scale for pain intensity and unpleasantness in pediatric acute postoperative pain: sensitivity to change over time. *J Pain.* 2012;13(4):359-369.

22. Pasero C, Quinlan-Colwell A, Rae D, Broglio K, Drew D. American Society for Pain Management nursing position statement: prescribing and administering opioid doses based solely on pain intensity. *Pain Manag Nurs.* 2016;17(3):170-180.

23. Seifert F, Maihöfner C. Functional and structural imaging of pain-induced neuroplasticity. *Curr Opin Anaesthesiol.* 2011;24:515-523.

24. Sieberg CB, Simons LE, Edelstein MR, et al. Pain prevalence and trajectories following pediatric spinal fusion surgery. *J Pain.* 2013;14(12):1694-1702. doi:10.1016/j.jpain.2013.09.005.

25. Stanley M, Pollard D. Relationship between knowledge, attitudes, and self-efficacy of nurses in the management of pediatric pain. *Pediatr Nurs.* 2013;39(4):165-171.

26. Stinson J, Yamada J, Kavanagh T, Gill N, Stevens B. Systematic review of the psychometric properties and feasibility of self-report pain measures for use in clinical trials in children and adolescents. *Pain.* 2006;125(1-2):143-157.

27. Taylor DM, Dhir R, Craig SS, et al. Complementary and alternative medicine use among paediatric emergency department patients. *J Paediatr Child Health.* 2015;51(9):895-900. doi:10.1111/jpc.12898. [Epub 2015].

28. Tomlinson D, von Baeyer CL, Stinson JN, Sung L. A systematic review of faces scales for the self-report of pain intensity in children. *Pediatrics.* 2010;126(5):e1168-e1198.

29. von Baeyer CL, Spagrud LJ, McCormick JC, et al. Three new datasets supporting use of the Numerical Rating Scale (NRS-11) for children's self-reports of pain intensity. *Pain.* 2009;143(3):223-227.

CHAPTER 35

PAIN IN THE OLDER PATIENT

Salim Hayek and Nidhi Sondhi

1. **Who is the "older patient"?**
   In general, the older adult is considered to be age 65 and older, and this age group is currently the fastest growing age group worldwide. By 2030 this age group is estimated to make up approximately 20% of the total population, and by 2040 they are estimated to have a population of 1.3 billion worldwide.

2. **Why is there a growing need for pain management in this population?**
   Traditionally, pain was believed to be an inevitable consequence of aging; however, this thought process has changed. Currently, pain in the elder population often remains undiagnosed and undertreated—50% of older patients in the community and 80% of nursing home residents report chronic daily pain.

   In addition, undiagnosed chronic pain in the elderly has significant social and financial impacts. This is due to chronic pain being a multidimensional syndrome with physical, psychological, and social consequences. Lack of diagnosis and treatment leads to impaired activities of daily living (ADLs), decrease in ambulation, falls, malnutrition, increased risk of frailty, and mood/cognitive changes.

3. **What are the challenges/barriers to effective pain management in the older patient?**
   The effective treatment of pain in the elder population is multifactorial, and barriers/challenges exist at many levels from the patients themselves, health care professionals, to the health care system.
   Patient Barriers: Many elder patients have the misconception that pain is untreatable and a normal part of aging, and therefore do not seek treatment. In addition, some older individuals whose pain may cause significant limitations avoid treatment, secondary to fear that their independence may be taken from them or that the medications prescribed will cause side effects or addiction. For others, comorbidities such as depression or dementia, sensory impairments such as vision and hearing loss, and memory impairment can make compliance and effective management challenging.
   Provider Barriers: Lack of adequate knowledge, training, and education on assessment, diagnoses, and pain medications used in elder individuals may limit many health care professionals from providing optimal care to elderly individuals in chronic pain. Many health care professionals have difficulty assessing patients, given the factors listed previously, while others, untrained in medication management in the elderly, may be in fear of polypharmacy, overdose, adverse reactions, and managing need for dose escalation. Failure to understand the physiologic changes that occur in the elderly that predispose them to increased risk for medication adverse reactions and at lower dosages is the main reason for apprehension among health care providers dealing with elderly individuals suffering from chronic pain.
   System Barriers: Lastly, systemic factors also affect access to care and treatment in the elderly. Many older patients have limited access to treatment secondary to health insurance, cost of medications and interventions, and transportation to office visits.

4. **What is the pathophysiology of pain in the older patient?**
   Although the pathophysiology of pain in the older patient continues to be studied, there are some known physiologic changes in both pain signaling and perception that influence pain in the elder population.

   First, there are age-related functional and structural changes to the peripheral nerves. Many studies in the elder population have shown a decrease in the number of myelinated and unmyelinated fibers, as well as an increase in the number of damaged fibers, both of which can alter pain conduction. In addition, there is a decrease in substance P and calcitonin gene-related peptide (CGRP), and a decrease in the rate of CGRP transport through neuronal axons. Substance P and CGRP are neurotransmitters for primary afferent nociceptive fibers, and these findings suggest age-related deterioration of afferent sensory neurons.

In the central nervous system, there are degenerative changes in dorsal horn sensory neurons in the spinal cord. These changes include axonal involution, demyelination, decreased CGRP, substance P, and somatostatin, and increased loss of noradrenergic and serotonergic neurons, all of which are found to cause altered pain processing and function of descending modulatory pathways. These age-related changes also impair the pain inhibitory systems of the nervous system. There are two endogenous inhibitory systems, opioid-dependent, and non-opioid dependent, both of which show age associated deterioration in many studies. It is suggested that the decreased effectiveness of endogenous pain systems may cause an increase in severity of pain due to noxious stimulation.

5. **How does the pain threshold change with age?**
Overall, multiple studies analyzed through a meta-analysis have shown that pain threshold generally increases with age. In studying the effect of stimulus-specific pain, as it affects the pain threshold in the elderly, an increase in pain threshold with age was noted for non-noxious stimuli; however, there was a decrease in threshold for pressure-like pain and no change for thermal pain.

6. **What are the physiologic changes that occur in the elderly patient?**
See Table 35.1.

7. **What are the pharmacokinetic and pharmacodynamic changes that occur in the elderly patient?**
Pharmacokinetic changes are those that affect the absorption, distribution, protein binding, metabolism and bioavailability, and elimination of a drug. Pharmacodynamic changes relate to alterations in drug-receptor interactions. See Table 35.2.

8. **How can adverse events related to medications be prevented?**
The elderly population is highly vulnerable to medication-related problems manifesting in adverse events including falls, depression, confusion, constipation, and hip fractures. Studies suggest a 6% to 30% incidence of adverse drug events (ADEs) in the elderly. These ADEs are undesirable, harmful, and in many cases preventable by following some basic principles when prescribing medications to the elderly.

Polypharmacy remains a significant risk factor for adverse drug events, especially in the elderly population due to the presence of multiple comorbidities. For this reason, it is advised that the number of providers prescribing medication is limited. In addition, when starting a new medication, it is best to start only one at a time and use the least invasive route of delivery and to start at a low dose that is slowly titrated to effect. When titrating medications and/or changing medication, adequate time intervals should be given in order to prevent adverse drug events or overdosage. Knowing the half-life of a drug can allow a provider to confidently make adjustments while minimizing the risk of harm.

Prior to starting a patient on a new medication, it is essential to determine the quality of the pain the patient is suffering from (i.e., nociceptive vs. neuropathic vs. mixed) in order to choose a medication best suited for that type of pain.

9. **What tools are available to assist prescribers when treating the elderly?**
To help providers minimize the risk of medication-related negative outcomes, multiple screening tools as well as a list of medications with known potential for greater risk than benefit in the elderly have been developed.

The Screening Tool of Older People's Potentially Inappropriate Prescriptions (STOPP) and Screening Tool to Alert Doctors to Right Treatments (START) consist of 114 evidence-based criteria (80 STOPP and 34 START) that are categorized by physiologic system and assist prescribers in preventing inappropriate prescribing and polypharmacy.

The American Geriatrics Society Beers Criteria, recently updated in 2015, provide prescribers with evidence-based tables of reference. Table 1 lists medications that are potentially inappropriate for use in older adults, independent of specific medical conditions. Table 2 considers specific diagnoses and lists certain common medical conditions and medications that may be potentially inappropriate due to drug-disease interactions. In the 2015 update, two additional tables were added, one with common drug-drug interactions seen in the elderly, and another with medications that require dose adjustment based on renal function/creatinine clearance.

Table 35.1. Physiologic Changes With Aging and Their Effects

	CHANGES	EFFECT	EFFECT ON DRUG USE
General	Increased body fat Decreased total body water Decreased muscle mass	Increased V_d for lipophilic drugs Decreased V_d for hydrophilic drugs	*Lipophilic:* Delayed onset of action Prolonged half life *Hydrophilic:* Increased plasma levels Higher frequency of ASEs
Cardiovascular	Decreased cardiac index	Rapid and high drug peak	Increased toxicity risk
Gastrointestinal	Altered secretions Decreased gastric emptying Decreased gastric acid secretion Decreased splanchnic blood flow Decreased absorptive capacity	Increased transit time Decreased drug absorption	Altered oral bioavailability
Liver	Decreased liver blood flow Decreased liver mass Decreased protein synthesis Decreased hepatic enzyme function	Decreased serum albumin Decreased first pass metabolism Decreased liver clearance	Increased bioavailability of drugs with extensive first pass metabolism Decreased bioavailability of prodrugs requiring activation by liver Increased toxicity risk Decreased clearance of high extraction ratio drugs
Renal	Decreased GFR Decreased renal blood flow Decreased size	Decreased renal clearance	Dose adjustment
Nervous system	Decreased cerebral blood flow Decreased neurotransmitters Neuronal atrophy Altered receptor density/affinity	Decreased descending inhibitory pain control Altered pain processing	Altered response to pain Increased pain with noxious stimuli Altered response to CNS/PNS drugs

ASEs, Adverse side effects *CNS,* central nervous system; *GFR,* glomerular filtration rate; *PNS,* peripheral nervous system; V_d, volume of distribution.

Rastogi R, Meek BD. Management of chronic pain in elderly, frail patients: finding a suitable, personalized method of control. *Clin Interv Aging.* 2013:37, Web.

Table 35.2. Pharmacokinetic and Pharmacodynamic Changes With Aging and Their Effects

	CHANGES	EFFECT	EFFECT ON DRUG USE
Absorption	Decreased gastric emptying Decreased gastric acid secretion Decreased splanchnic blood flow Decreased absorptive capacity of the small intestine	Decreased drug absorption	Altered oral medication absorption
Distribution	Decreased total body water Decreased lean muscle mass Increased body fat	Increased V_d for lipophilic drugs Decreased V_d for hydrophilic drugs	*Lipophilic:* Delayed onset of action Prolonged half life *Hydrophilic:* Increased plasma levels Higher frequency of ASEs
Protein binding	Decreased liver mass Decreased protein synthesis	Decreased albumin levels	Increased free drug availability Increased drug-drug interaction
Metabolism/ bioavailability	Decreased liver mass Decreased liver blood flow Decreased CYTP450 and hepatic enzyme function	Decreased first pass metabolism	Increased bioavailability of drugs with extensive first pass metabolism Decreased bioavailability of prodrugs requiring activation by liver Increased toxicity risk
Elimination	*Liver:* Decreased liver blood flow *Kidney:* Decreased GFR Decreased renal blood flow Decreased size	*Liver:* Decreased liver clearance *Kidney:* Decreased renal clearance	*Liver:* Decreased clearance for drugs with high extraction ratio *Kidney:* Dose adjustment
Pharmacodynamic	Decreased receptor density Increased receptor affinity	Altered sensitivity to CNS/PNS drugs	Increased sensitivity to centrally acting drugs Decreased sensitivity to adrenergic/cholinergic receptor-specific drugs Increased drug-drug and drug-disease interaction

ASEs, Adverse side effects; CNS, central nervous system; CYTP450, cytochrome P450; GFR, glomerular filtration rate; PNS, peripheral nervous system; V_d, volume of distribution.

10. **What methods can be used to assess pain in the elderly?**

    There are a number of pain assessment instruments used throughout medicine. Many of the most commonly used instruments are unidimensional and measure only pain intensity. Examples of these include the visual analog scale (VAS) and the Wong-Baker Faces Pain Rating Scale, which provide a visual with a series of faces with varying levels of discomfort from a happy face to a crying face that a patient can identify with. Alternatively, there is the pain thermometer, variations of which include visual factors such as gradual color scales from blue to red or yellow to red, with red identifying severe pain.

    Although these instruments can be useful, pain is a multidimensional experience with sensory and emotional components that further impact a patient's psychological and functional abilities, especially in the elderly population. It is therefore more valuable to perform a complete pain assessment in which unidimensional scales are used in conjunction with multidimensional pain instruments, known as Verbal Descriptor Scales (VDS) to measure pain experience. The McGill Pain Questionnaire (MPQ) is one such multidimensional scale that uses subjective word descriptors as well as a five-point pain intensity scale to evaluate the sensory, affective, and evaluative components of pain. In addition, there is the West Haven-Yale Multidimensional Pain Inventory (WHYMPI), which is divided into three parts. The first part measures the chronic pain experience, including perceived interference of pain, spousal concern, distress, life control, and severity. The second part assesses the patient's perceptions on the degree to which spouses display negative behaviors in response to the pain, and the third part assesses a patient's self-report on their ability to perform everyday activities.

11. **What methods can be used to assess pain in the cognitively impaired elderly?**

    The use of VAS and VDS scales can be limited in a patient with dementia or cognitive impairment, placing this elder population at an even higher risk for underdiagnosis and treatment. In a study of elderly patients with dementia, 84% were not receiving pain medication, despite diagnoses likely to elicit pain.

    In the cognitively impaired, observation for vocalizations or changes in function/behavior patterns can provide insight toward underlying pain. The Hierarchy of Pain Assessment is a tool that can provide a framework for assessment, diagnosis, and treatment in the cognitively impaired. It begins with self-report in those with mild to moderate dementia, progresses to considering common pain etiologies and searching for potential causes of pain, observing behaviors, considering proxy reports by caregivers and family, and lastly an analgesic trial with close follow-up on results.

NONPHARMACOLOGICAL MODALITIES

12. **What nonpharmacological modalities can be used for pain control?**

    Given the multifactorial nature of pain, nonpharmacological modalities are often used for the psychological and functional components of the pain experience. Relaxation and biofeedback training are two methods that teach a patient to have a greater sense of awareness of their pain, with the intent to use techniques that allow them to manipulate their psychological, emotional, and physical response. Behavioral training is a similar technique which focuses on extinguishing pain enhancing behaviors such as talking about pain and rather re-focuses attention on behaviors not related to pain. Cognitive behavioral therapy (CBT) coaches patients on how to change negative thoughts and behaviors that prevent coping into behaviors that allow for greater control over one's pain. Studies have shown mixed results for these pain coping strategies in the elderly; however, when used in a multidisciplinary approach, these methods have been beneficial in helping reduce pain intensity and medication intake.

    Physical therapy and occupational therapy are important modalities for preventing frailty, as well as maintaining independence and function. Goals of therapy include stabilizing the primary condition, preventing secondary injuries, changing pain perception, assessing and treating for functional deficits, and fostering modifications around existing disabilities. Physical therapy allows for evaluation of mobility, strength, endurance, and range of motion, whereas occupational therapy evaluates activities of daily living, safety, and independent living skills.

NON-OPIOIDS

13. **What non-opioid pharmacological agents are available for the elderly?**

    Acetaminophen and nonsteroidal anti-inflammatory drugs (NSAIDs) are the most common non-opioid pain medications prescribed. Acetaminophen potentiates the effects of opioids and is therefore a useful co-analgesic; however, it does have a ceiling effect, and therefore dose escalation is limited. It is metabolized by the liver and excreted by the kidneys, and therefore caution must be taken in cases of altered liver/kidney function. The maximum recommended dose for the elderly is 2000 mg a day. Overall, acetaminophen is considered a safe drug with demonstrated effectiveness and should be used as a first line as well as ongoing medication if not contraindicated.

NSAIDs, on the other hand, are considered high risk for cardiac, gastrointestinal, and renal side effects, drug-disease, and drug-drug interactions in the elderly, and should therefore be avoided in long-term management. Effects include dose- and time-dependent increased risk for GI bleeding and ulcers, renal vasoconstriction, and increased tubular sodium reabsorption, contributing to hypertension, fluid retention, renal failure, myocardial infarcts, and heart failure. If NSAIDs are to be used, topical NSAIDs are preferred; however, if systemic NSAIDs are used, a proton pump inhibitor is suggested for gastrointestinal protection.

ADJUVANTS

14. What are pharmacologic adjuvants, and which are used in the treatment of chronic pain?
Pharmacologic adjuvants are medications used as analgesics that were originally developed for other indications. These are commonly used in conjunction with analgesics for chronic and refractory pain. Most commonly, antiepileptics, antidepressants, corticosteroids, local anesthetics, and muscle relaxants are used in pain.

Commonly used antiepileptics include gabapentin, pregabalin, and topiramate, as these have been found to be effective analgesics in the management of neuropathic pain. Titration of these medications in the elderly should be slow, as sedation and cognitive impairment are known side effects. Dose adjustment is also required for patients with renal dysfunction.

Antidepressants that are commonly used as analgesics include those in the category of tricyclic antidepressants (TCAs) or serotonin norepinephrine reuptake inhibitors (SNRIs). TCAs include nortriptyline and amitriptyline. In the elderly population, however, caution should be taken, as side effects include cardiac dysrhythmias, cognitive impairment, and anticholinergic effects such as hypotension, urinary retention, and sedation. SNRIs on the other hand, such as duloxetine, are efficacious in neuropathic pain and better tolerated than TCAs.

Local anesthetics are often used in the form of topical patches and are therefore easy to use, and also have a decreased risk of toxicity and drug interactions. Muscle relaxants, in general, have very limited efficacy, if any, as analgesics in chronic pain.

OPIOIDS

15. What opioid pharmacologic agents are available?
Patients with moderate to severe pain or pain related functional impairment not controlled with non-opioids should be considered for opioid therapy. Typically milder and short-acting opioids are attempted prior to the use of stronger opioids. These consist usually of oxycodone, hydrocodone, and tramadol. Tramadol, a weak opioid agonist and monoamine uptake inhibitor, is considered a safer drug with less respiratory and gastrointestinal effects. Care should be taken in patients with a history of seizures, as tramadol lowers the seizure threshold, and with patients on serotonergic drugs due to concern for serotonin syndrome.

Stronger opioids such as morphine, oxymorphone, fentanyl, hydromorphone, and methadone may be indicated in cases where less potent opioids fail to provide adequate pain relief. Many of these stronger opioids come in immediate release and extended release formulations.

16. What are the opioid considerations for patients with hepatic and renal dysfunction?
With hepatic and renal dysfunction being common comorbidities in the elderly, it is essential to take into the account the severity of dysfunction when prescribing opioids. Hydromorphone, oxycodone, and methadone metabolism is dependent on the function of the liver and should therefore be avoided in patients with significant liver impairment. Fentanyl is therefore the opioid of choice with liver dysfunction.

Morphine undergoes hepatic metabolism and is broken down into two metabolites: morphine-6-glucoronide (M6G) and morphine-3-glucoronide (M3G). These metabolites undergo enterohepatic circulation and are then excreted through the bile/feces and the urine. M3G has neuroexcitatory effects and therefore has detrimental effects secondary to accumulation in patients with renal impairment with potential for inducing convulsions. M6G, on the other hand, is a potent opioid analgesic.

17. **Do opioid concerns differ in the elderly?**
In general, opioid tolerance is less likely to set in the elderly compared to younger people. As such, it is not unusual to observe elderly individuals with chronic pain on stable doses of opioids for years. While elder individuals with chronic pain often cite fear of addiction for refusing opioids, the risk for dependence or addiction appears to be smaller than the general population. Risk factors for dependence or addiction include history of previous personal or family history of substance abuse, or alcohol abuse as well as some personality and psychological disorders. While evidence supports the use of opioid analgesics in acute pain and end-of-life care, limited evidence exists in support of opioid use in chronic noncancer pain. In general, use of opioids in the management of chronic pain in the elderly should be undertaken with the same precautions as their use in the general population.

18. **How should opioids be titrated in the elderly?**
Due to the extensive side effects associated with opioids, patients should be monitored closely and frequently for efficacy and side effects. Opioids should be started low and titrated slowly, taking into account kidney and liver function.
When starting an opioid, it is recommended to start an immediate release opioid at the lowest effective dose with slow titration as needed. As a generalization, starting at a dose 25% to 50% less than the dose that would be given to a younger patient is recommended. When titrating opioids, practice guidelines suggest increasing dosages by 25% to 50% in those with mild to moderate pain and by 50% to 100% in those with moderate to severe pain. Once effective analgesia is obtained, the immediate release opioid dose may be converted to extended release formulations, if appropriate.
In the case of opioid rotation and converting from one opioid to another, the new opioid should be initiated at 50% to 67% of the current total opioid dose.

19. **How should opioid side effects be managed?**
Common side effects of opioids include constipation, nausea/vomiting, sedation, dizziness, impaired cognition, and respiratory depression. These adverse effects can be exaggerated in the elderly population, and therefore close monitoring and early management is required by the prescriber. Management can be in the form of symptomatic medication management, opioid rotation/changing the opioid used, altering the dose, or altering the route of delivery (transdermal vs. oral).
In the case of constipation, the most common side effect, prophylaxis with a stool softener or laxative is recommended. Opioid induced nausea can be effectively managed with antiemetic agents that target the chemoreceptor trigger zone such as droperidol and prochlorperazine, serotonin antagonists such as ondansetron, gastric motility agents such as metoclopramide, and antihistamines/anticholinergics to reduce vestibular sensitivity. Sedation, impaired cognition, and respiratory depression usually require a reduction in opioid dosage. It is important to avoid combining opioids and benzodiazepines, given synergistic effects on respiratory depression. Other central nervous system depressants may have similar effects when combined with opioids and should be avoided.

INTERVENTIONAL MODALITIES

20. **What interventional modalities are available for pain control in the older patient?**
In cases where pharmacologic and nonpharmacologic interventions may be limited in achieving adequate analgesia, interventional modalities that target the pain pathways may be beneficial. There are limited studies on the effectiveness of interventional procedures specifically in the elderly population; however, it is believed that a combination of medications and interventional procedures helps to overall reduce medication intake and decrease the risk for side effects.
Various interventions exist that use either chemical or electrical means to either destroy or alter the pain signals. These include nerve blocks, chemical neurolysis, cryoneurolysis,

radiofrequency ablation, and neuraxial interventions, such as epidurals and intrathecal drug delivery, and spinal cord stimulation.

Epidural steroid injections have been useful for the treatment of spinal stenosis, degenerative disease, and sciatica. Studies are again limited, but in general a combination of epidural steroid injections, medication, and physical therapy affords the patient a good chance to reduce pain and increase function.

Spinal cord stimulation (SCS) and intrathecal drug delivery (IDD) are other options. Although no specific studies have been performed in the elderly specifically, studies that have included patients over the age of 65 have supported the use of IDD and SCS for patients with chronic pain uncontrolled by medication.

KEY POINTS

1. The older adult is aged 65 years and older and this age group is the fastest growing age group worldwide.
2. Patient, provider, and systemic barriers exist in providing effective pain management to this population.
3. Understanding the physiologic and pharmacokinetic/pharmacodynamic changes that occur in the elderly are essential for optimal management and preventing adverse drug events.
4. A multidisciplinary approach including nonpharmacologic modalities, non-opioids, adjuvants, opioids, and interventional modalities is best to improve pain control, reduce medication intake, decrease risk for side effects, and increase function.

BIBLIOGRAPHY

1. "American geriatrics society 2015 updated beers criteria for potentially inappropriate medication use in older adults". *J Am Geriatr Soc.* 2015;63(11):2227-2246, Web.
2. Argoff CE, Cranmer KW. The pharmacological management of chronic pain in long-term care settings: balancing efficacy and safety. *Consult Pharm.* 2003:4-18, Print.
3. Chau DL, et al. Opiates and elderly: use and side effects. *Clin Interv Aging.* 2008;3:273-278, Web.
4. Gagliese L, Melzack R. Chronic pain in elderly people. *Pain.* 1997;70(1):3-14, Web.
5. Gibson SJ, Farrell M. A review of age differences in the neurophysiology of nociception and the perceptual experience of pain. *Clin J Pain.* 2004;20(4):227-239, Web.
6. "Guidance on the management of pain in older people". *Age Ageing.* 2013;42(suppl 1):i1-i57, Web.
7. Herr K, et al. Pain assessment in the patient unable to self-report: position statement with clinical practice recommendations. *Pain Manag Nurs.* 2011;12(4):230-250, Web.
8. Kaye AD, Baluch A, Scott JT. Pain management in the elderly population: a review. *Ochsner J.* 2010;10(3):179-187, Print.
9. Mangoni AA, Jackson SHD. Age-related changes in pharmacokinetics and pharmacodynamics: basic principles and practical applications. *Br J Clin Pharmacol.* 2003;57(1):6-14, Web.
10. O'Mahony D, et al. STOPP/START criteria for potentially inappropriate prescribing in older people: version 2. *Age Ageing.* 2014;44(2):213-218, Web.
11. "Pharmacological management of persistent pain in older persons". *J Am Geriatr Soc.* 2009;57(8):1331-1346, Web.
12. Rastogi R, Meek BD. Management of chronic pain in elderly, frail patients: finding a suitable, personalized method of control. *Clin Interv Aging.* 2013:37, Web.

TOPICAL ANALGESICS

Claire Collison and Charles E. Argoff

CHAPTER 36

OVERVIEW

1. What is the history of topical medications as analgesics?

   For centuries, topical analgesics have been used to treat various medical conditions and pain. One of the most famous books in the history of medicine, Avicenna's *Canon of Medicine*, originally published in 1025, provides an extensive list of substances to treat headache. Most of these substances included topical analgesics derived from plants, animals, and minerals. There are topical formulations of plant-derived products created centuries ago that are still used today, including camphor, capsaicin, and menthol. Topical medications for pain have had a critical role in alleviating painful syndromes and will continue to do so as we learn more about their underlying mechanisms and uses.

2. How is a topical medication different from a transdermal drug?

   Both topical (topiceutical) and transdermal medications are applied locally to the skin. However, once transdermal preparations are absorbed through the skin, the bloodstream distributes the medication throughout the body for a systemic effect. To be effective, the transdermal analgesic requires a systemic analgesic concentration. Transdermal drugs provide the same effect, as if the same active ingredient was taken orally. These kinds of patches can be placed to any skin area (according to the product instructions), since the medication will be delivered through the bloodstream to the targeted area in the body. One example is the Durogesic patch (Janssen Pharmaceutica, Titusville, New Jersey).

   In comparison, a topical patch produces more local effects. Once the medication penetrates skin, it takes its effect on tissues (muscles, ligaments, tendons, nerves) that lie directly underneath the area where it was applied on the skin application. These medications do not reach the bloodstream, so they do not result in any significant systemic concentration of analgesic. However, topical medications must be used according to the package instructions, because excessive application for extended periods of time over a larger area can promote increased medication penetration, leading to accumulation in the bloodstream, which may cause side effects. Topical patches include but are not limited to the Bengay spa cream (Pfizer, New York), Lidoderm patch (Endo Pharmaceuticals, Chadds Ford, Pennsylvania), and EMLA cream (2.5% lidocaine and prilocaine 2.5%) (AstraZeneca, Wilmington, Delaware).

   Topical agents that are delivered directly to targeted tissues under the skin are advantageous over systemic pain medications for several reasons. One reason is that there is a lower risk of unwanted side effects in the body. For example, topical nonsteroidal antiinflammatory agents (NSAIDs) for controlling pain with osteoarthritis and rheumatic diseases were found to be effective and avoided the gastrointestinal adverse effects of oral NSAIDs like peptic ulcers and hemorrhage. Since topical agents do not result in bodywide (systemic) concentrations or lead to drug-drug interactions, these medications can be safely added to an existing pain treatment plan without worry. Patients with chronic pain conditions may be receiving other pharmacological therapies for their comorbid conditions, so the ability to add a topiceutical to their existing regiment is clinically helpful.

3. What are the various topical formulations available for the treatment of pain?

   Topical pain medications can be taken as both a prescription and nonprescription (e.g., over-the-counter [OTC]) drugs. Prescription topical pain preparations are administered as a patch or a cream. For example, the lidocaine patch has an adhesive material containing the active ingredient applied to a polyester felt backing that is covered with a release liner, which is removed before applying to the skin. Current prescription topical medications include the Lidoderm patch, EMLA cream, the 8% capsaicin patch, diclofenac sodium gel patch and solution, and doxepin cream. Current OTC topical formulations include lidocaine creams, benzocaine creams, menthol creams, gels, and patches, as well as combination products that can combine menthol, camphor, salicylate, and capsaicin.

4. **What are the advantages and disadvantages of using topical medications?**
Topical medications offer few systemic adverse effects and drug-drug interactions. They have a clinical advantage in that they can be added to a patient's current list of medications for pain or other comorbid conditions. There is extensive evidence showing their effectiveness and safety in treating a range of conditions like neuropathic pain and chronic pain syndromes that may otherwise be refractory to prior traditional treatments. The benefits to patients are clear; they are generally easy and nonpainful to apply on the skin and take effect relatively quickly. The possible side effects of topical analgesics that may include erythema or rash are often minimal and self-limited. Topical anesthetics are a helpful alternative for patients who fear needles or who are unable to take oral tablets and capsules. Some skin patches can be shaped to cover the painful area.

The disadvantages of topical medications vary on the specific dosage formulation used. Sometimes ointments, creams, and lotions can stain clothing. Careful attention must be used with children who may remove the medication and accidentally eat it or put it in the ears or eyes. Some formulations require measurement or are dosed according to weight (e.g., for use on children). Skin patches may lead to localized reactions, causing the skin area to become pale, itchy, red, or inflamed. Long-term adherence to the skin is difficult if the skin is oily or hairy. Patients may not be able to shower or swim while wearing the skin patch. One newly available type of skin patch, Synera, contains a built-in heating element to improve drug delivery that may cause thermal burns if the top cover is removed. Another skin patch requires a device that creates a mild electrical current to run through the patch and skin to increase the permeability and absorption of the drug through the skin. This drug, however, should only be applied by a health care professional at the office, clinic, or hospital.

OVER-THE-COUNTER PAIN RELIEVERS

5. **What topical analgesics are currently available in the United States without a prescription? How are they being used?**
There are four broad categories of nonprescription (OTC) topical medications used to treat pain.
1. Local anesthetics, such as lidocaine (e.g., ELA-Max), work by inhibiting the sodium-channel in nociceptive peripheral nerves, thus blocking the signal from traveling to the brain to produce a painful sensation.
2. Counterirritants, medications containing menthol or camphor (e.g., Bengay spa cream), are used to treat conditions such as osteoarthritis or injuries such as sprains or strains by blocking the painful signal from reaching the brain. Specifically, menthol activates the transient receptor potential cation channel subfamily M member 8 (TRPM8), an ion channel in cold-sensitive peripheral sensory neurons, which has a role in pain control.
3. Antiinflammatory medications, such as methyl salicylate (e.g., Myoflex or Aspercreme), are hydrolyzed in the tissues to salicylic acid, which has antiinflammatory actions. By reducing the inflammation in the affected area, these compounds reduce the ongoing irritation of local nerves, thereby blocking the pain signals from reaching the brain.
4. Capsaicin, the main ingredient in a relatively new group of OTC topical analgesics, originates from hot chili peppers and can be found in products such as Zostrix and Capzasin-HP. Capsaicin selectively binds to the transient potential vanilloid subfamily member 1 found on sensory neurons. Initially capsaicin excites the nerve and there may be an initial increase in pain. Then, as the medication empties the chemical substance required by the nerve to transmit the pain, the sensation generally subsides within a few minutes after application. Hence, these particular medications containing capsaicin should be applied carefully, and patients should wash hands thoroughly after application to prevent spreading of the medication and a burning sensation over other areas of the body.

Finally, certain OTC topical analgesic preparations may contain various combinations of the ingredients mentioned previously in an attempt to improve clinical efficacy by combining medications that have different mechanisms.

6. **What are specific examples of over-the-counter pain relievers?**
Table 36.1 lists examples of OTC pain relievers and includes information about their active ingredients, proper use, and side effects.

Table 36.1. Available Nonprescription (Over-the-Counter) Topical Analgesics

EXAMPLE PRODUCTS (MANUFACTURER)	ACTIVE INGREDIENT	USE	INFORMATION FOR PROPER USE	COMMON SIDE EFFECTS	ADDITIONAL TIPS FOR USE
Local Anesthetic-Containing Products					
ELA-Max (Ferndale) Xylocaine (Astra) Solarcaine (Schering-Plough) DermaFlex (Zila) Nupercainal (Ciba) Lanacane (Combe) Hurricaine (Beutlich)	4% lidocaine in a topical cream 0.5%–2.5% lidocaine in gels, creams, ointments, depending on the product. Many generic lidocaine products also available. 0.5%–1.0% dibucaine 5%–20% benzocaine in gels, ointments, creams, lotions, and sprays. Many generic benzocaine products also available.	Relief of local pain caused by minor cuts and burns, abrasions, sunburn, insect bites, needle sticks for blood draws, and needle insertion into veins	Apply to affected areas no >3 or 4 times per day Apply only to intact skin For external use only	Irritation, redness, itching, rash	Not recommended for use on mucous membranes Not for use in patients <2 years old without consulting a physician Avoid contact with eyes, mouth, or nose and inside of ears Dressing recommended for children to prevent accidental ingestion Do not use in large amounts over raw skin or blistered areas; do not use more often than 3 or 4 times per day
Menthol- or Camphor-Containing Products					
Bengay Spa Cream (Pfizer) Therapeutic Mineral Ice Gel (Bristol-Myers)	1.25%–16% menthol in creams, gels, patches	Relief of pain of muscular aches, neuralgia, rheumatism, arthritis, sprains and like conditions	Apply to affected areas no more than 3 or 4 times per day Apply only to intact skin For external use only	Irritation, rash, burning, stinging, swelling	Not recommended for use on mucous membranes Avoid contact with eyes, mouth or nose and inside of ears

Continued on following page

Table 36.1. Available Nonprescription (Over-the-Counter) Topical Analgesics (*Continued*)

EXAMPLE PRODUCTS (MANUFACTURER)	ACTIVE INGREDIENT	USE	INFORMATION FOR PROPER USE	COMMON SIDE EFFECTS	ADDITIONAL TIPS FOR USE
Capsaicin-Containing Products					
Capzasin-HP & Capzasin-P (Thompson Medical) Zostrix, Zostrix-HP (GenDerm)	0.025%–0.075% capsaicin in creams, gels, lotions	Temporary relief of pain from rheumatoid arthritis, osteoarthritis, and relief of neuralgias such as the pain following shingles or diabetic neuropathy	Apply to affected areas no more than 3 or 4 times per day Apply only to intact skin For external use only	Burning, redness, stinging, cough	Not for use on mucous membranes Avoid contact with the eyes Wash hands immediately after application Use caution when handling contact lenses after application Do not bandage tightly
Salicylate-Containing Products					
Myoflex (Fisons) Sportscreme (Chattem) Infrarub (Whitehall) Aspercreme (Chattem) Arthritis Formula Bengay (Pfizer)	Many products available, ranging from 83%–55% methyl salicylate in creams, gels, ointments, and lotions	Relief of pain of muscular aches, neuralgia, rheumatism, arthritis, sprains, and like conditions	Apply to affected areas no more than 3 or 4 times per day Apply only to intact skin For external use only	If applied to large areas may cause tinnitus, nausea, or vomiting	Not recommended for use on mucous membranes Avoid contact with eyes, mouth, or nose and inside of ears
Combination Products					
Flexall Ultra Plus Gel (Chattem) Icy Hot Chill Stick (Chattem) Arthritis Hot Cream (Chattem) Banalg Lotion (Forest)	Many different products that combine menthol or camphor with a salicylate or capsaicin in creams, gels, liquids, or patches	Relief of pain of muscular aches, neuralgia, rheumatism, arthritis, sprains, and like conditions	Apply to affected areas no more than 3 or 4 times per day Apply only to intact skin For external use only	See information above for each of the various ingredients' side effects Not recommended for use on mucous membranes	Avoid contact with eyes, mouth, or nose and inside of ears

PRESCRIPTION PAIN RELIEVERS

7. What are the most commonly prescribed topical analgesics in the United States? How are they used?

There has been increasing interest in developing topical medications for the treatment of various pain conditions over the past 5 years. Examples of prescription topical analgesics available in the United States can be found in Table 36.2, which includes information concerning their use, directions for use, and side effects.

One subcategory of prescription topical analgesics includes the Lidoderm patch and EMLA cream. In 1999, the Lidoderm patch (lidocaine 5%; Endo Pharmaceuticals, Chadds Ford, Pennsylvania) was approved by the Food and Drug Administration to treat pain caused by damaged nerves following a shingles infection. Several randomized controlled trials show that the lidocaine patch 5% is significantly effective and safe at reducing pain in patients with postherpetic neuralgia and allodynia, and in patients with peripheral neuropathic pain syndromes. In addition to treating postherpetic neuralgia and allodynia, lidocaine has been shown to be therapeutically useful to relieve pain associated with diabetic neuropathy, carpal tunnel syndrome, and postmastectomy pain, as well as nonnerve conditions such as joint and low back, myofascial, osteoarthritis, and sports injury pains.

Lidoderm is applied as a 10-by-14-cm, white, polyester felt patch that contains an adhesive with 5% lidocaine (700 mg) and a clear, film-release liner that is removed prior to patch application to the most painful area of intact skin (e.g., no blisters or open skin ulcers). One of the advantages is that topical lidocaine patches can be used as a first-line treatment and can also be added to current therapies for peripheral neuropathic pain syndromes The patch can also act as a barrier for patients who have a painful skin area extra sensitive to touch.

The mechanism of action is by reducing peripheral processing of pain from the affected or injured nerves to the central processing, or brain. Since injured peripheral sensory nerves are extremely sensitive to the blocking effects of lidocaine, absorption of the drug into the bloodstream is not necessary for its effect. This topical formulation releases an amount of lidocaine sufficient to block pain signals in the local tissues but not enough to cause complete numbness of the area.

EMLA cream (AstraZeneca Pharmaceuticals, Wilmington, Delaware) is a cream or a topical adhesive disc system that contains a mixture of lidocaine and procaine. Unlike the Lidocaine 5% patch, which only produces analgesic effects, the EMLA cream produces both analgesia and anesthesia, so it can be used in adults and children to provide pain relief from a surgical procedure. EMLA cream can provide transient anesthesia for procedures such as arterial or venous puncture, placement of intravenous catheters, lumbar puncture, minor superficial surgeries (e.g., circumcision, genital wart removal), dermatological procedures (e.g., biopsies, laser treatments), and wound care. The mechanism of action is that the mixture of lidocaine and procaine inhibit nerve signals from traveling to the brain. To provide anesthesia for minor dermal procedures, EMLA cream is placed over the skin surface for at least 1 hour. For major dermal procedures, the cream is applied to the affected area, and then wrapped in an occlusive dressing for 1.5 to 2 hours before the procedure. EMLA also comes as single-use transdermal patch form; the disc contains the medication and is placed over the skin area (10 cm^2) to be anesthetized, and an adhesive tape ring keeps the patch in place. There are several disadvantages to the EMLA cream. The research on EMLA for pain control has mixed findings, and some studies show that EMLA cream is less effective for relieving postherpetic neuralgia. Further, EMLA cream requires repeated applications 2 or 3 times daily, while the Lidocaine patch is applied once daily.

FUTURE DEVELOPMENTS

8. What new topical analgesics are available, and what topical analgesics are now in development that may become available in the United States over the next few years?

Recently, various formulations of topical NSAIDs products are available in the United States for acute and chronic musculoskeletal conditions. These antiinflammatory medications reduce the inflammation (i.e., swelling), thereby relieving pain. Recent research shows that topical NSAIDs provide more pain relief for chronic musculoskeletal pain than other treatments that use lidocaine, capsaicin, and rubefacients. These topical NSAIDs include diclofenac creams/patches/gels, ketorolac gels/drops/foams, ibuprofen cream, ketoprofen gel, and indomethacin ointments/sprays/gels. The American College of Rheumatology recommends topical NSAIDs for hand and knee osteoarthritis for patients

Table 36.2. Available Prescription Topical Analgesics

	FORMULATION	USE	INFORMATION FOR PROPER USE	COMMON SIDE EFFECTS	ADDITIONAL TIPS FOR USE
Lidoderm Patch (lidocaine patch 5%) Endo Pharmaceuticals (Chadds Ford, Pennsylvania)	Lidocaine 5% in a nonwoven, polyester felt patch	Relief of pain persisting after a shingles infection	Apply up to three patches (after removing the protective liner) to the site of pain for 12 h in a 24 h period Apply only to dry, intact skin Cut the patch if needed to fit the area of painful skin	Mild redness or swelling of skin in area of patch application; generally clears up after patch removal	Avoid contact with eyes Fold the patch onto itself and discard in trash; keep away from children and pets Store in envelopes until use so the patches do not dry out Do not apply in conjunction with other creams, ointments, lotions, or heating pads
—	Lidocaine 70 mg and tetracaine 70 mg in a patch containing a heating element	Relief of local pain caused by needle insertion into veins, needle sticks for blood draws, or skin procedures of the upper skin layers (e.g., biopsy of the skin where tissue is removed for further examination)	For needle insertion or vein puncture, apply one patch for 20–30 min For skin procedures involving the upper layers of the skin, apply patch for 30 min prior to the procedure Apply only to intact skin	Mild redness, swelling, paleness of skin, or abnormal feeling in area of patch application; generally clears up after patch removal Remove patch if irritation or burning sensation occurs with patch application	Do not cut the patch or remove the top cover—the patch could heat to temperatures that could cause burns Do not block the holes on the top of the patch—the patch may not properly heat Fold the patch onto itself and discard in trash; keep away from children and pets

LidoSite Topical System (lidocaine HCl/epinephrine topical iontophoretic patch 10%/0.1%) and the LidoSite Controller B. Braun (Bethlehem, Pennsylvania)	Lidocaine 10% and epinephrine 0.1% in a circular reservoir, single-use patch; the treatment side and return reservoir on the other side complete the electrical circuit	Relief of local pain caused by needle insertion into veins, needle sticks for blood draw, lasers used to burn skin lesions away in upper skin layers	One patch should be applied by a health care professional in a health care setting for 10 min Apply only to intact skin	Electric current may cause skin irritation, burning feeling, or burns Skin under the patch may show short-lived skin whitening or redness, rash, or pain/burning sensations	For use in patients 5 years old and older Uses electric current to help the drug cross the skin; not for use in someone with electrically sensitive devices (e.g., pacemakers) Contains a sulfite (sodium metabisulfite) that can pose allergic reactions of varying degrees Not tested for use on mucous membranes
EMLA Cream (lidocaine 2.5% and procaine 2.5%) AstraZeneca (Wilmington, Del.)	Lidocaine 2.5% and procaine 2.5% in a cream (may use with Tegaderm skin dressing)	For use on normal intact skin for local pain relief or on genital mucous membranes for minor surgery involving the upper skin layers and as a pretreatment for more extensive skin numbing procedures Used in adults for blood draw needle sticks, genital wart removal; in children for blood draw needle sticks; in newborns prior to circumcision	Apply a thick layer of cream and use a dressing to cover the cream Cream amount required, size of application area, and length of application time vary depending on the type of procedure and the age of the patient (e.g., adult, child, newborn)	Skin paleness, redness, burning, alterations in temperature sensation, edema, itching, and rash in the area of patch application	Dressings are recommended to keep the cream in place and to protect clothing Avoid contact with the eye Use care when applying cream over large areas or leaving it on the skin for longer than 2 h Acutely ill, debilitated, older, or severe liver disease patients may be more sensitive to body-wide effects of lidocaine/procaine

older than 75 years old or with gastrointestinal risk. Since topical NSAIDs do not cause gastrointestinal and other systemic side effects seen with oral NSAIDs, they are useful for patients with osteoarthritis who cannot tolerate oral NSAIDs. Further, topical NSAIDs can be used for sprains, strains, and contusion.

There are also novel formulations of another class of medications called *N*-methyl-D-aspartate (NMDA)-antagonists that may be able to help treat some neuropathic pain disorders. While ketamine, an NMDA-antagonist, is effective for treating neuropathic pain, research shows that it may have a future role in treating conditions including inflammatory pain and nociceptive pain. A study on the uses of amitriptyline and ketamine (AmiKet 4%/2%) supports future development of this drug for treatment of postherpetic neuralgia and in other neuropathy conditions. Research is being done on the combination of AmiKet with an oral formulation for enhanced analgesia for neuropathic pain.

There are new formulations of local anesthetics being developed to treat headaches and neuromas, and recent studies are opening up new avenues of research on topical analgesics for these types of pain.

9. **What is the role of compounded non-Food and Drug Administration-approved topical agents in the treatment of chronic pain?**
Compounded topical agents are prepared by pharmacists and are being used with an increased frequency to treat conditions including postherpetic neuralgia, joint pain, arthritis, fibromyalgia, and other pain conditions. While there is some evidence that these compounded formulations are efficacious, there are few preclinical or human studies on the actual efficacy of these drugs in topical/transdermal formulations. The four most common compounded analgesic drugs, formulated in combination as 5% topical creams or gels, are baclofen, cyclobenzaprine, gabapentin, and amitriptyline. One study showed that a combination of topical baclofen and amitriptyline with ketamine may relieve pain from chemotherapy-induced neuropathy. The research on compounded topical agents is complex; another double-blind randomized, placebo-controlled study found that a combination of amitriptyline and ketamine did not provide pain relief for patients with neuropathic pain. A systematic review of current research on compounded topical agents suggests that most of the drug formulations inhibit pain locally, and the study calls for future work to determine if these drugs are also systemic acting or have localized peripheral effects.

KEY POINTS

1. Topical analgesics exert their effect via a local mechanism and do not have any systemic activity, in contrast to transdermal agents, which require a systemic concentration of analgesic.
2. The advantages of topical analgesics include the following: minimal risk for systemic side effects, reduced drug-drug interactions, fast acting relief, and a simple analgesic treatment option for patients who are already on several other medications, cannot swallow pills, and/or are fearful of needles.
3. The disadvantages of topical analgesics include the following: risk of accidental eye exposure and subsequent irritation, restriction of activities while using the topical agent (e.g., showering or swimming), and various unpleasant skin reactions seen more with capsaicin.
4. Future development of topical analgesics in the United States includes the development of topical NSAIDs, NMDA receptor antagonists, and new formulations of topical agents to treat conditions including headache and neuroma.

BIBLIOGRAPHY

1. Gorji A, Khaleghi Ghadiri M. History of headache in medieval Persian medicine. *Lancet Neurol*. 2002;1(8):510-515.
2. Heyneman CA, Lawless-Liday C, Wall GC. Oral versus topical NSAIDs in rheumatic diseases: a comparison. *Drugs*. 2000;60(3):555-574.
3. Galer BS, Rowbotham MC, Perander J, Friedman E. Topical lidocaine patch relieves postherpetic neuralgia more effectively than a vehicle topical patch: results of an enriched enrollment study. *Pain*. 1999;80(3):533-538.
4. Meier T, Wasner G, Faust M, et al. Efficacy of lidocaine patch 5% in the treatment of focal peripheral neuropathic pain syndromes: a randomized, double-blind, placebo-controlled study. *Pain*. 2003;106(1-2):151-158.
5. Argoff CE. Topical agents for the treatment of chronic pain. *Curr Pain Headache Rep*. 2006;10(1):11-19.
6. Galer BS, Gammaitoni A. Use of topiceuticals (topically applied, peripherally acting drugs) in the treatment of chronic pain. *Curr Drug Ther*. 2006;1:273-282.

CHAPTER 37

NONSTEROIDAL ANTIINFLAMMATORY DRUGS AND ACETAMINOPHEN

Robert A. Duarte, Charles E. Argoff and Andrew Dubin

1. List the indications for treatment with aspirin, acetaminophen, and nonsteroidal antiinflammatory drugs.

   Aspirin, acetaminophen, and other nonsteroidal antiinflammatory drugs (NSAIDs) are generally considered to be the drugs of choice for mild to moderate pain. They represent the first step in the analgesic ladder proposed by the World Health Organization. These agents have a relatively low abuse potential and are primarily used in nociceptive somatic pain syndromes (e.g., arthritis). They do, however, have a ceiling effect. Pure opioid analgesics such as hydromorphone and morphine do not. The ceiling effect refers to the dose after which additional quantities of an analgesic no longer provide additional analgesia.

2. Describe the mechanism of action of the nonsteroidal antiinflammatory drugs.

   The antiinflammatory effect of nonsteroidal antiinflammatory agents is due mainly to inhibition of the enzyme cyclooxygenase (COX), which is required for synthesis of prostaglandins and thromboxanes. There are two COX isoforms: COX1, which is expressed constitutively in most tissues and is thought to protect the gastric mucosa and platelets, and COX2, which is expressed constitutively in the brain and kidney but can be induced at sites of inflammation. Traditional NSAIDs are nonselective COX1 and COX2 inhibitors, whereas celecoxib is a selective COX2 inhibitor.

3. What are the major pharmacokinetic differences among the nonsteroidal antiinflammatory drugs?

   All the NSAIDs possess similar absorption characteristics. In general, they are rapidly absorbed after oral and rectal administration. They are highly protein-bound and metabolized primarily in the liver. However, durations of action vary markedly. Some drugs, such as ibuprofen, require dosing every 4 to 6 hours, whereas piroxicam can be given once a day. The newer COX2 inhibitors also require only once or twice daily dosing. NSAIDs encompass a broad group of medications. Salicylates have a long history in the management of both rheumatoid arthritis as well as osteoarthritis. Proprionic acid derivatives including but not limited to ibuprofen, flurbiprofen, naproxen, and ketoprofen have also been used for years. Acetic acid derivatives such as sulindac, indomethacin, and tolmetin can also be used. Failure to respond to one class of NSAID does not mean that they are ineffective. Changing class from an acetic acid derivative to a proprionic acid derivative or vice versa may at times prove effective.

4. List the most common side effects associated with the traditional nonsteroidal antiinflammatory drugs.

   Gastrointestinal (GI) irritation, nausea, and impairment of platelet aggregation are the most common side effects associated with the traditional NSAIDs. These side effects may lead to dyspepsia, GI ulcers, and bleeding. Some of the nonacetylated salicylates (e.g., choline magnesium trisalicylate) do not inhibit platelet function. Other known side effects include peripheral edema and elevated blood pressure. Risk for renal toxicity is further increased in patients with underlying diabetes and hypertension. COX inhibitors may be associated with fewer GI risks compared to classic NSAIDs, but this has only been demonstrated in short-term studies. There are no well-controlled studies to show this holds for long-term use. The risk for renal toxicity does not appear to be any different. COX inhibitors carry the same black box warning as NSAIDs. As such caution should be the watch word with the long-term use of NSAIDs, including COX inhibitors

5. Describe the clinical presentation for acute acetaminophen overdose.
   Symptoms of acetaminophen overdose include vague abdominal pain during the first week, followed by signs of hepatic failure. Acetaminophen, at doses of 400 mg/kg, can be fatal.

6. What are the risks of combining nonsteroidal antiinflammatory drugs with acetaminophen?
   The risk of analgesic nephropathy appears to increase when different NSAIDs are used together or in combination with acetaminophen. This effect is generally seen in long-term use. The primary lesion is papillary necrosis with secondary interstitial nephritis.

7. What is the risk of nephrotoxicity with nonsteroidal antiinflammatory drugs?
   Aspirin and NSAIDs at therapeutic doses generally do not cause renal disease in patients with normal renal function. However, problems such as nephrotic syndrome, acute interstitial nephritis, and acute renal failure have been observed when aspirin and other nonsteroidals are given to patients with abnormal renal function. This can occur as a result of the inhibition of renal prostaglandin production by NSAIDs and the coxibs. Congestive heart failure, hepatic cirrhosis, collagen vascular disease, intravascular volume depletion, and arthrosclerotic heart disease are known contributing factors that may increase the risk of renal failure.

8. Which groups of nonsteroidal antiinflammatory drugs are available in the United States?
   - Traditional, or nonselective, COX1 and COX2 inhibitors
   - Salicylate (salsalate, diflunisal, and choline magnesium trisalicylate)
   - Proprionic (ibuprofen, ketoprofen, naproxen, fenoprofen)
   - Indole (indomethacin, sulindac, tolmetin)
   - Fenamate (mefenamic, meclofenamate)
   - Mixed (piroxicam, ketorolac, diclofenac)
   - Selective COX2 inhibitors
   - Celecoxib (Celebrex)

9. Which agent is considered to be the drug of choice for pain control?
   There is no conclusive evidence supporting one NSAID over another for analgesia. Frequency of dosing, cost, and side-effect profile should be considered when deciding on a specific NSAID agent for pain control. Following a review of the overall efficacy of the NSAIDs and their potential risk for cardiovascular disease, the US Food and Drug Administration (FDA) Arthritis Panel currently suggests Naprosyn, or Celebrex if there are risk factors that mitigate against the use of Naprosyn, as the preferred agents for the treatment of arthritis pain.

10. Describe an adequate trial of nonsteroidal antiinflammatory drugs for pain control.
    An analgesic should not be considered a failure unless it has been given an adequate trial. For non-cancer-related pain, 2 weeks of treatment with a maximum scheduled dose constitutes an adequate trial. For cancer-associated pain, a 1-week duration of continuous dosing is considered sufficient. However, ketorolac is not recommended for more than 5 days' duration because of the risk of serious GI and other side effects.

11. If one nonsteroidal antiinflammatory drug fails to provide sufficient pain relief, how should a clinician proceed?
    If an adequate trial of one class of NSAID does not cause analgesia, the clinician should switch to an alternative class of NSAID. For example, if an agent from a salicylate group is considered ineffective, it is recommended to change to a proprionic or indole group. On the other hand, when one group of NSAID is effective but produces intolerable side effects, the clinician should first search for another agent in the same class before switching to another group of NSAIDs.

12. List the potential risk factors for the traditional nonsteroidal antiinflammatory drug-associated gastrointestinal toxicity.
    - Advancing age
    - Concomitant administration of corticosteroids
    - History of either ulcer disease or prior GI complications from NSAIDs

13. **What is the role of protective therapies in association with administration of traditional nonsteroidal antiinflammatory drugs?**
To date, only misoprostol has been proved to reduce the risk for serious GI toxicity. Misoprostol diminishes the incidence of endoscopically detectable lesions. However, no evidence has confirmed that misoprostol diminishes the risk of complications from the lesions when they occur. Protective agents may be indicated in patients over the age of 60 years of age and patients with predisposition to GI problems.

14. **Do the selective COX2 inhibitors have a lower risk for gastrointestinal toxicity compared to the traditional nonsteroidal antiinflammatory drugs?**
Yes. The COX2 inhibitors were associated with a lower incidence of symptomatic ulcers compared with traditional NSAIDs at standard doses. The decrease in upper GI toxicity was strongest among patients not taking aspirin concomitantly.

15. **What are the major distinctions among the mechanisms of action of aspirin, acetaminophen, nonsteroidal antiinflammatory drugs, and the COX2 inhibitors (coxibs)?**
Aspirin is an irreversible inhibitor of the COX enzymes. The exact mechanism of action of acetaminophen is not known. However, it is a weak nonselective inhibitor of both the COX1 and the COX2 enzymes. NSAIDs inhibit the activity of both COX1 and COX2 enzymes. The coxibs selectively inhibit the COX2 enzyme.

16. **Which COX2 inhibitor(s) are currently available in the United States?**
Originally, there were three selective COX2 inhibitors in the United States. Presently, celecoxib is the only oral selective coxib available in the United States approved for osteoarthritis and rheumatoid arthritis. The FDA removed rofecoxib from the US market because of increasing evidence that it increased risk for cardiovascular disease. Of note, valdecoxib was removed by the FDA primarily because of the high risk of skin lesions (i.e., Stevens-Johnson syndrome) attributed to it.

17. **What are the documented precautions with celecoxib?**
Celecoxib is contraindicated in patients who have had an allergic-type reaction to sulfonamide drugs. This agent is not recommended for patients with severe hepatic insufficiency or advanced renal disease. In postmarketing studies, patients receiving celecoxib concurrently with warfarin experienced bleeding events in association with an increase in prothrombin time. Therefore, if celecoxib therapy is initiated or changed, the international normalized ratio (INR) should be monitored, especially in the first few days. In addition, the clinician should be aware of the potential interaction with lithium and cytochrome P450 inhibitors when patients are taking celecoxib.

18. **Discuss some cardiovascular issues associated with selective COX2 inhibitors.**
NSAIDs and coxibs do not provide the same protective effects as low-dose aspirin. Coxibs (selective COX2 inhibitors) decrease vascular prostacyclin (PGI2) production and may affect the balance between prothrombotic and antithrombotic eicosanoids. However, the available studies can suggest only that there is a potential increase in cardiovascular events compared to the traditional NSAIDs. In patients taking a coxib agent, the recommendation is to maintain low-dose daily aspirin in patients who are at significant risk of a cardiovascular event. However, the use of low-dose acetyl salicylic acid (ASA) does not consistently negate the potential cardiovascular risk of COX2 inhibitors.

19. **List the potential central nervous system side effects associated with nonsteroidal antiinflammatory drugs.**
All NSAIDs have the potential to produce central nervous system side effects, including sedation, dizziness, and headaches. Headaches occur in about 10% of patients taking indomethacin. Usually side effects are mild and transient.

20. **What are the only parenteral nonsteroidal antiinflammatory drugs available in the United States?**
Ketorolac and diclofenac are the only parenteral NSAIDs available in the United States. Doses of parenteral 30 mg ketorolac is equivalent to 12 mg of parenteral morphine. However, the risks of bleeding limit its use to no more than 5 days. Contraindications to ketorolac and diclofenac include a history or current risk of GI bleeding, risk of renal failure, compromised homeostasis, hypersensitivity to aspirin or other NSAIDs, labor, delivery, and nursing. There are ongoing trials of parenteral forms of COX-2 inhibitors.

KEY POINTS

1. Multiple NSAIDs, including both nonselective agents and one selective agent, are commercially available. Unlike opioid analgesics, these medications appear to have a ceiling effect.
2. The risk for nephrotoxic effects appears to be increased when different NSAIDs are used in combination with each other or with acetaminophen.
3. If an adequate trial of one type of NSAID does not result in adequate pain relief, the clinician should consider switching the patient to a different type of NSAID.
4. The clinician should prescribe these drugs cautiously, especially in view of the potential for cardiovascular, GI, and renal adverse effects.

BIBLIOGRAPHY

1. Bombardier C, Laine L, Reicin A, et al. Comparison of upper gastrointestinal toxicity of Rofecoxib and Naproxen in patients with rheumatoid arthritis. *N Engl J Med*. 2000;343:1520-1528.
2. Crofford LJ. Rational use of analgesic and anti-inflammatory drugs. *N Engl J Med*. 2000;345(25):1844-1846.
3. Giovanni G, Giovanni P. Do NSAIDs and COX 2 inhibitors have different renal effects? *J Nephrol*. 2002;15(5):480-488.
4. Macario A, Lipman AG. Ketorolac in the era of cyclo-oxygenase 2 selective nonsteroidal anti-inflammatory drugs: a systemic review of efficacy, side effects, and regulatory issues. *Pain Med*. 2001;2(4):336-351.
5. Mukherjee D, Nissan SE, Topol EJ. Risk of cardiovascular events associated with selective COX 2 inhibitors. *JAMA*. 2001;286:954-959.
6. Nikles CJ, Yelland M, Del Mar C, Wilkinson D. The role of paracetamol in chronic pain: an evidence-based approach. *Am J Ther*. 2005;12(1):80-91.
7. Olsen NJ. Tailoring arthritis therapy in the wake of the NSAID crisis. *N Engl J Med*. 2005;352:2578-2580.
8. Scheiman JM, Fendick AM. Practical approaches to minimizing gastrointestinal and cardiovascular safety concerns with COX 2 inhibitors. *Arthritis Res Ther*. 2005;7(suppl 4):523-529.
9. Silverstein FE, Faich G, Goldstein GL. Gastrointestinal toxicity with celecoxib vs. nonsteroidal anti-inflammatory drugs for osteoarthritis and rheumatoid arthritis, the class study. *JAMA*. 2000;284(10):1247-1255.

CHAPTER 38

OPIOID ANALGESICS

Jeffrey Fudin, Jacqueline H. Cleary and Steven Sparkes

1. **What is the most common side effect of opioids?**
   The most common side effect of opioids is opioid-induced constipation (OIC). The rate of constipation with chronic use of opioids for noncancer pain may be as high as 90%, and remains an issue even with intermittent regular use. Prevalence is no doubt elevated, because OIC is the only opioid side effect that does not improve over time with development of tolerance. Moreover, as tolerance develops, doses of opioids are often escalated, which serves to further enhance OIC.

2. **Is opioid-induced constipation readily treatable in the majority of patients using over-the-counter (OTC) laxatives?**
   In many patients, OIC can be treated with OTC stimulant laxatives, with or without emollient laxatives (stool softeners). OIC is caused when opioid agonists combine with and activate mu-opioid receptors within the gastric mucosa. This results in reduced peristalsis, decreased fluid resorption, increased fluid absorption, and decreased rectal sphincter tone. Therefore, emollients such as docusate which does not promote peristalsis, will not generally be effective as single agents—in layman's terms, "mush with no push." Therefore, a stimulant laxative will be the most likely OTC agent to successfully treat OIC.

   OIC does not resolve in up to 54% of patients treated with OTC agents. Peripherally acting mu-opioid receptor antagonist (PAMORA) provides targeted relief that pharmacologically is specific to the pathology of OIC. These drugs block the intestinal mu receptors from mu-agonists, but do not cross into the central nervous system (CNS) and therefore do not detract from the analgesic effects of opioids. The first PAMORA approved for OIC in the United States was subcutaneous methylnaltrexone (Relistor) in 2008, intended for palliative care patients; however, in 2014 naloxegol (Movantik) was approved for OIC in the noncancer patient requiring chronic opioid therapy.

3. **What is a narcotic?**
   The word "narcotic" refers to an agent capable of inducing sleep, which includes opioids. Over time the term "narcotic" has become a derogatory term for opioids and other drugs of abuse. Naming police units that deal with illicit drugs "narcotics divisions" and the name of the group "narcotics anonymous" both place negative implications on the word. Moreover, the slang term "narc" or "nark" is associated with a person that reports any misbehavior to an authority, similar to "tattletale" or "squealer." Therefore, the term "opioid" is now preferred. The term "opioid" is also more accurate, as the term "narcotics" may apply to many agents other than opioids.

4. **Are poppies the only naturally occurring source for opiates?**
   Historically, poppies have been thought to be the only naturally occurring source of opiates, specifically opium and derived products morphine and codeine. Recently kratom has become a popular designer drug of abuse. Kratom is indigenous to areas of Southeast Asia. Although the US Drug Enforcement Administration (DEA) warns kratom has no legitimate medical use and a high potential for abuse, it is not scheduled under federal law and is legal in most states. The alkaloid mitragynine is responsible for kratom's natural opiate activity, and so like the poppy, kratom is an opioid source in nature. At low doses kratom blocks reuptake of neuroamines, including dopamine, serotonin, and norepinephrine, but as doses escalate, opiate agonist properties are also noted.

5. **What is the difference among a pure agonist, partial agonist, and an agonist/antagonist?**
   Pure agonists are opioid drugs that bind to mu-opioid receptors in the body. That binding then produces naturally occurring endorphins, analgesia, euphoria, and other well-known opioid properties. Examples of full agonists include morphine, oxycodone, hydrocodone, fentanyl, methadone, and several others. Partial agonists are opioids that bind to mu-opioid receptors; however, they produce endorphins to a much lesser extent than previously discussed full agonists.

When the dosage of a partial agonist is increased, the production of endorphins is not proportionately increased. There is only a small increase, and with receptor saturation these medications begin to take on properties of antagonists. The term "partial agonist" should not be interpreted to be equivalent to partial analgesic effect—the term refers to receptor pharmacology.

An example of a partial agonist is buprenorphine. An antagonist is a medication that binds to the opioid receptor but does not stimulate endorphin production at all. Examples of opioid antagonists are naltrexone and naloxone. An antagonist/agonist is a product that can stimulate the opioid receptors in both ways. Buprenorphine can act as both for reasons previously discussed; it is a partial agonist at mu receptors and antagonist at kappa receptors. Nalbuphine is an opioid agonist at kappa receptors and an antagonist or partial agonist at mu receptors. There are also co-formulated products such as buprenorphine/naloxone (Suboxone) that contain both a partial agonist and an antagonist. However, at most doses the buprenorphine has a higher mu-receptor affinity compared with naloxone, therefore it will not be displaced by naloxone.

6. Which opioids are hepatically activated or inactivated?

Almost all opioids are metabolized in the liver. Some are metabolized to inactive compounds, some to active compounds, and some to both. For example, hydrocodone is metabolized to the more active hydromorphone by cytochrome 2D6 (CYP2D6) and by CYP3A4 to inactive norhydrocodone. Likewise, oxycodone is metabolized to the more potent oxymorphone by CYP2D6 and to inactive noroxycodone by CYP3A4. Codeine is basically inactive as an analgesic until CYP2D6 converts it to morphine. When providing a separate drug that enhances production of certain hepatic enzymes (inducers) or diminishes production (inhibitors), problems can arise in terms of potential opioid overdose. Depending on genetic phenotype, some patients have more or less of various hepatic isoenzymes. The only opioids that do not rely on CYP enzymes for metabolism are morphine, oxymorphone, hydromorphone, levorphanol, and tapentadol.

7. Are extended release opioids *always* more dangerous than immediate release opioids?

No. In fact, if used properly, extended release opioids may be a safer option of treatment over immediate release opioids but only if taken as intended. Use of certain extended release (ER) opioid preparations may actually result in less total daily opioid dose than use of short acting opioids. Therefore, the prescriber must be knowledgeable about the specific preparation being prescribed to prescribe safely and effectively. Potential benefits of extended release opioids include less sedation, decreased fall risk, and less end-of-dose failure. Despite these known benefits, use of extended release opioids is also a known risk factor for opioid-induced respiratory depression (OIRD) if misused or abused, *but* also even if used appropriately. Furthermore, despite relatively low prescribing rates, methadone is responsible for up to 30 percent of overdose deaths, likely due to prescribing by inexperienced providers unfamiliar with its complex pharmacokinetics, and extensive risk for both drug interactions and variable half-life due to interpatient variability by genetic phenotype. Although methadone is classified as a "long-acting" drug by the US Food and Drug Administration (FDA), it in fact has only 6 to 8 hours of analgesic activity, but does have a long and variable half-life with a large volume of distribution.

8. How does medicinal chemistry or structure activity relationship impact opioid tolerability?

Medicinal chemistry can absolutely be used to a clinician's advantage when predicting how a patient may respond to a specific opioid. There are five chemical classes of opioids: phenanthrenes, benzomorphans, phenylpiperidines, diphenylheptanes, and phenypropylamines (Fig. 38.1).

Semisynthetic dehydroxylated phenanthrenes such as hydrocodone, hydormorphone, levorphanol, oxycodone, buprenorphine, butorphanol, and others lack the 6-OH group contained in the morphine molecule. This seems to diminish side effects otherwise seen with morphine and codeine, such as pruritis and nausea. More importantly, if a patient has a true allergy (which is extremely rare) to one phenanthrene, they will be allergic to the entire phenanthrene class. Conversely, it is not possible to be allergic to one dehydroxylated phenanthrene and not another. For example, if a patient claims to be allergic to oxycodone but not hydrocodone, or vice versa, this is in fact impossible and is more likely a result of a pseudoallergy. The distinction between a pseudo-allergy versus a true allergy is that a pseudoallergy is related to histamine release and therefore not life threatening, while a true allergy is related to immunoglobulin activity and could be life threatening. If a patient is grossly intolerant to one opioid chemical class, they may tolerate another.

Phenanthrenes	Benzomorphans	Phenylpiperidines	Diphenylheptanes	Phenylprpyl amines
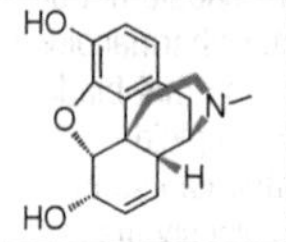	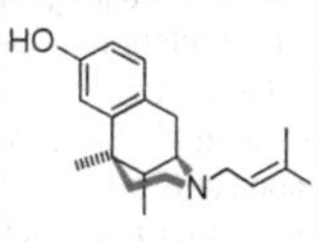	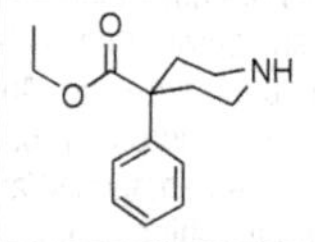	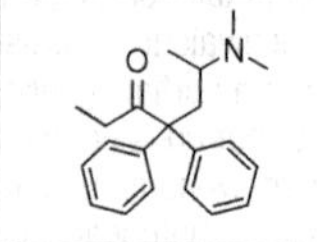	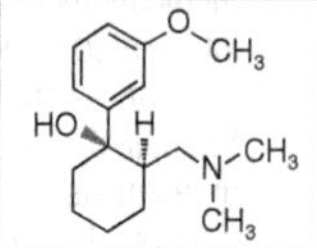
Morphine	Pentazocine	Meperidine	Methadone	Tramadol
Buprenorphine* Butorphanol* Codeine Dextromethorphan* Heroin (diacetyl- morphine) Hydrocodone* Hydromorphone* Levorphanol* Methylnaltrexone** Morphine (Opium, conc) Nalbuphine* Naloxone* Naloxegol* Naltrexone** Oxycodone* Oxymorphone*	Diphenoxylate Loperamide Pentazocine	Alfentanil Fentanyl Meperidine Remifentanil Sufentanil	Methadone Propoxyphene	Tapentadol Tramadol
Cross-sensitivity risk				
Probable	Possible	Low risk	Low risk	Low risk

* Agents lacking the 6-OH group of morphine, possibly decrease cross-tolerability within the phenanthrene group.
** 6-position is substituted with a ketone group and tolerability is similar to hydroxylation.

Figure 38.1. Chemical classes of opioids. (*Reprinted and revised with permission from Dr. Jeffrey Fudin. From Gudin, J, Fudin J, Nalamachu S. Levorphanol use: past, present and future. Postgrad Med. 2016;128(1):46–53.*)

For example, if a patient claims only to tolerate meperidine, then fentanyl may be a viable option because both are phenylpiperidines, especially given fentanyl is the only opioid with little to no histaminergic activity.

9. **Are there any extended release opioids that can be crushed without causing harm?**
Until recently, there were no extended release opioid products that were safe to crush. In fact, there is a black box warning to caution against crushing or splitting all ER or long acting (LA) dosage units, with the exception of one product as of the publication date. A new microsphere-in-capsule technology known as DETERx is now available for patients with dysphagia or feeding tubes that allows the powdery wax-based content of each capsule to be dispersed in soft foods or drinks, or emptied into feeding tubes. Crushing or any mechanical manipulation does not affect the dosage form or cause rapid release of the product. The DETERx technology is also abuse deterrent in individuals who deliberately attempt to bypass extended-release technology by crushing contents for the euphoric effects from dose dumping. Even with snorting, the DETERx technology does not allow for rapid bioavailability of opened capsules. Oxycodone ER is already available as Xtampza, and a similar dosage form of hydrocodone is on the way.

10. **Are opioids useful in the treatment of neuropathic pain?**
There are four unique opioids that are presumed to have enhanced efficacy for neuropathic pain syndromes. They include methadone, levorphanol, tramadol, and tapentadol. Each medication

exhibits opioid agonist activity; however, each also inhibits the reuptake of norepinephrine in a similar fashion to certain antidepressants that is useful for treating neuropathic pain. Norepinephrine has demonstrated efficacy in the treatment of neuropathic pain. Methadone and levorphanol additionally inhibit N-methyl-D-aspartate (NMDA) receptors. Pure NMDA antagonists, such as ketamine, can improve neuropathic pain, and consequently medications such as methadone and levorphanol are presumed to have similar benefits. Opioids with multiple mechanisms of action should most certainly be considered in the treatment of neuropathic pain after nonopioid therapies have been exhausted, and/or as part of a rational polypharmaceutical regimen and after carefully assessing for drug interactions. In addition, studies support the use of extended release oxycodone for the treatment of neuropathic pain.

11. Are any opioids contraindicated in opioid naïve patents?

Fentanyl is absolutely contraindicated in opioid naïve patients in the outpatient setting. It can be used in a controlled environment for patients that present for ambulatory procedures, where intravenous (IV) access and intubation is available. Fentanyl is 100 times more potent than morphine and even the lowest dose transdermal patch of 12 µg/hour may result in OIRD. Fentanyl is only indicated for use in patients who are opioid tolerant and have chronic pain. There are also a number of new buccal, sublingual, transmucosal, and nasal formulations FDA approved for cancer patients inadequately managed by higher dose opioid maintenance regimens. These are highly regulated through the Transmucosal Immediate Release Fentanyl Risk Evaluation and Mitigation Strategy program. This helps avoid use of these products in those at high risk for abuse or misuse, and for patients that are not sufficiently opioid tolerant. It should also help reduce the chances of improper interchange between these transmucosal products. With respect to extended release opioids, all doses of transdermal fentanyl and hydromorphone should only be prescribed for opioid tolerant (not naïve) patients. The FDA defines someone as opioid tolerant if he or she has used 60 mg of oral morphine daily (total dose) or an equianalgesic amount of another opioid for 1 week or greater.

12. Is tapentadol a glorified tramadol?

Tapentadol is a mu-opioid agonist and also blocks reuptake of norepinephrine, the latter of which is particularly useful for the treatment of neuropathic pain. Additionally, tramadol blocks reuptake of serotonin; hence it is a serotonin norepinephrine reuptake inhibitor (SNRI) of sorts. Tramadol is metabolized by CYP 2D6 via O-demethylation to the active analgesic compound O-desmethyl-tramadol (M1). Tramadol also undergoes N-demethylation via CYP 3A4 and 2B6. M1 is more potent than its parent compound tramadol; however, M1 has difficulty penetrating the central nervous system. Comparatively, tapentadol does not require a CYP enzyme for analgesic activation. Tramadol requires renal and hepatic dosage adjustment, but there is no renal data currently published for tapentadol; however, the renal metabolite was found to be nonactive in preclinical trials. The mu-opioid binding affinity of tramadol at the receptor is 6000 times less than that of morphine compared to tapentadol, whose binding affinity at that same receptor is 18 times less than that of morphine.

13. Does naloxone reverse buprenorphine?

Buprenorphine has a much higher binding affinity for the mu-opioid receptor compared with naloxone. Buprenorphine has a longer elimination half-life than naloxone. The half-life of buprenorphine is between 24 and 42 hours, depending on the patient. Comparatively, the half-life of naloxone is only 2 to 12 hours. Therefore, buprenorphine binds to the mu receptor longer, and it also remains at the receptor site 4 to 12 times longer than naloxone. Naloxone reversal of buprenorphine therefore would not be effective, especially at moderate to high doses of buprenorphine. The good news is, the higher the dose of buprenorphine, the higher the antagonist properties become as previously discussed.

14. What buprenorphine products are FDA approved specifically as an analgesic?

Butrans is a transdermal patch formulation, and Belbuca is a twice-daily buccal formulation. Butrans and Belbuca are FDA approved for the management of chronic "pain requiring around-the-clock, long-term opioid treatment not adequately controlled by alternatives." Buprenex is the IV or intramuscular (IM) formulation of buprenorphine approved for relief of moderate to severe pain. Of note, Buprenex is a viable perioperative option for patients managed with buprenorphine as outpatients chronically, since buprenorphine will block the effect of other opioids.

15. Can Suboxone and methadone be legally prescribed for pain, and if so, is this considered off-label?

Methadone carries two FDA labeled indications: (1) chronic pain and (2) detoxification. Initial inpatient detoxification of opioids by a licensed trained provider with methadone and supportive care is appropriate. A methadone maintenance provider must have special credentialing and training as required by state and federal governments. Methadone can be written for pain management purposes; however, any outpatient prescription for pain should indicate "for pain" on the prescription in order to avoid any miscommunication or misperceptions. Continuation of methadone maintenance from an outside provider while the patient is inpatient for another condition is appropriate.

Patients with a history of opioid abuse disorder can legally receive methadone by prescription for analgesic purposes if written and monitored appropriately. The provider should use risk mitigation strategies discussed in this chapter to help reduce the risk of abuse and/or misuse. Suboxone requires providers to register for a specific DEA number in order to prescribe Suboxone for the treatment of substance abuse. This required certification obtained through the medical boards, precludes unregistered practitioners from prescribing Suboxone for any other indication.

Specifically, according to 21 CFR § 1308.13(e)(2)(i), all controlled substances (including all of the buprenorphine products), may only be "prescribed, administered, or dispensed for a legitimate medical purpose by a DEA-registered practitioner acting in the usual course of professional practice and otherwise in accordance with the Controlled Substances Act (CSA) and DEA regulations." The general registration requirement applicable to all practitioners (registration under 2 1 U.S.C. § 823(t)) applies to a practitioner who prescribes buprenorphine for the legitimate treatment of pain in the usual course of professional practice. No additional DEA registration is required for such purpose.

Subutex is a sublingual tablet of single entity buprenorphine FDA approved for opioid abuse disorder. Bunavail and Zubsolv are other products available similar to Suboxone.

More specifically, if a buprenorphine product is prescribed for maintenance or detoxification, the prescribing practitioner must obtain an identification number that the DEA issues to the practitioner under 21 CFR § 1301.28(d). Unlike Suboxone, Bunavail, Zubsolv, and Subutex, both Belbuca and Butrans, and even injectable Buprenex (all three of which are specifically FDA approved for analgesia), do not require anything more than a DEA license and of course are all consistent with FDA labeling when prescribed for pain management. For maintenance and detoxification, however, certification requires that the prescribing clinician "hold a subspecialty board certification in addiction psychiatry from the American Board of Medical Specialties or a subspecialty board certification in Addiction Medicine from the American Osteopathic Association OR an addiction certification from the American Society of Addiction Medicine, and have the capacity to provide or to refer patients for necessary ancillary services, and agree to treat no more than the new limit of 275 patients at any one time in their individual or group practice."

16. Is methadone considered an extended release opioid?

Methadone is not considered an extended release opioid; however, its long serum half-life can sometimes lend it to being labeled that way. Methadone has a very long and variable serum half-life (24 to 36 hours, outliers as long as 60 to 150 hours). Methadone's onset of action is 30 minutes to 2 hours, and due to the long serum half-life, methadone can build up slowly in a patient's tissue. Methadone's unique pharmacokinetic and pharmacodynamic properties typically require multiple daily doses (usually 3 to 4 doses per day). Although the analgesic onset is similar to most opioids, the duration of analgesia is not (e.g., 6 to 12 hours).

17. Is there a validated and accepted schematic to determine morphine daily equivalent dose?

No. The concept of morphine equivalents was employed because the daily dose of various opioids may not reflect their clinical potencies. However, the daily dose of one opioid does not necessarily exhibit the same effects of the daily dose of another opioid. This distinction then creates a problem clinically when opioid use or transition to another opioid is being evaluated. The concept of morphine daily equivalents was created in order to convert between opioids; however, due to the variations in equivalence calculators and numerous sources having different potency equivalent estimators, these calculators are flawed. There is no consideration given to interpatient variability and attributes that differ among opioids. Other factors to be considered are pharmacogenetics, organ dysfunction, overall pain control, drug tolerance, drug-drug interactions, drug-food interactions, patient age, and body surface area. Single-dose studies, expert opinion, and observations are largely the source from which equianalgesic tables are derived.

18. Which opioids have the potential to prolong the QTc interval?
    Methadone and buprenorphine both have the potential to prolong the QTc interval.

19. Can tramadol and other opioids be used in combination with selective serotonin reuptake inhibitors?
    Tramadol, like selective serotonin reuptake inhibitors (SSRIs), inhibits reuptake of serotonin. Therefore, tramadol carries a risk for serotonin syndrome. Unlike tramadol, which inhibits reuptake of both norepinephrine and serotonin, tapentadol has limited interaction with serotonin transporter proteins and minimal effect upon serotonin reuptake. A compound without serotonergic activity would carry no risk of contributing to serotonin syndrome. Therefore, the risk of serotonin syndrome is drastically reduced and nearly non-existent with the use of tapentadol. Of note, methadone does inhibit reuptake of serotonin too, and therefore does in fact carry at least some elevated risk of serotonin syndrome when combined with SSRIs. Tramadol and methadone nevertheless can be used in combination with SSRIs or SNRIs; however, caution should be used with additive serotonergic agents. The lowest possible dosages should be used, and the patient and caregivers should be counseled on potential signs of serotonin syndrome: neuromuscular hyperactivity, autonomic hyperactivity, altered mental status, and seizures.

20. Which opioid should be avoided in mothers who are breastfeeding their babies?
    Codeine is a prodrug that is metabolized extensively to morphine. The parent compound codeine and its morphine metabolite are readily excreted into breast milk. Respiratory depression and death have occurred in children who received codeine and morphine through the breast milk but in particular from mothers that are phenotypic CYP 2D6 ultrarapid metabolizers.

21. Which opioids should be avoided in the setting of renal impairment?
    Morphine especially should be avoided in the setting of renal impairment. This is because about 75% of morphine is metabolized to morphine-3-glucuronide, which is inactive in the sense that it does not act on the mu receptor; however, it may be neurotoxic. Neurotoxic effects such as myoclonus have been documented. Also of concern is the morphine-6-glucuronide, which is a more potent mu-agonist than parent morphine. Elimination of morphine and its metabolites is primarily through renal excretion, and thus the issues of neurotoxicity with M3G and overdose with M6G are of concern in this special population. Meperidine also has a neurotoxic metabolite, normeperidine, which is known for causing seizures, and of important note, normeperidine is also renally cleared. For these reasons, morphine and meperidine should always be avoided in patients with renal insufficiency, particularly dialysis patients and geriatric patients. In clinical practice, meperidine is rarely used for pain, regardless of renal function, as much safer options are readily available.

22. Which opioid is contraindicated within 14 days of use of an monoamine oxidase inhibitor (MAOI)?
    Tapentadol is contraindicated within 14 days of an MAOI. While use of MAOIs for depression is now uncommon, the antibiotic linezolid has MAOI activity. Serotonin syndrome is one reason for this concern. However, the larger concern with the combination is additive norepinephrine activity that has led to adverse cardiovascular effects. Tapentadol has minimal serotonergic activity, and therefore serotonin syndrome is only a theoretical concern with its use. Meperidine is also contraindicated within 14 days of an MAOI, though its use is rare and its chronic use should be nonexistent due to the issues with the normeperidine metabolite mentioned earlier. Note that tramadol and methadone also should not be used within 14 days of an MAOI due to their reuptake blockade of norepinephrine.

23. Which opioid has a ceiling effect of accumulation of CO_2?
    Due to the unique pharmacology (partial mu-agonist, as discussed in Question 5), buprenorphine provides analgesia at therapeutic doses but also has a suggested "ceiling effect" on respiratory depression. As the medication dose increases, the activity that buprenorphine exhibits as a partial agonist plateaus regardless of subsequent increases. Opioids block the carbon dioxide feedback loop that is used to stimulate the brainstem to increase respiratory rate. The higher the dose, the more effect an opioid has on the feedback loop and the greater the risk of respiratory depression. Buprenorphine, due to its "ceiling effect" at the opioid receptor, has a much lower likelihood of respiratory depression. The risk is, however, still elevated in the presence of benzodiazepines and other sedating substances.

24. **Which OTC opioid has the same opioid binding affinity as tramadol?**
    Dextromethorphan, which is an ingredient available in multiple cough preparations.

25. **What is the role of the NMDA receptor? Which opioids block the NMDA receptors?**
    Methadone, levorphanol, and ketamine are three opioids that block the NMDA receptor. The role of the NMDA receptor is to cause sensitization of the neuron and heightened responses following glutamate activation. This sensitization is what can lead to spontaneous pain and allodynia long term. When the NMDA receptor is blocked from the glutamate receptor over time, the process of prolonged glutamate activation is stopped causing less neuronal sensitization.

26. **Is hyperalgesia a real thing?**
    Hyperalgesia is a phenomenon in which patients treated with opioids for pain or drug abusers using opiates for euphoria paradoxically become more sensitive to certain nociceptive stimuli. It typically occurs at high doses, so it may be more common in drug abusers using excessive doses than in legitimate patients using minimum effective doses. This is thought to be due to changes in the neurobiological systems that occur over time with high dose opioids. Both animal and human models have shown improvements in pain with tapering of high dose opioids, indicative of a hyperalgesic effect. The presumed phenomenon of hyperalgesia has been questioned among scientists, and there is limited evidence to support hyperalgesia. Many have hypothesized that it exists; however, there is no clear high-quality evidence to support this hypothesis.

27. **Describe "opioid rotation." What is the rationale behind it and what is meant by dose reduction for cross-tolerance?**
    Opioid rotation is a concept that takes advantage of the fact that there is incomplete cross-tolerance between the opioids. Periodically switching between opioids may benefit patients who inadequately respond to high doses of opioids due to tolerance, who are presumed to have "hyperalgesia," or who suffer from adverse effects of higher doses. Cross-tolerance can be incomplete between any opioids, but is more incomplete between different chemical classes (as discussed previously, there are four major chemical classes of opioids).

28. **What tools are available to risk stratify patients prior to initiating opioid therapy?**
    Several screening tools are available to help providers assess a patient's risk prior to initiating opioid therapy or determining misuse/abuse of an opioid medication. Some include the Opioid Risk Tool (ORT), Diagnosis Intractability Risk Efficacy (DIRE) Score, Prescription Drug Use Questionnaire (PDUQ), and Screener and Opioid Assessment for Patients With Pain—Revised (SOAPP-R), while examples of opioid misuse tools include the Addiction Behaviors Checklist (ABC), Current Opioid Misuse Measure (COMM), and the Pain Assessment and Documentation Tool (PADT). It is recommended that at least one tool be utilized before initiation of chronic opioid therapy. Additionally, Zedler et al. developed the risk index for overdose or serious opioid-induced respiratory depression (RIOSORD) score, a risk stratification tool that was validated in a veteran population of almost 2 million patients to determine probability of an overdose of serious opioid-induced respiratory depression qualifying patients for in home naloxone. A civilian score of similar design is also available. Urine drug screens, serum drug monitoring, state prescription drug monitoring, and pill counts are all also useful tools to help reduce risk of abuse and misuse while a patient is actively receiving opioid therapy.

29. **What factors contribute to a patient's risk of opioid-induced respiratory depression?**
    The RIOSORD analysis that is mentioned in the previous question is helpful in assessing risk for OIRD. The RIOSORD score is intended to determine probability of an overdose of serious opioid-induced respiratory depression. Each variable contributes a certain percentage to the score, and each RIOSORD score correlates with an average predicted probability of an opiate overdose or serious opioid-induced respiratory depression.
    Civilian RIOSORD score factors include history of substance abuse disorder, diagnosis of bipolar or schizophrenia, stroke or cerebrovascular disease, heart failure, chronic kidney disease, nonmalignant pancreatic disease, chronic pulmonary disease, chronic headache, fentanyl, morphine, methadone, hydromorphone, ER/LA formulation of opioid, benzodiazepine, antidepressant, or daily morphine equivalence >100 mg/day.

Veterans RIOSORD score factors include opioid dependence, chronic hepatitis or cirrhosis, diagnosis of bipolar or schizophrenia, chronic kidney disease, chronic pulmonary disease, sleep apnea, active traumatic injury (excluding burns), morphine equivalents per day, ED visit in the past 6 months, hospital admission in the past 6 months.

30. Are some urine drug tests more accurate than others? What is the risk of not confirming immunoassay drug testing?

There are two types of urine drug tests used in clinical practice. Typically a clinician will start by using an immunoassay test, as these are faster and less expensive versus other types, mass-spectrometry gas, or liquid-chromatography. However, immunoassay tests are subject to both false positive and negative results, and are considered "presumptive" tests. Some examples of false positives with immunoassay are quetiapine causing a methadone positive, venlafaxine causing a phencyclidine (PCP) positive, omeprazole causing a cannabis positive, bupropion causing an amphetamine positive, and sertraline causing a benzodiazepine false positive. Many other false positives are possible. Providers inexperienced with urine drug tests have hastily discharged or discontinued opioid therapy in legitimate patients. For this reason, careful assessment and definitive testing by chromatography are essential in certain cases, especially if there is a questionable or unexpected test outcome.

31. What is the only immunoassay test that is not subject to false positives?

False positives with the immunoassay cocaine test are virtually nonexistent. This is because the cocaine immunoassay test is testing for the metabolite benzoylecgonine, not cocaine agents such as lidocaine and benzocaine.

32. What is meant by a "cut-off" in a urine drug screen?

A "cut-off" or minimum level for detection is the minimum amount of drug (usually expressed in ng/mL) that must be present in urine to cause a positive presumptive test. Depending on the specific agent and test, lower doses of a prescribed agent may not always result in a positive test. However, a provider can typically ask their laboratory to quantify the test which will give them an exact quantified level within the sample, despite the "cut off" level.

33. Which opioids should never test negative on an immunoassay opiate screen, and which opioids may result in a negative test, depending on dose?

The two naturally occurring opiates, morphine and codeine, should always test positive on an immunoassay opiate screen. Synthetic and semisynthetic opioids including hydrocodone, oxycodone, and their metabolites plus oxymorphone and hydromorphone will often test negative, depending on the dose. However, lower doses may result in a positive test, and higher doses may result in a negative test, depending on factors such as urine concentration or hydration status.

Acknowledgment

All authors disclosed that their involvement with this article was not prepared as part of their official government duties.

KEY POINTS

1. It is critical to understand opioid metabolism to be able to identify potential drug-drug interactions, drug-food interactions, and pharmacogenetic population differences that may affect safety and efficacy of opioid medications.
2. Opioid medications that in particular affect norepinephrine can be useful in the treatment of neuropathic pain.
3. Buprenorphine exhibits a unique pharmacologic profile that can lend itself to the treatment of substance abuse or the treatment of pain in the setting of prior addiction.
4. There is no validated tool that is widely accepted to convert an opioid to a daily morphine equivalence. Clinical judgment and patient specific factors should always also be considered when converting a patient from one opioid to another.
5. Risk stratification tools should be used prior to starting opioid therapies to help determine misuse and abuse risk, addictive behaviors, as well as risks for OIRD.

BIBLIOGRAPHY

1. Anantharamu T, Sharma S, Gupta AK, et al. Naloxegol: first oral peripherally acting mu opioid receptor antagonists for opioid-induced constipation. *J Pharmacol Pharmacother.* 2015;6(3):188-192.
2. Bennett GJ. Update on the neurophysiology of pain transmission and modulation: focus on the NMDA-receptor. *J Pain Symptom Manage.* 2000;19(suppl 1):S2-S6.
3. Boyer E, Shannon M. The serotonin syndrome. *N Engl J Med.* 2005;352:1112-1120.
4. Eisenberg E, Suzan E, Pud D. Opioid-induced hyperalgesia (OIH): a real clinical problem or just an experimental phenomenon? *J Pain Symptom Manage.* 2015;49(3):632-636.
5. Fine PG, Portenoy RK. Establishing "best practices" for opioid rotation: conclusions of an expert panel. *J Pain Symptom Manage.* 2009;38(3):418-425.
6. Fleming AB, Carlson DR, Varanasi RK, et al. Evaluation of an extended-release, abuse-deterrent, microsphere-in-capsule analgesic for the management of patients with Chronic Pain with Dysphagia (CPD). *Pain Pract.* 2016;16(3):334-344.
7. Fudin J, Cleary JP, Schatman ME. The MEDD myth: the impact of pseudoscience on pain research and prescribing-guideline development. *J Pain Res.* 2016;9:153-156.
8. Fudin J, Levasseur DJ, Passik SD, Kirsh KL, Coleman J. Chronic pain management with opioids in patients with past or current substance abuse problems. *J Pharm Pract.* 2003;16(4):291-308.
9. Moaleji-Wafa N, Pangarkar S. Oral Methadone Dosing Recommendations for Treatment of Chronic pain. https://www.pbm.va.gov/PBM/clinicalguidance/clinicalrecommendations/Methadone_Dosing_Recommendations_for_the_Treatment_of_Chronic_Pain_July_2016.pdf. Accessed 10 April 2017.
10. Grissinger M. Inappropriate prescribing of fentanyl patches is still causing alarming safety problems. *Pharm Ther.* 2010;35(12):653-654.
11. Gudin J, Fudin J, Nalamachu S. Levorphanol use: past, present and future. *Postgrad Med.* 2016;128(1):46-53.
12. Hanson J, Ginman C, Hartvig P, et al. Clinical evaluation of oral methadone in treatment of cancer pain. *Acta Anaesthesiol Scand.* 1982;74:124-127.
13. Hartrick CT, Rozek RJ. Tapentadol in pain management: a μ-opioid receptor agonist and noradrenaline reuptake inhibitor. *CNS Drugs.* 2011;25(5):359-370.
14. Hoskin PJ, Hanks GW. Opioid agonist-antagonist drugs in acute and chronic pain states. *Drugs.* 1991;41(3):326-344.
15. Koren G, Cairns J, Chitayat D, et al. Pharmacogenetics of morphine poisoning in a breastfed neonate of a codeine-prescribed mother. *Lancet.* 2006;368(9536):704.
16. Kratom. 2013. http://www.deadiversion.usdoj.gov/drug_chem_info/kratom.pdf. Accessed 1 May 2015.
17. Lee M, Silverman SM, Hansen H, Patel VB, Manchikanti L. A comprehensive review of opioid-induced hyperalgesia. *Pain Physician.* 2011;14(2):145-161.
18. Lugo R, Satterfield K, Kern S. Pharmacokinetics of methadone. *J Pain Palliat Care Pharmacother.* 2005;19(4):13-24.
19. Moeller KE, Lee KC, Kissack JC. Urine drug screening: practical guide for clinicians. *Mayo Clin Proc.* 2008;83(1):66-76.
20. Panchal SJ, Müller-Schwefe P, Wurzelmann JI. Opioid-induced bowel dysfunction: prevalence, pathophysiology and burden. *Int J Clin Pract.* 2007;61(7):1181-1187.
21. Raffa RB, Buschmann H, Christoph T, et al. Mechanistic and functional differentiation of tapentadol and tramadol. *Expert Opin Pharmacother.* 2012;13(10):1437-1449.
22. Rowbotham MC, Twilling L, Davies PS, et al. Oral opioid therapy for chronic peripheral and central neuropathic pain. *N Engl J Med.* 2003;348:1223-1232.
23. Sawe J, Hansen J, Ginman C, et al. Patient-controlled dose regimen of methadone for chronic cancer pain. *Br Med J (Clin Res Ed).* 1981;282(6266):771-773.
24. Suboxone (buprenorphine/naloxone) [Canadian product monograph]. United Kingdom: Indivior UK Limited; 2015.
25. Vadivelu N, Timchenko A, Huang Y. Tapentadol ER for treatment of chronic pain, a review. *J Pain Res.* 2011;4:211-218.
26. Vallejo RV, Barkin RL, Wang VC. Pharmacology of opioids in the treatment of chronic pain syndromes. *Pain Physician.* 2011;14:E343-E360.
27. Vranken JH. Mechanisms and treatment of neuropathic pain. *Cent Nerv Syst Agents Med Chem.* 2009;9(1):71-78.
28. Walsh SL, Preston KL, Stitzer ML, Cone EJ, Bigelow GE. Clinical pharmacology of buprenorphine: ceiling effects at high doses. *Clin Pharmacol Ther.* 1994;55:569-580.
29. Zedler B, Saunders W, Joyce A, Vick C, Murrelle L (Venebio Group). Validation of a screening risk index for overdose or serious prescription opioid-induced respiratory depression. http://www.painmed.org/2015posters/posterIb010.pdf. Accessed 10 April 2017.
30. Zedler B, Xie L, Wang L, et al. Risk factors for serious prescription opioid-related toxicity or overdose among Veterans Health Administration patients. *Pain Med.* 2014;15(11):1911-1929.

CHAPTER 39

THE REGULATORY LANDSCAPE: OPIOIDS

Maya A. Babu

1. **What are "opioids," "opiates," and "narcotics?"**
   "Opiates" are agents derived from opium. Opioid agents bind to opioid receptors (protein molecules located on the membranes of some nerve cells) found in the central nervous system and gastrointestinal tract. There are four classes of opioids: endorphins (endogenous opioids naturally produced in the body), opium alkaloids (such as morphine and codeine), semisynthetic opioids (such as heroin, oxycodone, and buprenorphine), and fully synthetic opioids (such as methadone). "Narcotic" is a generic term that can be used to refer to opiate pain relievers.

2. **For a patient without a substance abuse history, does initiation of opioid treatment pose a risk?**
   A retrospective study that assessed opioid naïve patients at the time of hospital discharge found that chronic opioid use 1 year following discharge was more common among patients who received opioids at the time of discharge relative to those who did not. Receiving opioids at the time of discharge was associated with an almost fivefold increased risk of chronic opioid use and greater subsequent opioid refills. It was recommended by study authors that physicians inform patients of this risk prior to prescribing opioids at discharge.

3. **What is the federal legislation that governs opioid prescribing?**
   The Controlled Substances Act (CSA) stipulates that licensed medical practitioners can prescribe controlled substances for legitimate medical purposes in accordance with accepted standard medical practice. The CSA also assigns controlled substances to five classes, with differing penalties for unlawful uses, based on the potential for misuse. Schedule I substances have an extremely high potential for abuse, are deemed to have no medicinal benefit, and cannot be prescribed. Schedule II drugs also have an extremely high potential for abuse, yet are deemed to have medicinal benefit in limited circumstances. When the CSA was developed, schedule III drugs were believed to have less abuse potential than schedule II drugs. Schedule IV drugs are those that have less abuse potential than schedule III drugs. Schedule V drugs are those with the lowest abuse potential among the controlled substances within the CSA. The CSA stipulates that controlled substances must be made available for medical purposes, which is accomplished through a quota system that attempts to balance the medical need for these medications while discouraging overproduction, which could lead to diversion.

4. **What is the Controlled Substances Act?**
   Title I of the CSA provides authority and funding for prevention and treatment efforts through community mental health centers and certain hospitals. Title II of the CSA assigns regulated substances into one of five schedules based on medical value, harmfulness, and potential for abuse and dependence. Schedule I contains prohibited drugs, including heroin, lysergic acid diethylamide (LSD), and marijuana, judged to be of high abuse potential but no accepted medical use. Schedule II contains drugs with high abuse potential but recognized therapeutic value. Schedules III to V contain other prescription drugs—the higher the schedule number, the easier to gain access through telephone refills and so on.

5. **What is the Drug Enforcement Administration?**
   The mission of the Drug Enforcement Administration (DEA) is to enforce controlled substances laws and regulations in the United States.

6. **What is the Food and Drug Administration?**
   The US Food and Drug Administration (FDA) is responsible for protecting the public health by assuring the safety, efficacy, and security of human and veterinary drugs, biological products, medical devices,

our nation's food supply, cosmetics, and products that emit radiation. The FDA is also responsible for advancing public health by helping speed innovations that make medicines more effective, safer, and more affordable, and by helping the public get the accurate, science-based information they need to use medicines and foods to maintain and improve their health.

7 What is the prescription data monitoring program?

According to the National Alliance for Model State Drug Laws, a prescription data monitoring program (PDMP) is a statewide electronic database that collects data on substances dispensed in the state. The PDMP is used as a tool by states to address prescription drug abuse, addiction, and diversion. As of March 2014, 49 states had passed PDMP legislation to improve patient care and safety, and the one state without a program (Missouri) had introduced legislation to establish a PDMP as well.

8. How are opioids regulated in the United States?

Physicians must be registered with the DEA to prescribe controlled substances (or in very rare cases, receive an exemption from registration), which is dependent upon being licensed within a state. Registration must be renewed every 3 years, and the physician must be registered in every state in which he or she dispenses controlled substances. Regulation enforcing the CSA further requires that there be a legitimate medical purpose for prescriptions, the practitioner must be acting in the usual course of medical practice, and only a pharmacist can fill a prescription. All prescriptions have to be signed and dated on the day of prescribing (making presigning blank prescription pads illegal). There are additional regulations for e-prescriptions (online prescriptions) to minimize the chance of fraud or abuse. Penalties for violating law can include jail time, fines, and loss of DEA licensure. Physicians may lose their DEA registration if they lose their license to practice medicine in the state. The DEA itself can investigate and participate in the arrest and prosecution of physicians who violate controlled substance laws.

9. Why does the federal government regulate opioids (history)?

The first Congressional Act took place in 1890, which levied taxes on morphine and opium. In 1906, the Pure Food and Drug Act was passed, which prevented the manufacture, sale, or transportation of adulterated or misbranded or poisonous or deleterious foods, drugs, medicines, and liquors. In 1924 the Heroin Act was passed, which made the manufacture, importation, and possession of heroin illegal—even for medicinal use. In 1970 the Controlled Substance Act and the Controlled Substances Import and Export Act were passed. These laws consolidated numerous laws regulating the manufacture and distribution of narcotics, stimulants, depressants, hallucinogens, anabolic steroids, and chemicals used in the illicit production of controlled substances. The CSA places all substances that are regulated under existing federal law into one of five schedules. This placement is based upon the substance's medicinal value, harmfulness, and potential for abuse or addiction. Schedule I is reserved for the most dangerous drugs that have no recognized medical use, while schedule V is the classification used for the least dangerous drugs. In 1973 the Drug Enforcement Administration was created by an executive order. In 1988 the Anti-Drug Abuse Act established the Office of National Drug Control Policy (ONDCP) in the executive office of the president. This act authorized funds for federal, state, and local drug enforcement activities, school-based drug prevention efforts, and drug abuse treatment with special emphasis on injecting drug abusers at high risk for AIDS.

10. Who called pain the fifth vital sign?

In 1996 the American Pain Society deemed pain the "fifth vital sign," to be routinely measured in patients along with the four traditional ones: body temperature, blood pressure, heart rate, and breathing rate.

11. How are opioids and potential drugs of abuse classified?

Schedule I drugs, substances, or chemicals are defined as drugs with no currently accepted medical use and a high potential for abuse. Schedule I drugs are the most dangerous, with potentially severe psychological or physical dependence. Some examples of schedule I drugs are heroin, LSD, marijuana (cannabis), 3,4-methylenedioxymethamphetamine (ecstasy), methaqualone, and peyote. Schedule II drugs, substances, or chemicals are defined as drugs with a high potential for abuse, with use potentially leading to severe psychological or physical dependence. Some examples of schedule II drugs are oxycodone, morphine, codeine, amphetamines, methylphenidate (Corbin CB et al, 2014). Schedule III drugs, substances, or chemicals are defined as drugs with a moderate to low potential for physical and psychological dependence. Schedule III drug abuse potential is less than schedule I and schedule II drugs, but more than schedule IV. Some examples of schedule III drugs are drugs with less than 90 mg of codeine per unit (e.g., Tylenol with codeine), ketamine, and anabolic steroids. Schedule IV drugs, substances, or chemicals are defined as drugs with a low potential for abuse and low risk of dependence. Some examples of schedule IV drugs are Xanax, Soma, Darvon, Darvocet, Valium, Ativan, and Ambien. Schedule V drugs, substances, or chemicals are defined as drugs with lower potential for abuse than schedule IV and consist of preparations containing limited quantities of certain narcotics. Schedule V drugs are generally used for antidiarrheal, antitussive, or analgesic purposes. Some examples of schedule V drugs are medications with less than 200 mg of codeine (Robitussin AC), Lomotil, Motofen, or Lyrica.

12. How have federal laws impacted prescribing behavior?
The FDA initiated the Opioids Risk Evaluation and Mitigation Strategies program for long-acting opioid products, and anticipated that it will focus on educating prescribers regarding patient selection, risk stratification, monitoring, and other aspects of safe opioid analgesic prescribing. Although specific medical education is not mandatory, there has been discussion regarding the proposal of legislation to link mandatory training and certification to the DEA registration number that is required to prescribe controlled substances.

13. How have state laws impacted prescribing behavior?
Since 2007 states have increasingly used their authority to address inappropriate prescribing. There is general agreement that prescription painkiller abuse and overdoses are a complex problem and require a multifaceted solution. State strategies to address this complex problem have included establishing and strengthening prescription drug monitoring programs, regulating pain management facilities, and establishing dosage thresholds above which a consult for a pain specialist is required.

14. What are "pill mills"?
"Pill mill" is a term used primarily by investigators to describe a doctor, clinic, or pharmacy that is prescribing or dispensing powerful narcotics inappropriately or for nonmedical reasons. Pill mill clinics can be disguised as independent pain-management centers. They tend to open and shut down quickly in order to evade law enforcement. DEA officials believe the highest concentration of pill mills are in Florida and Texas. Some features of pill mills include: they accept cash only, no physical exam is rendered, no medical records or x-rays are needed, individuals pick their own medicine, these clinics treat pain with pills only, recipients receive a set number of pills, the clinic tells you a specific date to return for more, and there may be huge crowds of people waiting to be seen.

15. What legal risks do opioid prescribers face?
Physicians must be registered with the DEA to prescribe controlled substances, which is predicated on obtaining proper state licensing. Regulation enforcing the CSA further stipulates that there be a legitimate medical purpose for prescriptions, the practitioner must be acting in his or her usual medical course of practice, and that only a pharmacist can fill a prescription. All prescriptions have to be signed and dated on the day of prescribing (which makes presigning blank prescription pads illegal). There are additional regulations for e-prescriptions (online prescriptions) to minimize the chance of fraud or abuse, and registrants have to notify the DEA, in writing, of any significant loss or theft of a controlled substance. Penalties for violating various aspects of the law can include jail time, fines, and loss of DEA licensure. Physicians may lose their DEA registration if they lose their license to practice medicine in the state. The DEA itself can investigate and participate in the arrest and prosecution of physicians who violate controlled substance laws.

16. What is the doctrine of double effect?
The double effect doctrine forbids the achievement of good ends by wrong means, but it permits actions with a double effect, both good and bad, under certain conditions. These conditions include: the act performed is not itself morally evil, the good effect does not result from the evil effect, only the good effect is intended, or there is a proportionate reason for causing the harm.

17. What certifications are required to prescribe opioids?
Physicians must be registered with the DEA to prescribe controlled substances (or in very rare cases, receive an exemption from registration), which is predicated on obtaining proper state licensing. Registration must be renewed every 3 years, and the physician must be registered in

every state in which he or she dispenses controlled substances. Regulation enforcing the CSA further stipulates that there be a legitimate medical purpose for prescriptions, the practitioner must be acting in the usual course of medical practice, and only a pharmacist can legitimately fill a prescription.

18. **What is the role of state medical boards?**

Medical boards license physicians, investigate complaints, discipline those who violate the law, conduct physician evaluations, and facilitate the rehabilitation of physicians when appropriate. State medical boards also play a key role with physician behavior. The Federation of State Medical Boards' model policy to guide state medical boards in their review of physicians' pain management practices recommends proper medical evaluation of a patient, including a history and physical; a written treatment plan that clearly states the objectives of treatment; a discussion of the risks and benefits of treatment with the patient, including patient responsibilities like urine drug screening, reasons why therapy might be discontinued, and limits on refills; periodic review of efficacy and consideration of other treatment modalities; clear documentation in medical records; and compliance with applicable state and federal law.

19. **What is the Office of National Drug Control Policy?**

The ONDCP advises the president on drug-control issues, coordinates drug-control activities and related funding across the federal government, and produces the annual National Drug Control Strategy, which outlines administration efforts to reduce illicit drug use, manufacturing, and trafficking, drug-related crime and violence, and drug-related health effects.

20. **How often do prescription drug abusers obtain medications from family and friends?**

In 2011, 52 million people in the United States aged 12 and older had used prescription drugs nonmedically at least once in their lifetime, and 6.2 million had used prescription drugs nonmedically in the past month. According to a survey, 54.2% of those who used prescription drugs nonmedically obtained them from family and friends.

21. **What are the Centers for Disease Control and Prevention's new guidelines?**

On March 15, 2016, the Centers for Disease Control and Prevention released new guidelines utilizing the Grading of Recommendations Assessment, Development, and Evaluation method, for primary care clinicians who prescribe opioid medications to treat nonmalignant chronic pain. The guidelines are based on a systematic literature review with consideration of risk, benefits, and cost-effectiveness. Literature suggests that opioids have been moderately effective for pain relief, and a high percentage of patients discontinued opioid therapy due to unsatisfactory efficacy and adverse effects. They intend to facilitate communication between prescribers and patients to ensure opioids are the best possible treatment option available. These guidelines are accompanied by tools for physicians to utilize when implementing opioid therapy in this demographic, including fact sheets, mobile application, and a checklist for clinicians.

KEY POINTS

1. Opioids are classified from schedule I through V according to their medical use and their potential to be abused. Drugs, substances, or chemicals that are schedule I have little medical use and very high potential to be abused, compared to those that are schedule V, which are useful medically and have little to no potential to be abused.
2. The regulation of opioid use begins on both a state and federal level by requiring proper evaluation of patients and physician certification. If the physicians do not abide by federal and state law, there are legal consequences.
3. The United States has already attempted to reduce inappropriate prescriptions of opioids, but has yet to eliminate them completely.

BIBLIOGRAPHY

1. The National Alliance of Advocates for Buprenorphine Treatment. *Opiate Education.* 2016.
2. US National Library of Medicine. *Pain Medications—Narcotics.* 2015.
3. Calcaterra SL, Yamashita TE, Min SJ, et al. Opioid prescribing at hospital discharge contributes to chronic opioid use. *J Gen Intern Med.* 2016;31:478.

4. *Prescriptions.* 21 CFR Section 1306.04-06. 2013.
5. NIH. *National Institute on Drug Abuse.* http://www.nih.gov/about-nih/what-we-do/nih-almanac/national-institute-drug-abuse-nida. Accessed 20 February 2017.
6. DEA. *Drug Enforcement Administration Diversion.* 2016.
7. Silvey R. *Missouri PDMP NOW Coalition Applauds Sen. Sater and Rep. Engler for Sponsoring Bills to Combat Prescription Drug Abuse.* MPA; 2013. http://www.thepharmacyblog.com/missouri-pdmp-now-coalition-applauds -sen-sater-and-rep-engler-for-sponsoring-bills-to-combat-prescription-drug-abuse/.
8. DEA Diversion Control Division. Question: what does a practitioner/physician need to obtain before he/she can complete an application for a DEA registration?
9. *Practitioner Responsibilities.* 21 CFR 1311.102. 2013.
10. Federation of State Medical Boards of the United States, Inc. *Model Policy for the Use of Controlled Substances for the Treatment of Pain.* Washington, DC: The Federation; 2004. http://www.thepharmacyblog.com/missouri-pdmp -now-coalition-applauds-sen-sater-and-rep-engler-for-sponsoring-bills-to-combat-prescription-drug-abuse/.
11. Dowell D, Haegerich TM, Chou R. CDC guideline for prescribing opioids for chronic pain—United States, 2016. *MMWR Recomm Rep.* 2016;65:1-49. doi:10.15585/mmwr.rr6501e1.

CHAPTER 40

MUSCLE RELAXANTS, ANTICONVULSANTS AS ANALGESICS; ANTIDEPRESSANTS AS ANALGESICS

Charles E. Argoff and Nita Chen

1. **What is the mechanism of action of muscle relaxants?**
   The true mechanism of action of currently used muscle relaxants is poorly understood. Individual medications do have certain mechanisms of action associated with them, *but* whether a specific mechanism is responsible for their clinical effect is uncertain. Many of the available muscle relaxants also have sedating effects, and therefore it is somewhat difficult to determine whether their clinical effect is related to a direct effect on muscle or due to this sedating effect.

2. **How might quinine be used as a muscle relaxant?**
   Quinine increases muscle refractory time so that the muscle's response to continued stimulation is reduced. This property might be the reason quinine may be effective for the treatment of muscle cramps. Clinically, quinine is most commonly used to treat nocturnal muscle cramps at an oral dose of 200 to 300 mg at bedtime.

3. **What medications can be used to treat spasticity?**
   Baclofen, dantrolene, diazepam, and tizanidine are medications that can be used to control spasticity. Spasticity can be painful and is associated with congenital conditions such as cerebral palsy, as well as acquired conditions including multiple sclerosis, spinal cord injury, and cerebrovascular accidents. There is no clear evidence that one agent is better than another for an individual person.

4. **Describe how baclofen might be used to treat spasticity.**
   Baclofen is believed to act on presynaptic mechanisms to enhance gamma-aminobutyric acid (GABA) activity as well as to reduce the release of various excitatory neurotransmitters. Although originally developed in the United States for spasticity associated with multiple sclerosis, it has been prescribed for many other conditions associated with spasticity. Up-to-date recommends for spasticity: Oral: Initial: 5 mg 3 times daily; may increase by 5 mg per dose every 3 days (i.e., 5 mg 3 times daily for 3 days, then 10 mg 3 times daily for 3 days, etc.), until optimal response is reached. Usual dosage range: 40 to 80 mg daily. Do not exceed 80 mg daily (20 mg 4 times daily). Side effects include drowsiness, insomnia, dizziness, weakness, and confusion.

5. **Describe how dantrolene might be used to treat spasticity.**
   Dantrolene is believed to act primarily in the peripheral nervous system rather than centrally through a direct effect on muscle contraction. Clinical trials have suggested its benefit in reducing spasticity associated with cerebrovascular accidents, spinal cord injury, multiple sclerosis, and cerebral palsy. It may be hepatotoxic and therefore needs to be carefully monitored, especially in older patients. It has been reported to cause generalized weakness in some patients. Therapy is initiated with one 25 mg tablet daily. Benefits should be noted within 4 to 6 weeks.

6. **Describe how diazepam might be used to treat spasticity.**
   Diazepam is believed to potentiate the action of GABA. It has been used as monotherapy or in combination with other treatments for people with spinal cord injuries or other conditions associated

with spasticity. Somnolence, dizziness, and weakness are adverse effects of diazepam; because this is a benzodiazepine, special caution needs to be noted with respect to its potential respiratory depressant effects and for its potential increased risk of harm when combined with opioid therapy. Doses should be minimized and long-term treatment avoided if possible.

7. Describe how tizanidine might be used to treat spasticity.
   Tizanidine is an alpha 2 agonist agent that has been prescribed for spasticity, as an analgesic and as a muscle relaxant for many years. Multiple studies have suggested its benefit for spasticity, low back pain, fibromyalgia, neuropathic pain, and headache. One might consider capitalizing on its sedating effect by dosing initially at night—typically a 2-mg starting dose at bedtime may be well-tolerated. In many instances, titrating every 3 to 5 days to 4 to 8 mg at bedtime may be effective. Daytime doses are not always tolerated due to its sedating effect. Sedation, dizziness, and dry mouth are the three most common side effects, and liver functions should be periodically monitored if used on a long-term basis.

8. Describe additional muscle relaxants that are commonly prescribed.
   The medications that are often prescribed as muscle relaxants include metaxalone, cyclobenzaprine, chlorzoxazone, carisoprodol, methocarbamol, and orphenadrine. None of these medications has been proven to be superior in effect over others, and several have distinct properties that justify concern and warning. None of these agents has been proven to be effective for chronic use, although in my experience, many are prescribed long term.

9. Describe specific concerns of certain muscle relaxants.
   Cyclobenzaprine: The prescriber should be aware that cyclobenzaprine is in fact a tricyclic compound nearly identical in structure to amitriptyline. Among tricyclic compounds, it is known to have among the highest risks of cardiac arrhythmias, including those resulting in fatal outcomes. Thus, caution is advised when using this agent, especially in older patients and/or in combination with other relevant medications.
   Carisoprodol: The prescriber should be aware that carisoprodol is metabolized to the sedative-hypnotic agent meprobomate, a medication with a known risk for abuse. Carisoprodol has been taken off the market in Europe due to concerns regarding dependence.
   Orphenadrine: This medication is similar in mechanism of action to diphenhydramine, and therefore may be associated with sedating and anticholinergic side effects.

10. Describe the role of anticonvulsants (AEDS) for the treatment of chronic pain.
    Anticonvulsants are commonly used and have been widely accepted for the management of various types of chronic pain, including neuropathic pain, migraine, and other headache disorders and fibromyalgia, for example. As a class, these agents with various mechanisms of action are believed to result in their analgesic effect by reducing ectopic neuronal discharges. As these agents are described further in specific syndromes in other chapters, only general comments will be covered in this chapter. Phenytoin and carbamazepine were the first anticonvulsants to have demonstrated analgesic efficacy on the basis of controlled clinical trials. Although many of the trials have been conducted as monotherapy versus placebo, several recent trials have explored the role of certain AEDS in combination with other pharmacologic agents (opioid or non-opioid). The prescriber should consider not only the mechanism of action, potential for drug-drug interactions, and adverse effect profile of the AED being considered, but also the evidence for its use in a specific chronic pain condition prior to prescribing.

11. Describe the role of gabapentin and pregabalin for the treatment of chronic pain.
    Although originally developed as an add-on therapy for the treatment of epilepsy, gabapentin quickly became used off-label for the management of chronic pain. From an analgesic viewpoint, it is FDA approved only for postherpetic neuralgia. It is nevertheless widely prescribed off-label for many other chronic pain states, including diabetic neuropathy, complex regional pain syndrome, fibromyalgia, and various headache types. From an analgesic viewpoint, pregabalin is FDA approved for the treatment of postherpetic neuralgia, neuropathic pain associated with diabetic neuropathy, pain associated with spinal cord injury, and fibromyalgia. Gabapentin and pregabalin are believed to act as a neuronal calcium channel $\alpha 2$-δ ligand, dampening hyperexcitablity in excited neurons. Side effects for each are similar, including sedation, dizziness, peripheral edema, and weight gain. Unlike pregabalin, gabapentin demonstrates nonlinear pharmacokinetics, so as doses of gabapentin are increased, the bioavailability of the medication actually decreases. Pregabalin, on the other hand, demonstrates linear bioavailablity. There are currently two forms of gabapentin that have been

approved, in addition to the original form, that were designed in part of improve upon the bioavailability and to reduce the incidence of the side effects of gabapentin. These include a gastroretentive form of gabapentin taken once daily with dinner, as well as gabapentin enacarbil, a prodrug of gabapentin with more favorable bioavailability and adverse effects. Each of the forms of gabapentin as well as pregabalin have a low potential for pharmacokinetic drug interactions.

12. **Describe the role of carbamazepine and oxcarbazepine for the treatment of chronic pain.**
Carbamazepine has established efficacy for the treatment of trigeminal neuralgia, as well as for painful traumatic neuropathy. Its side effect profile and potential for bone marrow suppression and hepatic side effects have resulted in it typically being used second line for neuropathic pain. General side effects include sedation, dizziness, unsteadiness, and rash, and blood monitoring is required to check for evidence of bone marrow suppression as well as hepatic effects.

     Oxcarbazepine has been offered to patients who may have become refractory to treatment for carbamazepine for trigeminal neuralgia. Although not specifically FDA approved for trigeminal neuralgia, clinical experience and several studies have suggested that for certain patients, oxcarbazepine may be more effective and better tolerated than carbamazepine.

13. **Describe the role of lamotrigine for the treatment of chronic pain.**
While very few controlled studies have been conducted and/or shown that lamotrigine may be effective in the treatment of chronic pain, there is some evidence to support its use as an add-on therapy for the treatment of trigeminal neuralgia. In addition, there is some evidence to support its use in central or poststroke pain.

14. **Describe the role of topiramate for the treatment of chronic pain.**
Topiramate's use in the treatment of migraine is described elsewhere in this book. Clinical experience, along with a few published studies and case series, suggest that there may be a role for its use in the treatment of neuropathic pain. Common side effects often preclude its use, including paresthesias and cognitive dysfunction. It is also associated with weight loss, which for some may be a desired effect, as well as several serious side effects, including acute visual loss associated with glaucoma and nephrolithiasis.

15. **Describe the role of lacosamide for the treatment of chronic pain.**
Lacosamide is a novel sodium channel modulator. While animal studies have suggested that this AED may be helpful for the treatment of neuropathic pain, the FDA did not approve this drug for such in humans when presented with the clinical trial data. Nevertheless, there are published studies to support its use in painful diabetic neuropathy, as well as fibromyalgia. I have used this medication successfully for select patients who had not responded well to other AEDs.

16. **Describe the role of valproic acid for the treatment of chronic pain.**
Similar to topiramate, the use of valproic acid to treat migraine is described elsewhere in this book. Controlled trials for neuropathic pain are lacking.

17. **Describe the role of antidepressants in the treatment of chronic pain.**
Antidepressants are among the most commonly prescribed medications for chronic symptoms. More than 30 placebo-controlled, double-blind studies suggest the effectiveness of antidepressants in the treatment of various types of chronic pain. Antidepressants may be clinically effective in treating for chronic pain through a direct analgesic effect, through their effect on treating a comorbid psychiatric condition, through the treatment of pain related symptoms such as insomnia, or through its enhancement of opioid or non-opioid analgesics. Certain antidepressants may modulate pain perception through their action on descending noradrenergic and serotonergic pathways, and in addition, certain antidepressants have demonstrated inhibition of sodium channel activity, another possible analgesic effect.

18. **Describe the role of the tricyclic antidepressants in the treatment of chronic pain.**
Multiple tricyclic antidepressants including amitriptyline, imipramine, doxepin, desipramine, and nortriptyline have consistently shown analgesic effects at doses typically lower than required to treat depression. Amitriptyline, doxepin, and imipramine tend to have a greater side effect burden than desimpramine and nortriptyline. However, it is extremely important to recognize that *despite* the reduced side effects associated with those agents, the *analgesic* benefit was not compromised. This should be considered when prescribing these agents. These agents have been used for the

treatment of neuropathic pain, chronic headache, chronic low back pain, fibromyalgia, and various other chronic pain states. Side effects of these agents include anticholinergic side effects such as dry mouth, urinary retention, and constipation, as well as sinus tachycardia, blurred vision, confusion, hallucinations, cognitive dysfunction, orthostatic hypotension, and weight gain. Dangerous drug-drug interactions may occur with monoamine oxidase inhibitors, as with other medications whose use could result in increasing central serotonin (serotonin specific reuptake inhibitor [SSRI] agents, for example). The prescriber should consult the pharmacist and other sources for any questions regarding drug-drug interactions. Although widely used, no tricyclic antidepressants (TCA) are FDA approved for the treatment of chronic pain.

19. Describe the role of antidepressant serotonin-norepinephrine reuptake inhibitors (SNRI) in the treatment of chronic pain.
Duloxetine is perhaps the most well-known serotonin-norepinephrine reuptake inhibitor (SNRI) agent used in the treatment of chronic pain. This medication and other SNRI agents have a dual mechanism of action (e.g., inhibition of both the reuptake of norepinephrine as well as serotonin). From an analgesic viewpoint, duloxetine is FDA approved for the treatment of fibromyalgia, painful diabetic neuropathy, and chronic musculoskeletal pain. Nausea and sedation are among the more common side effects. Other reported side effects of note include impaired glucose control, hypertension, and rare hepatic toxicity. Venlafaxine has a dual mechanism of action *only* at higher doses (>150 mg). At lower doses, it is primarily a SSRI drug, and its analgesic benefit is not as great as documented in clinical trials. This is very important to consider, as many patients placed on venlafaxine for chronic pain have not been titrated to doses likely to be effective in my experience. The most common side effects include nausea, sedation, dizziness, sexual dysfunction, insomnia, and increases in diastolic blood pressure. Minalcipran is FDA approved for the treatment of fibromyalgia only in the United States (not depression).

Preclinical studies suggested that blocking the reuptake of central serotonin alone was not as effective as blocking the reuptake of both central serotonin and norepinephrine for analgesic purposes. These preclinical observations have held true in human clinical trials. Therefore, while there may be published trials showing some benefit of SSRI agents for chronic pain treatment and individual patients who experience benefit, in general, these are not as effective for most patients as the medications described previously.

20. Describe the role of the atypical antidepressants in the treatment of chronic pain.
Buprorion, trazadone, and mirtazapine are among the atypical antidepressants that have shown benefit in limited studies to support their use in chronic, primarily neuropathic, pain.

KEY POINTS

1. The term *muscle relaxant* comprises a large heterogeneous group of medications with various drug interactions and side effects; thus the prescriber should carefully consider the specific needs of the patient when prescribing such medications for patients.
2. AEDs similarly comprise a heterogeneous group of medications. The prescriber needs to be aware of the specific indications of the medication being prescribed, as well as the specific pharmacokinetic and pharmacodynamic properties of the AED being considered.
3. Although commonly referred to generally as antidepressants, only the TCAs and SNRI agents have strong evidence for their use in chronic pain. Other antidepressant medications including SSRIs and the atypical antidepressants either have not been shown to be as effective or have less robust data to support their use in chronic pain.
4. Given the common practice of multidrug therapy for chronic pain, the prescriber must be aware of the differences and similarities among the various agents described previously, as well as using those together that are least likely to result in drug-drug interactions and/or serious side effects.

BIBLIOGRAPHY

Dworkin RH, O'Connor AM, Backonja M, et al. Pharmacologic management of neuropathic pain: evidence based recommendations. *Pain.* 2007;132(3):237-251.
Harden RN, Argoff C. A review of three commonly prescribed skeletal muscle relaxants. *J Back Musculoskelet Rehabil.* 2000;15(2):63-66.
Onghena P, Van Houdenhove B. Antidepressant-induced analgesia in chronic non-malignant pain: a meta-analysis of 39 placebo-controlled studies. *Pain.* 1991;49:205-219.

CHAPTER 41

NOVEL ANALGESICS FOR ACUTE AND CHRONIC PAIN

Mark S. Wallace and R. Carter W. Jones III

1. **What new and emerging therapies exist to treat acute postoperative pain?**
   Opioids continue to be the standard for treating moderate to severe postoperative pain. However, with the current emphasis on multimodal and nonopioid therapies, there has been a recent emergence of new nonopioid therapies, including intravenous acetaminophen and liposomal encapsulated bupivacaine. In addition, a sublingual sufentanil tablet system delivered via a patient controlled delivery device is in clinical development. With the widespread surge in opioid abuse and overdose in the United States over the past decade, there are efforts to develop abuse-deterrent, short-acting opioids for acute pain management.

2. **Is intravenous acetaminophen any better than oral delivery?**
   The effector site of action for acetaminophen is mainly located in the central nervous system (CNS); therefore, rapid and consistent penetration into the CNS should improve analgesia. Up until 2001, only oral and rectal delivery of acetaminophen was available. Since 2001, an intravenous (IV) preparation has been used in Europe. Surgery often leads to gastric stasis due to many systemic disturbances that will result in poor or erratic gastrointestinal absorption of acetaminophen. The intravenous delivery results in a rapid and consistent CNS penetration and better pain control. Intravenous acetaminophen can also be better tailored to specific needs of the patient.

3. **What are the advantages of liposomal-bupivacaine over regular bupivacaine?**
   The duration of action of bupivacaine is approximately 4 to 6 hours. Pain from surgery lasts well beyond the duration of bupivacaine, making it ineffective for most postoperative pain patients. The solution for this deficiency is to provide continuous infusion via a catheter; however, peripheral catheters are difficult to place, require high nursing maintenance, and the patients often cannot go home with them in place. Formulating bupivacaine so that it has an extended duration without increasing peak plasma levels is an attractive option over continuous infusions in selected patients. The liposomal delivery of bupivacaine extends the local residence time at the effector site, resulting in a 7-fold increase in T_{max} and a 10-fold extension of the terminal half-life without increasing peak plasma concentrations. Clinical studies comparing liposomal-bupivacaine with standard bupivacaine has had mixed results, likely due to underpowering.

4. **How does the pharmacokinetics of the sufentanil sublingual tablet system differ from intravenous morphine?**
   The effector site of action for all opioids is in the CNS, requiring penetration and pharmacokinetics (PK) that match the needs of the patient. Most of the commonly used opioids have inconsistent CNS penetration due to differences in PK or mismatched pharmacokinetic/pharmacodynamics (PD) profiles. An important cause of the PK/PD mismatch is the inability of certain opioids to penetrate the blood-brain barrier into the CNS effector site, resulting in high plasma drug levels that do not represent PD effects. The transit time from plasma to CNS effector site is termed the plasma: CNS equilibration half-life (TT). The TT for lipophilic drugs such as fentanyl or sufentanil is very fast, within 6 minutes. The TT for hydrophobic drugs such as morphine or hydromophone is very long (about 2.8 hours for morphine), resulting in a PK/PD mismatch and delayed analgesic effect, as well as delayed side effects such as respiratory depression. In addition, there are other factors that increase morphine's PK/PD mismatch, as it is a substrate for efflux transporters and has active metabolites with even longer TT (morphine-6-glucuronide). A sufentanil sublingual tablet system (SSTS; Zalviso; AcelRx Pharmaceuticals, Redwood City, California) has completed phase III trials. The SSTS allows for the self-administration of a 15-μg sublingual sufentanil tablet via a preprogrammed, handheld device. Like an intravenous patient-controlled analgesic device, the SSTS has a 20-minute lockout before the next dose can be administered. Due to the high lipid solubility, sufentanil is

rapidly absorbed transmucosally, resulting in a rapid and reliable intravenous uptake. Compared to intravenous sufentail, the sublingual delivery results in a 10-fold lower C_{max} and a greatly extended plasma half-time (time from C_{max} to 50% C_{max} = 2.61 hours vs. 0.18 hours). As sufentanil has a very short TT and no active metabolites, effector site activity is fast, reliable, and with fewer delayed side effects. A phase III study showed that SSTS was superior to IV PCA morphine in patient global assessment method of pain control.

5. What are some of the emerging novel analgesics in the pipeline for chronic pain?
   There are a number of pharmacological agents with novel mechanisms in both preclinical and clinical development. These agents target mechanisms that modulate pain at various levels of the nervous system. Table 41.1 lists the most promising emerging analgesics.

6. How is nerve growth factor related to pain, and what evidence exists for its efficacy and safety?
   Nerve growth factor (NGF) is a neuropeptide primarily involved in the regulation of growth, maintenance, proliferation, and survival of certain target neurons. It is important in early human development and becomes less important as we age. NGF is upregulated in painful conditions, and binding to the tyrosine receptor kinase A receptor is thought to activate nociceptors; inhibition reverses pain in animal models. Tanezumab and fulranumab are two different monoclonal antibodies to NGF currently in clinical trials. Tanezumab has positive trials in osteoarthritis, chronic low back pain, and cancer. Trials in diabetic peripheral neuropathy, postherpetic neuralgia, and pancreatitis failed to show any effect. A phase III trial in cancer-related pain is currently being conducted outside the United States. Fulranumab has had negative trials in low back pain and osteoarthritis. However, differences in trial design may have resulted in false-negative results, and development is still continuing. The main side effect reported with this class is some abnormal peripheral sensations. Reports of avascular necrosis in the early trials of these drugs resulted in a US Food and Drug Administration (FDA) hold on development. However, it was determined that these adverse events were nonsteroidal antiinflammatory drug (NSAID)-dependent; the hold was lifted and clinical trials have resumed.

7. How do the angiontensin II type 2 receptors modulate pain, and what clinical evidence exists for pain modulation?
   Angiotensin II is a potent vasopressor hormone important in controlling blood pressure and volume in the cardiovascular system. It binds and stimulates at least two types of receptors: AT1 and AT2.

Table 41.1. Emerging Novel Analgesics for Chronic Pain

NGF Inhibitors
PAP
T-type Calcium Channel Blockers
N-type Calcium Channel Blockers
Angiotensin II type 2 Receptor Antagonists
Selective Sodium Channel Blockers
TRPV1 Channel Antagonists
AMPA/Kainate Antagonists
Cannabinoids
p38 Kinase Inhibitors
CCR2 Antagonists
KCNQ Agonists
P2X Purinoreceptor Antagonists

NGF, Nerve growth factor; *PAP*, prostatic acid phosphatase; *TRPV1*, transient receptor potential cation channels, subfamily 1.

AT2 is a G-protein-coupled receptor that plays a role in CNS function. AT2 receptors are expressed on small diameter nerve fibers and dorsal root ganglion cells. Angiotensin converting enzyme (ACE) converts angiotensin I to angiotensin II. However, studies on ACE inhibitors have failed to show an effect on pain. Therefore, AT2 receptor antagonists have been developed for pain relief. A phase II study in postherpetic neuralgia randomized 183 patients to placebo or an AT2 receptor antagonist (EMA-401). The study met the primary endpoint of reduction in pain intensity. Secondary outcomes of onset, 30%/50% responder rate, McGill and Patient Global Impression of change were also met. The drug was safe and well tolerated.

8. **What is prostatic acid phosphatase?**
Adenosine has been shown to activate adenosine receptors in the nervous system resulting in analgesia. However, adenosine has a very short half-life, making it ineffective for chronic pain management. Nervous system injury results in the release of adenosine triphosphate (ATP) that is known to induce painful sensations. ATP is rapidly broken down into adenosine monophosphate (AMP) which prostatic acid phosphatase breaks down into adenosine. This pathway results in a much longer duration of analgesia (up to 3 days in animal studies) and has been shown to be 8 times more effective than morphine.

9. **How does sodium channel blockade reduce pain?**
Voltage-gated sodium channels are upregulated after nervous system injury and disease, resulting in spontaneous and elicited pain. In addition, gain- and loss-of-function mutations in a specific sodium channel subtype, Nav 1.7, have been linked to the pain syndromes primary erythromelalgia and congenital insensitivity to pain, respectively. Sodium channels blockers have been used for decades to treat chronic neuropathic pain (lidocaine, mexilitine, lamotrigine). However, they have not been very successful due to nonselectivity for sodium channel subtypes, resulting in dose limiting side effects. There is emerging interest in selective blockers to sodium channel subtypes specific to the pain pathways. As these subtypes are not present in heart tissue or the CNS, they are better tolerated and likely will provide better analgesia. Nav 1.3, Nav 1.7, Nav 1.8, and Nav 1.9 are specific channels that have been implicated in pain signaling. The most promising channels are the Nav 1.7 and Nav 1.8 subtypes. Both systemic and intrathecal agents are being developed that affect the function of these Nav channel subtypes.

10. **Are there any other voltage-gated ion channels that are targets for pain modulation?**
Potassium voltage-gated channel subfamily Q members are potential targets for pain management. The M potassium channel is a slowly activating and deactivating channel that regulates neuronal excitability. A defect in the KCNQ3 gene results in neonatal convulsions; therefore, activators of the M channel have the potential to treat seizures and reduce neuropathic pain. Retagabine activates the M channel and is a leading candidate.

11. **What are transient receptor potential cation channels, subfamily 1, and what role do they play in pain transmission?**
The transient receptor potential cation channels, subfamily 1 (TRPV1) channel is a capsaicin and vanilloid receptor 1 that is expressed on pain fibers. TRPV1 provides a sensation of scalding heat and pain when activated. It also functions in the detection and regulation of body temperature. The channel is activated by capsaicin, causing an influx of intracellular calcium. High levels of intracellular calcium will overwhelm the mitochondria, resulting in axonal death. A high-dose capsaicin patch (8%) is currently marketed for the treatment of postherpetic neuralgia. A single 60-minute application can result in 3 months of pain relief, due to the axonal death of TRPV1-expressing peripheral nerve fibers. Clinical effectiveness has been mixed, but a recent study suggested that patients with cold and pinprick hyperalgesia had a positive predictive value for response to high-dose capsaicin patch application. There has been interest in the systemic delivery of TRPV1 channel antagonists; however, systemic delivery results in hyperthermia and increased thermal sensation thresholds. A phase II study was stopped early due to futility.

12. **Are there any new calcium channel modulators in the pipeline?**
There are several N-type calcium channel blockers (intrathecal ziconotide) and modulators (pregabalin and gabapentin) currently on the market. Clinical effectiveness has been mixed with both positive and negative clinical trials. Mirogabalin is a new promising N-type calcium channel modulator. Pregabalin and gabapentin bind the alpha-2-delta subunit of the N-type calcium channel

and reduce the amount of time the channel is in the open state. This reduces the amount of calcium influx, resulting in less presynaptic neurotransmitter release and dampening of pain signaling. Whereas pregabalin and gabapentin are nonspecific alpha-2-delta subunit ligands, mirogabalin is specific to the alpha-2-delta type II subunit. It is thought that the type I subunit is responsible for the side effects seen with N-type calcium channel modulators. Thus there appears to be fewer side effects with mirogabalin, resulting in the ability to achieve higher doses and improved efficacy. A recent study in painful diabetic neuropathy showed significant pain reductions at 15, 20, and 30 mg doses versus placebo. In the same study, an active comparator (pregabalin 300 mg) was not effective.

T-type Ca 3.2 calcium channels are thought to play a crucial role in pain signaling at central and peripheral endings of primary afferent neurons. Unlike antagonism of the T-type Ca 3.1 and 3.3 subtypes, the 3.2 subtype does not produce any sedation and is likely better tolerated. Preclinical studies have demonstrated efficacy in capsaicin-induced pain, models of arthritis, and neuropathic pain models. However, a recent study in a healthy volunteer pain model failed to show any effect whereas an active comparator (pregabalin) was effective. This discrepancy may be due to different locations of action between the two drugs. Pregabalin is thought to act mainly at the level of the spinal cord dorsal horn, whereas the T-type calcium channels antagonists may work at the thalamic level. Therefore, the T-type calcium channel antagonists may act through modulation of the affective component of pain.

13. What are some of the new ways to modulate the postsynaptic *N*-methyl-D-aspartate ionophore?
Presynaptic release of glutamate binds to the postsynaptic glutamate receptor of the *N*-methyl-D-aspartate (NMDA) ionophore, resulting in channel opening and influx of sodium and calcium. This in turn results in postsynaptic depolarization and pain transmission. There have been many studies evaluating the analgesic effects of NMDA antagonists; however, there are dose-limiting side effects associated with these agents. There are several other binding sites within the ionophore channel that will modulate channel opening when glutamate binds and attempts have been made to utilize these sites to reduce side effects (Fig. 41.1). A glycine binding site must be occupied in order for the channel to open. A phase II clinical trial with a glycine antagonist for neuropathic pain showed a reduction in evoked allodynia but no effect on spontaneous pain. Noncompetitive channel antagonists such as ketamine prevent channel opening but are still associated with side effects. A magnesium binding site will prevent channel opening when occupied by magnesium. The AMPA/kainate channel is linked to the NMDA ionophore and, when activated, results in a rapid influx of sodium, which will remove the magnesium block, thus allowing glutamate to open the NMDA channel. A study in healthy volunteers showed promising analgesia without side effects of an AMPA/kainate channel blocker.

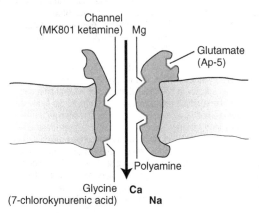

Figure 41.1. Schematics of the *N*-methyl-D-aspartate (NMDA) ionophore. Glutamate binds to the glutamate receptor and opens the channel. Noncompetitive NMDA antagonists, such as ketamine, bind to intrachannel sites and reduce opening. Also, there is a magnesium binding site that deactivated the channel. The glycine binding site must be occupied by glycine in order for the channel to open in response to glutamate.

14. **What is the current status of the cannabinoids to treat pain?**
There are two cannabinoid receptors, CB1 and CB2. Both receptors are G protein coupled positively to potassium channels and negatively to N-type and P/Q-type calcium channels, resulting in postsynaptic membrane hyperpolarization and a presynaptic reduction in neurotransmitter release. CB1 receptors are located peripherally and centrally in the nervous system. CB2 receptors are found mainly on inflammatory cells, and activation has potent antiinflammatory effects. There are two families of naturally occurring endocannabinoids, anandamide and 2-arachidonyl glycerol. Both have degrading enzymes, and there have been attempts at developing inhibitors of these enzymes that would theoretically result in higher levels of circulating endocannabinoids and analgesia. An inhibitor of anandamide, fatty acid amino hydrolase, was being developed by Pfizer but failed in clinical trials. However, other companies continue to develop these inhibitors. Cannabidiol (CBD) is a cannabinoid that is promising in that it is a cannabinoid receptor agonist that is void of psychoactive effects seen with tetrahydrocannabinol (THC). Due to the high lipid solubility of the cannabinoids, both transdermal and transmucosal delivery is feasible. Both synthetic and cannabis-based medicinal extracts are being developed for transdermal and transmucosal delivery. Nabixomols is a sublingual spray of a THC: CBD combination approved to treat multiple sclerosis pain in Canada. It was being developed in the United States to treat cancer pain. A phase II study met the primary efficacy endpoint for the low and medium dose, but not the high dose. A phase III trial failed to meet the primary endpoint, and further development is in question.

There is a rapid movement across the United States for the legalization of marijuana for medicinal purposes. Currently 23 states and the District of Columbia have legalized medicinal marijuana, with at least 16 states having ballots for the next elections. Although synthetic and cannabis based extracts are important, they may not completely meet the effects that the whole plant provides, in that there are many active compounds in the plant with medicinal properties. This is a strong argument of many medicinal marijuana advocates. This recently led the American Pain Society to commission the first white paper on medical marijuana, which will hopefully provide physicians with needed guidelines for patients using medical marijuana.

15. **What are p38 kinase inhibitors?**
The p38 mitogen-activated protein kinases are responsive to stress stimuli, such as cytokines, resulting in inflammation. Inhibition of these kinases is antiinflammatory. They have potential utility in autoimmune disease and inflammatory states; however, clinical trials to date have not been successful. Inhibition may result in prolonged QTc interval and will be contraindicated in patients at risk for arrhythmias.

16. **What are chemokine receptors, and how do they modulate pain?**
Chemokine receptor type 2 is a chemokine receptor that mediates monocyte chemotaxis. Antagonism results in a reduced monocyte infiltration and is thought to have potential in disease, such as rheumatoid arthritis and other autoimmune diseases. However, there was a recent negative phase II posttraumatic neuralgia study by AstraZeneca, placing further development in question. Although there were trends favoring the primary efficacy endpoint of the Neuropathic Pain Symptom Inventory score, it did not reach significance.

17. **Are there any agents being developed specifically for visceral pain?**
Linaclotide, a guanylate cyclase inhibitor, and lubiprostone, a chloride channel activator, have demonstrated analgesic efficacy in both animal models of visceral pain and patients with constipation-predominant irritable bowel syndrome. In humans, the analgesic efficacy of these drugs is closely tied to their promotility effects. Serotonin receptor subtype 3 (5HT3R) antagonists, like alosetron, have similar visceral analgesic effects; however, severe restrictions have been placed on its use due to adverse effects of ischemic colitis. Eluxadoline, a mixed agonist/antagonist at mu-, delta-, and kappa-opioid receptors, has recently been demonstrated to be effective for both pain and diarrhea in patients with IBS diarrhea-predominant subtypes. P2X purinoreceptor 3 antagonists are undergoing animal studies. The P2X3 receptor functions as a ligand-gated ion channel that may transduce ATP-evoked nociceptor activation, thought to be involved in visceral pain mediation. Antagonism results in pain relief in mouse models of visceral pain.

KEY POINTS

1. Both new and early development agents exist for the treatment of acute and chronic pain.
2. Most of the pipeline agents for chronic pain are either preclinical or in early phase studies.
3. Pipeline novel agents exist for a variety of pain mechanisms both neuropathic and nonneuropathic.

BIBLIOGRAPHY

1. Palmer P. Novel pharmaceuticals in the management of postoperative pain. *Expert Rev Clin Pharmacol.* 2015;8(5):511-513.
2. Melson TI, Boyer DL, Minikowitz HS, et al. Sufentanil sublingual tablet system vs. patient-controlled analgesia with morphine for postoperative pain control: a randomized, active-comparator trial. *Pain Pract.* 2014;14:679-688.
3. Watson JJ, Allen SJ, Dawbarn AD. Targeting nerve growth factor in pain. What is the therapeutic potential. *Biodrugs.* 2008;22:349-359.
4. Rice AS, Dworkin RH, McCarthy TD, et al. EMA401, an orally administered highly selective angiotensin II type 2 receptor antagonist, as a novel treatment for postherpetic neuralgia: a randomized, double-blind, placebo-controlled phase 2 clinical trial. *Lancet.* 2014;383:1637-1647.
5. Zylka MJ, Sowa NA, Taylor-Blake B, et al. Prostatic acid phosphatase is an ectonucleotidase and suppresses pain by generating adenosine. *Neuron.* 2008;60:111-122.
6. Allerton C, Fox D. *Pain Therapeutics: Current and Future Treatment Paradigms.* Cambridge: Royal Society of Chemistry; 2013:146-148.
7. Main MJ, Cryan JE, Dupere JR, et al. Modulation of KCNQ2/3 potassium channels by the novel anticonvulsant retigabine. *Mol Pharmacol.* 2000;58:253-262.
8. Wallace M, Pappagallo M. Qutenza: a capsaicin 8% patch for the management of postherpetic neuralgia. *Expert Rev.* 2011;11:15-27.
9. Rowbotham MC, Nothaft W, Duan WR, et al. Oral and cutaneous thermosensory profile of selective TRPV1 inhibition by ABT-102 in a randomized healthy volunteer trial. *Pain.* 2011;152:1192-1200.
10. Vinik A, Rosenstock J, Sharma U, et al. Efficacy and safety of mirogabalin (DS-5565) for the treatment of diabetic peripheral neuropathic pain: a randomized, double-blind, placebo- and active comparator-controlled, adaptive proof-of-concept phase 2 study. *Diabetes Care.* 2014;37:3253-3561.
11. Wallace MS, Duan R, Liu W, Locke C, Nothaft W. A randomized, double-blind, placebo-controlled, crossover study of the T-type calcium channel blocker ABT-639 in an intradermal capsaicin experimental pain model in healthy adults. *Pain Med.* 2015;17:551-560.
12. Wallace MS, Rowbotham MC, Katz N, et al. A randomized, double-blind, placebo-controlled trial of a glycine antagonist in peripheral neuropathic pain. *Neurology.* 2002;59:1694-1700.
13. Wallace MS, Lam V, Schettler J. NGX426, an oral AMPA-kainate antagonist, is effective in human capsaicin-induced pain and hyperalgesia. *Pain Med.* 2012;13:1601-1610.
14. Goldstein DM, Gabriel T. Pathway to the clinic: inhibition of p38 MAP kinase. A review of ten chemotypes selected for development. *Curr Top Med Chem.* 2005;5:1017-1029.
15. Kalliomaki J, Attal N, Jonzon B, et al. A randomized, double-blind, placebo-controlled trial of a chemokine receptor 2 (CCR2) antagonist in posttraumatic neuralgia. *Pain.* 2013;154:761-767.
16. Chizh BA, Illes P. P2X receptors and nociception. *Pharmacol Rev.* 2001;53:553-568.
17. Andresen V, Montori VM, Keller J, et al. Effects of 5-hydroxytryptamine (serotonin) type 3 antagonists on symptom relief and constipation in nonconstipated irritable bowel syndrome: a systematic review and meta-analysis of randomized controlled trials. *Clin Gastroenterol Hepatol.* 2008;6:545-555.
18. Chey WD, Lembo AJ, Lavins BJ, et al. Linaclotide for irritable bowel syndrome with constipation: a 26-week, randomized, double-blind, placebo-controlled trial to evaluate efficacy and safety. *Am J Gastroenterol.* 2012;107:1702-1712.
19. Drossman DA, Chey WD, Johanson JF, et al. Clinical trial: lubiprostone in patients with constipation-associated irritable bowel syndrome-results of two randomized, placebo-controlled studies. *Aliment Pharmacol Ther.* 2009;29:329-341.
20. Lembo AJ, Lacy BE, Zuckerman MJ, et al. Eluxadoline for irritable bowel syndrome with diarrhea. *N Engl J Med.* 2016;374:242-253.
21. Rao S, Lembo AJ, Shiff SJ, et al. A 12-week, randomized, controlled trial with a 4-week randomized withdrawal period to evaluate the efficacy and safety of linaclotide in irritable bowel syndrome with constipation. *Am J Gastroenterol.* 2012;107:1714-1724.

COMMON NERVE BLOCKS FOR HEADACHES AND FACIAL PAIN

Sarah Narayan and Andrew Dubin

Peripheral nerve blocks will use local anesthetic to block (provide pain suppression) in sensory nerve fibers and/or mixed superficial nerves. Local anesthetics in the amide family (i.e., lidocaine and bupivacaine) are more tolerable to patients and have a longer half-life. They limit neural activity by inhibiting the sodium and potassium channels that promote depolarization of nerves. Common anesthetics used are lidocaine, prilocaine, mepivacaine, and bupivacaine. Lidocaine takes effect in 4 to 8 minutes and lasts 1 to 2 hours. Bupivacaine lasts a bit longer, taking effect in 8 to 12 minutes and lasting 4 to 8 hours. Bupivacaine is the most cardiotoxic. Great care needs to be taken in order to prevent intravascular injection. Common side effects include pain, minor bleeding, and sensation changes at the injection site. Although nerve blocks administered to the head require small amounts of local anesthetic, rare side effects include seizures and cardiac arrhythmia. Other adverse responses related to the injection include infections, direct injection in to the peripheral nerve, and hematoma formation. On rare occasions one may inject steroid such as triamcinolone and methylprednisolone. When injecting steroid medication, hair loss, skin discoloration, and loss of fatty tissue may occur. There is no proven benefit to using steroids, although use of steroids may be beneficial for greater occipital nerve blocks. The effects of these injections can be very short or can last for weeks.

What are common nerve blocks that can be used for headaches or facial pain?

The greater occipital nerve is the medial branch of the dorsal primary ramus that comes off the C2 (second cervical) nerve root. It innervates sensation along the posterior scalp to the vertex. The nerve is located at one-third the length from the external occipital protuberance to the mastoid process. This nerve can be located approximately 2 cm lateral to the external occipital protuberance. The occipital artery runs alongside this nerve.

The lesser occipital nerve is derived from the C2 and C3 nerve roots. This nerve supplies sensory innervation to the base of the skull and posterior superior aspect of the neck. This nerve is located a third of the way from the mastoid process to the greater occipital protuberance.

The auriculotemporal nerve stems from the mandibular division of the trigeminal nerve. It provides sensations along the temporal area and ear. This nerve is located just anterior to the tragus.

The supratrochlear (STN) and supraorbital (SON) nerves stem from the ophthalmic division of the trigeminal nerve. The STN injection involves injecting 1 to 2 cc of anesthetic above the medial eyebrow. The SON is located 2 cm lateral to the STN.

The sphenopalatine ganglion harbor bodies of the maxillary branch of the trigeminal nerve as well as sympathetic and parasympathetic fibers. This nerve can be accessed along the posterior nasal mucosa.

Degenerated C2 to C3 facet joints and C2 or C3 nerve roots may refer pain along the distribution of the skull. Fluoroscopic injections to the facet joint can provide relief for the facet-mediated pain.

Transforaminal epidural steroid injections under fluoroscopic guidance may provide relief for radicular pain in the head and neck.

What are indications for the above nerve blocks?

Greater occipital nerve blocks (GON blocks) have been found to be effective in alleviating occipital neuralgia and acute migraines, and alleviating the allodynia associated with it. GON blocks have been effective in managing acute pain in those suffering from cluster headaches. GON blocks may be beneficial in those with postlumbar puncture headaches. GON blocks have not proven beneficial for those with tension headaches.

STN and the SON nerves are superficial nerves that can be injured with anterior head trauma. Frontal pain postinjury can suggest neuralgia. STN and SON are nerve blocks that can be performed for diagnostic and therapeutic reasons. SON block is a treatment for SON neuralgia. SON neuralgia is marked by pain in the distribution of the SON, and pain along the supraorbital notch and alleviated with SON.

The lesser occipital nerve block may be beneficial when injecting a trigger point around this vicinity of the nerve. Injecting 2 to 3 cc of lidocaine or bupivicaine can be beneficial.

The auriculotemporal nerve block may typically be performed by injecting 2 to 3 cc of lidocaine or bupivicaine, providing anesthetic relief to the temporal region of the head.

The sphenopalatine ganglion block is a simple though somewhat invasive way to approach anesthesia, by applying a cotton swap with 4% lidocaine intranasally along the lateral aspect of the nasal mucosa. The patient's head is tilted upward toward the side of discomfort to access the right location intranasally. If effective, patients can even self-administer this technique.

The greater occipital nerve block is the most common nerve block performed, and it may provide several weeks of improvement with infrequent risk.

Indications for nerve blocks include acute pain despite standard medication management for migraines. The theory behind pain relief is not based solely on the fact that the medication injected will anesthetize the affected nerves. If that were the case, the effects would be extremity short term. There may be influence on synaptic transmission. Above procedures seem to be more successful in those suffering from occipital neuralgia, cluster headaches, and cervicogenic headaches.

KEY POINTS

1. Nerve blocks involving the head have been proven to be effective using local anesthetic only. Use of steroid may be beneficial for greater occipital nerve blocks.
2. Risks of the injection include infection, direct trauma to the nerve, and bleeding.
3. On very rare occasion, intravascular injection of local anesthetic can cause seizures or cardiac arrhythmia.
4. The most common nerve block performed to the head is the greater occipital nerve block for occipital neuralgia.

BIBLIOGRAPHY

1. Levin M. Nerve blocks in the treatment of headache. *Neurother.* 2010;7:197-203.
2. Blumenfeld A, Ashkenazi A, Napchan U, et al. Expert consensus recommendations for the performance of peripheral nerve blocks for headaches—a narrative review. *Headache.* 2013;53:437-446.

CHAPTER 43

NERVE BLOCKS: SPINE

Sarah Narayan and Andrew Dubin

Nerve blocks can be performed for regional anesthesia, but also executed for pain management purposes. Common sites for nerve blocks are at the levels of the cervical and lumbar spine. These procedures can be performed in the thoracic spine, but these injections are less often performed, as nerve injury to the thoracic spine is less common. This may be attributed to the protected structure for the ribs at the level of the T-spine.

We will be discussing common nerve blocks performed for pain management. The injections are performed for both diagnostic and therapeutic treatments. A majority of the injections are performed outpatient—in the clinic or a same-day procedural facility. Some nerve blocks, such as epidurals, can be performed blind (without guided imaging) or under CT imaging, though most injections are performed under fluoroscopic guidance, utilizing x-rays. Injections should not be performed in those suffering an active infection. Precautions should be made—with consideration of possibly withholding injection—for those susceptible to infection. Patients should not be receiving an injection if they are receiving active anticoagulation or high dose blood thinning agents. There are specific American Society of Regional Anesthesia and Pain Medicine (ASRA) and American Society of Interventional Pain Physicians (ASIPP) guidelines to hold such medications prior to an intervention. Those with an allergy to contrast dye should not receive contrast confirmation during the injection, or the treating physician should withhold the injection altogether. Those pregnant should not receive an injection under x-ray exposure.

What are epidural steroid injections?

This type of injection involves injecting glucocorticoids into the epidural space in order to administer antiinflammatory relief to the spine. The objective of this injection is to decrease inflamed nerves that may contribute to pain in conditions of radiculopathy, radiculitis, or spinal stenosis with back pain with neurogenic claudication. Some practitioners will perform injections for nonspecific back pain or discogenic pain (causing localized back pain). There is little research to support the use of epidural injections for spinal stenosis, discogenic pain, or nonspecific back pain. A common indication for epidural steroid injection treatment is for disc herniations causing radicular pain. A high level of phospholipase A2 has been found in herniated disc matter. In animal studies it has been shown that the detection of this substance is associated with demyelinating nerve roots. The intention of injecting glucocorticoids, or "steroids," into the epidural or transforaminal space would be to inhibit inflammation causing the production of phosphoslipase A2, to inhibit neural transmission of nociceptive C fibers, and to decrease capillary permeability.

Adverse responses from the injection include postural headaches, nausea, dizziness, hyperglycemia, vasovagal syncope, infection, epidural hematoma, nerve injury, and adrenal suppression (though there is limited research on this last adverse response). It is advised that no more than three to four epidurals be performed each year, to minimize steroid exposure.

The epidural can be approached in the interlaminar space between the ligamentum flavum and dura, or approached into the transforaminal space just posterior to the nerve root near the neuroforamina. For the interlaminar approach, the needle must penetrate skin, fat, subcutaneous tissue, supraspinous ligament, interspinous ligament, and ligamentum flavum to get to the epidural fat in the epidural space. This space is on average 5 to 6 mm deep. One must be familiar with spinal anatomy to avoid vascular structures, especially when using the transforaminal approach. These injections can be performed in the cervical, thoracic, and lumbar segments. A caudal epidural also may be approached through the sacral hiatus.

What are facet joint injections?

Glucocorticoids or steroids have been injected in spinal facet or zygapophyseal joints for joint related arthritis of the spine. These joints are diarthrodial joints covered by synovial lining, and whose bony interior is covered by hyaline cartilage. Although there is less supportive literature backing the effectiveness of injecting facet joints, these interventions have been standard practice in many interventional pain clinics and institutions for joint mediated or arthritic pain. Using fluoroscopy, the needle is visualized and guided into the joint space. These injections can be performed for diagnostic purposes using an anesthetic, or for therapeutic purposes using glucocorticoid medications.

Medial nerve branch blocks target the medial branch of the dorsal rami. These medial branches innervate the facet joints. Injections targeting this nerve can be performed for diagnostic and therapeutic reasons. Each joint is innervated by two medial branches; for example, the L2 and L3 medial branches innervate the L3 to L4 facet joints, and the L4 and L5 medial branches innervated the L5 to S1 joint. A similar approach to medial branch blocks or steroid injections is radiofrequency ablation, which is a procedure that may provide more sustained relief without involving steroid administration.

What are sacroiliac joint injections?

Sacroiliac joints are diarthrodial joints made up of synovial fluid. The bony wall of the sacrum is made up of hyaline cartilage, although the pelvic side is lined by fibrocartilage. These injections are relatively safe, so long as the needle does not advance beyond the anterior wall of the sacrum to hit viscera. Performing a thorough history and physical examination aids in the diagnosis of SI joint dysfunction. Confirmation of the source of a patient's pain can be accomplished with a diagnostic sacroiliac joint injection. Often these injections are performed using fluoroscopy to assist in visualizing the inferior pole of the joint. This is often the site for a steroid injection.

What are Sympathetic nerve blocks?

Sympathetic nerve blocks are often performed for patients who present with pain in the limbs related to sympathetic mediated pain, an example being complex regional pain syndrome type I. These injections target the sympathetic chain. A positive injection will cause a temperature increase in the limb by 2°C, a decrease of pain, and vasodilation. The lumbar sympathetic change is comprised of the first four spinal nerves exiting the lumbar segments. Larger segments of the ganglia are located along the anterior level of the L2 and L3 vertebrae, which are sites often targeted for lumbar sympathetic nerve blocks. It is important that an effective nerve block is followed by a rigorous therapy program to optimize functional return in the affected extremity.

What are celiac plexus blocks?

This type of block is typically reserved for cancer patients experiencing abdominal pain. A posterior approach is used to infuse anesthetic into the celiac plexus. The blocks are intended for diagnostic reasons only. A therapeutic procedure could also be performed, injecting various medications from clonidine to steroid. Risks of this injection include injury to organ structures such as the kidneys, lungs, bowels, bladder, or vascular structures.

What are stellate ganglion blocks?

Stellate ganglion blocks are performed for patients who present with complaints of sympathetic mediated pain; refractory angina pain to the limb; or head, neck, and upper limb postherpetic neuralgia. This injection is approached at the level of the C6, and sometimes C7, vertebrae. There may be a slightly higher risk of pneumothorax or vertebral artery puncture at the C7 level. Visualization through fluoroscopic guidance should be used. Patients will experience Horner syndrome with successful blocks, which is marked by ptosis (lid lag), miosis, (pupillary constriction), and anhidrosis (diminished sweating on the unilateral face). An increase in facial temperature and nasal congestion may also occur.

KEY POINTS

1. Layers needle must penetrate for an interlaminar epidural injection: skin, fat, subcutaneous tissue, supraspinous ligament, interspinous ligament, and ligamentum flavum to get to the epidural fat.
2. Positive response directly after a sympathetic nerve block includes a temperature increase in the limb by 2°C, a decrease of pain and vasodilation.
3. There are two medial nerve branches off the dorsal rami that innervate each joint. For example, the L4 and L5 medial branches innervate the L5 to S1 zygapophyseal (facet) joint.

BIBLIOGRAPHY

1. Horlocker TT, Wedel DJ, Rowlingson JC, et al. Regional anesthesia in the patient receiving antithrombotic or thrombolytic therapy: American Society of Regional Anesthesia and Pain Medicine Evidence-Based Guidelines (Third Edition). *Reg Anesth Pain Med.* 2010;35(1):64-101.

2. Berkwits L, Davidoff SJ, Buttaci CJ, Furman MB. Lumbar transforaminal epidural steroid injection, supraneural (traditional) approach. In: Furman MB, Lee TS, Berkwits L, eds. *Atlas of Image-Guided Spinal Procedures*. Philadelphia: Elsevier, Saunders; 2012:93-103.
3. Davidoff SJ, Furman MB. Lumbar interlaminar epidural steroid injection, paramedian approach. In: Furman MB, Lee TS, Berkwits L, eds. *Atlas of Image-Guided Spinal Procedures*. Philadelphia: Elsevier, Saunders; 2012:111-117.
4. Lee TS, Furman MB. Lumbar zygapophysial joint intraarticular joint injection, posterior approach. In: Furman MB, Lee TS, Berkwits L, eds. *Atlas of Image-Guided Spinal Procedures*. Philadelphia: Elsevier, Saunders; 2012:119-131.
5. Stone JB, Gilhool JJ, Furman MB. Lumbar sympathetic block. In: Furman MB, Lee TS, Berkwits L, eds. *Atlas of Image-Guided Spinal Procedures*. Philadelphia: Elsevier, Saunders; 2012:149-154.
6. Fox KW, Furman MB. Stellate ganglion block. In: Furman MB, Lee TS, Berkwits L, eds. *Atlas of Image-Guided Spinal Procedures*. Philadelphia: Elsevier, Saunders; 2012:309-314.

CHAPTER 44

PERIPHERAL NERVE BLOCKS

Andrew Dubin

Before one can discuss the role of peripheral nerve blocks in the management of pain syndromes, one must address the question of the role of the peripheral nerve block. A block could potentially be therapeutic, but more often than not may be diagnostic.

Instances where nerve blocks may be of diagnostic utility include but are not limited to elucidation of a source generator of pain, or possibly establishing whether or not a loss of range of motion and an associated increase in pain or loss of function in a patient with underlying upper motor neuron syndrome (UMN) is secondary to fixed contracture or spasticity.

Diagnostic nerve blocks are typically done with short acting local anesthetics, as the goal is to assess a response. If the response is affirmative and there is a reduction in pain, improvement in function, or range of motion, then one can address and consider a trial of more long-term intervention.

Consider the case of lateral dorsal foot pain, as well as medial arch pain, in a patient status postankle fracture that was treated with open reduction internal fixation (ORIF) and plate fixation of the fibula and distal tibia. This patient may present with burning, tingling type pain in the previously noted areas. Examination will reveal two well-healed surgical scars, and minimal to no ankle swelling. From an orthopedic perspective, the ankle is healed and there has been a successful outcome, despite the pain complaints noted.

Examination will further reveal that percussion over the scar sights at the level of the lateral malleolus and just anterior to the medial malleolus replicates the patient's pain. The pain is in the distribution of the sural nerve as it crosses behind the lateral malleolus and becomes the dorsal sural nerve laterally, and the saphenous nerve medially. In both instances a diagnostic block with a short acting local anesthetic will have profound diagnostic value. A markedly positive response confirms the source generator and now guides treatment. Failure to respond effectively rules out these two nerves as source generators and allows one to focus more on structural mechanical issues.

Distal radius fracture or Colles fracture can also be associated with pain syndrome. Given that this is a distal radius wrist fracture, an acute median nerve neuropathy or carpal tunnel syndrome can develop secondary to swelling. In this scenario early electrodiagnostic testing (EDX) testing with nerve conduction studies may elucidate the problem and allow for early carpal tunnel injection and resolution of symptoms. Radial sensory nerve injury can also occur with these factures in the elderly, either as a direct result of an angulated fracture or secondary to cast fixation in a patient with minimal subcutaneous tissue and underlying issues of diabetes, which increases the risk of compressive neuropathies. In this scenario, once again a diagnostic radial sensory nerve block done distally approximately 10 to 14 cm proximal to the base of the thumb can give excellent diagnostic information and guide further treatment.

UMN, where diagnostic nerve block can be of utility, include finger flexor and wrist flexor "contracture" poststroke. With the advent and popularity of botulinum toxin in the management of UMN syndromes, there is a tendency to lose focus on the problem and not fully appreciate the underlying pathophysiology. As such, a failure to respond to botulinum toxin injections is described as the patient being a nonresponder, when in fact they may have been better served with another form of intervention. In the case of the clenched fist poststroke, the first question that must be answered is whether or not this is spasticity versus fixed contracture. One can do progressive escalating doses of botulinum toxin injections into the finger and wrist flexors; however, this is expensive, time consuming, and may be ultimately a singularly unsatisfying experience for both the patient and the provider. A more focused approach to this problem would be to do proximal nerve block to both the median and ulnar nerves with local anesthetic. If after perineural injection with the local anesthetic the hand can be passively opened, proceeding forward with botulinum toxin injections may be very helpful. If, however, the hand remains fisted, this confirms contracture is the etiology of the problem, and at that point referral to hand surgery for consideration of tendon lengthening procedures can be contemplated after discussion with the patient and caregivers.

Another (UMN) syndrome is the equino-varus postured foot poststroke. In this scenario the ankle plantar flexors as well as the ankle invertors and toe flexors are overactive. Once again the question of spasticity versus contracture must be answered. The best approach to this problem is to perform a diagnostic tibial nerve block at the level of the popliteal space. This can be done under ultrasound imaging or under needle electromyography guidance—whatever the practitioner's experience and preference is. Once again this block will give very important data that will help determine the next steps in the long-term management of this patient.

In all instances, an appreciation for potential complications must be held when performing peripheral nerve blocks. Realize there is always the potential with injection around a sensory nerve, or a mixed nerve with a large sensory component, to worsen the pain when the anesthetic wears off. This is a small risk but can happen and must be explained to the patient. Typically the increase in pain is transient and subsides back to baseline in days, but it may require a course of gabapentanoids, or other neuromodulators such as a short course of oral steroids.

KEY POINTS

1. Understand that peripheral nerve blocks can be used for diagnostic as well as therapeutic purposes.
2. Understand the potential complication of increasing pain postprocedure and its management.
3. Understand where peripheral nerve blocks fit into the armamentarium of pain management and evaluation.

BIBLIOGRAPHY

1. Anderson JG, Bohay DR, Maskill JD, et al. Complications after popliteal block for foot and ankle surgery. *Foot Ankle Int.* 2015;36(10):1138-1143.
2. Fisker AK, Iversen BN, Christensen S, et al. Combined saphenous and sciatic catheters for analgesia after major ankle surgery: a double-blinded randomized controlled trial. *Can J Anaesth.* 2015;62(8):875-882.
3. Lam NC, Petersen TR, Gerstein NS, et al. A randomized clinical trial comparing the effectiveness of ultrasound guidance versus nerve stimulation for lateral popliteal-sciatic nerve blocks in obese patients. *J Ultrasound Med.* 2014;33(6):1057-1063.
4. López AM, Sala-Blanch X, Magaldi M, et al. Ultrasound-guided ankle block for forefoot surgery: the contribution of the saphenous nerve. *Reg Anesth Pain Med.* 2012;37(5):554-557. doi:10.1097/AAP.0b013e3182611483.
5. Sala-Blanch X, López AM, Pomés J, et al. No clinical or electrophysiologic evidence of nerve injury after intraneural injection during sciatic popliteal block. *Anesthesiology.* 2011;115(3):589-595. doi:10.1097/ALN.0b013e3182276d10.

CHAPTER 45

INTRATHECAL THERAPY

R. Carter W. Jones III and Mark S. Wallace

1. **Why is intrathecal drug delivery an attractive option for the treatment of pain?**
   The dorsal horn of the spinal cord is a major site for pain control. Nociceptive information from the peripheral nervous system is conveyed to the central nervous system by primary afferent neurons. These are primarily myelinated and unmyelinated small-diameter neurons with cell bodies located in the dorsal root ganglia (DRG). The DRG extends central processes through the dorsal roots to synapse on neurons in the superficial and deep laminae of the spinal cord dorsal horn. Inhibitory and facilitatory nociceptive pathways composed of neurons located in the brainstem send axons that descend the neuraxis to synapse on and modulate the function of dorsal horn neurons. Many targets of analgesic drugs (e.g., opioid receptors, voltage-gated calcium channels, adrenergic receptors, and gamma-aminobutyric acid [GABA] receptors) are found in high concentrations in the spinal cord dorsal horn. Consequently, delivery of analgesic drugs directly into the intrathecal space places them in close proximity to their target sites for nociceptive transmission and modulation.

2. **What are the advantages of using intrathecal drug delivery compared to systemic drug administration?**
   There are several advantages of intrathecal drug delivery over systemic medication administration. Delivery of analgesic drugs (e.g., opioids) to the intrathecal space eliminates first pass metabolism that occurs with oral administration and the larger volume of distribution that occurs with systemic administration, resulting in a much higher effective drug concentration at the site of action. This leads to greater potency and improved side-effect profile compared to systemic administration. In addition, clonidine, bupivacaine, and ziconotide are potent analgesic medications commonly administered by intrathecal administration, but either are ineffective or produce intolerable side effects without significant analgesia when given by systemic administration. Lastly, intrathecal drug delivery is achieved by continuous delivery of concentrated drug stored in an implanted pump; therefore patients with severe, chronic pain treated with intrathecal drug delivery do not necessarily need to rely on self-administration of medications on a frequent, repetitive basis.

3. **What are some disadvantages of intrathecal drug delivery?**
   The delivery of intrathecal analgesics is an invasive technique that requires surgical implantation of a drug delivery system, including an intrathecal catheter and drug reservoir/pump, that may be contraindicated in some patients based on their medical comorbidities. It also requires continuous follow-up because the drug reservoir will eventually empty and require refilling to prevent drug withdrawal, which may preclude use in patients who have limited access to medical care. The initial costs of intrathecal drug delivery are high compared to oral or parenteral analgesic administration; however, studies show cost savings over time.

4. **Which patients are potential candidates for intrathecal drug delivery?**
   Intrathecal drug delivery is appropriate to consider in patients with severe pain refractory to systemic medications, those with intolerable side effects from systemic medications, and those who fail to respond to less invasive interventions. A lack of significant psychosocial abnormalities is also an important consideration. While most practitioners agree that it should be considered for patients with cancer-related pain that meet these criteria, more controversy exists in the general medical community regarding whether it is appropriate for patients who have chronic nonmalignant pain.

5. **What drugs can be given intrathecally for the treatment of pain?**
   Medications approved in the United States for intrathecal analgesia by the US Food and Drug Administration (FDA) include two drugs: morphine and ziconotide. Baclofen is FDA approved for intrathecal therapy for spasticity. It is common clinical practice to use other unapproved medications (e.g., other opioids and bupivacaine), and to mix different drugs together in an off-label manner. Theoretically, any soluble analgesic medication can be given intrathecally for the treatment of pain;

however, many can be toxic to neural tissue and should be avoided, especially in higher doses and for chronic administration (e.g., ketamine). The Polyanalgesic Consensus Conference published guidelines on drugs, doses, and combinations considered appropriate for intrathecal analgesic therapy that can serve as a guide for practitioners. These recommended drugs are divided into first line, second line, third line, etc. agents and combinations based on clinical experience with efficacy and safety.

6. **What is the role of an intrathecal drug trial in considering intrathecal analgesic therapy, and how does one conduct a trial?**
   The concept of trialing a patient on an intrathecal medication is based on the premise that a test dose of intrathecal medication will permit identification of patients who are likely to respond to this mode of drug delivery and therefore warrant permanent implantation of an intrathecal drug delivery system. There are primarily two ways that intrathecal drug trials are currently done. They can consist of (a) a single intrathecal or even epidural injection of a test drug (e.g., ziconotide), done in the outpatient setting, or (b) continuous infusion of a test drug via a percutaneous intrathecal catheter in the inpatient setting. There is no consensus on which method is most appropriate, and all have advantages and disadvantages. Importantly, none accurately reflect how drug will be delivered via currently available implantable systems. In addition, it is impossible to test all drugs, drug combinations, and drug doses so a negative trial does not necessarily predict lack of treatment response to intrathecal drug delivery. Lastly, each method of trialing is subject to a placebo response that may produce a false positive trial. There are methods proposed to attempt to reduce this effect (e.g., alternating active drug delivery with saline administration in a blinded manner); however, this is still problematic for the reasons stated previously. The lack of agreement on best approach for trialing, limitations of each method, and high likelihood of successful intrathecal therapy in appropriate patients have led some experts to argue for careful patient selection and proceeding directly to system implantation, eliminating drug trialing altogether. No matter what method is used, it cannot replace a thorough patient selection process based on a biopsychosocial model.

7. **How does one determine the starting dose and drug concentration when initiating intrathecal therapy?**
   The factors to consider when initiating intrathecal therapy in a patient include patient-related factors (e.g., reactions to systemic medications, medical comorbidities) and device-related factors. Conservative dosing regimens should be used for patients with multiple and/or severe comorbidities. All drug delivery systems have a finite volume and delivery rate; some systems have rates that can be adjusted. Drug reservoir volume, drug delivery rate, and drug dose are the device-related factors to consider when formulating intrathecal drugs to be administered to the patient. For example, with a 20-mL pump reservoir volume, a delivery rate of 0.5 mL/day will produce a reservoir refill interval of approximately 40 days compared to a delivery rate of 1 mL that will require a refill of approximately 20 days. Higher delivery rates will negatively impact the life span of intrathecal systems that rely on battery-powered modes of delivery. Ideally, the drug should be delivered at a rate of between 0.25 mL/day and 0.5 mL/day to maximize efficacy, system life-span, and patient convenience. When a desired drug dose is determined (typically measured as dose/day), a delivery rate is chosen, and these two will dictate the drug concentration to be formulated to fill the pump reservoir.

8. **What are the different modes of intrathecal drug delivery?**
   Intrathecal drugs can be delivered in one of three modes—simple continuous infusion, "flex" dosing, or continuous infusion plus patient administered boluses. Simple continuous infusion is achieved either through peristaltic delivery or administration of sequential delivery of small microboluses, depending upon the delivery system used. "Flex" dosing is possible with the Medtronic Synchromed II intrathecal pump system, and involves a background rate of drug delivery plus periods of increased delivery that are preprogrammed to occur on a daily basis. Patient administered boluses are also possible with the Synchromed II system, and can be programmed to deliver a specific dose of drug at a specified interval and maximum doses per day.

9. **Does location of the catheter tip within the intrathecal space or mode of delivery affect the efficacy of intrathecal therapy?**
   There is no definitive evidence supporting close proximity of the catheter tip to the spinal level corresponding to the patient's painful area or one method of drug delivery over another. However,

research studies and clinical experience indicate that intrathecal administration does not result in drug distribution throughout the neuraxis—rather drug concentrates in close proximity to where it exits the catheter, particularly with slow, continuous infusion. Factors that influence the intrathecal spread of drug include lipophilicity of the drug, rate and volume of delivery, mode of delivery (e.g., continuous vs. microbolus), patient anatomy, patient activity levels, and patient positioning. Consequently, attempts to place the catheter at the appropriate dermatome for each patient depending upon the location of pain should be made to maximize the efficacy of intrathecal therapy.

10. **What side effects can occur from intrathecal analgesics?**
Intrathecal delivery of analgesic medications carries with it the potential for all side effects of systemic administration, with a few additional risks specific to the intrathecal route. For example, intrathecal opioids can cause pruritus, urinary retention, and respiratory depression, while intrathecal local anesthetics can cause weakness, numbness, arrhythmias, and seizures. These side effects tend to occur less frequently with intrathecal administration than with systemic administration, because of the much lower doses that are required for analgesia. Ziconotide, a peptide antagonist of voltage-gated calcium channels, is only approved for intrathecal use. Common side effects of this medication include dizziness, nausea, altered mental status, nystagmus, and urinary retention. Lastly, catheter-tip associated inflammatory masses ("granuloma") are an uncommon but potentially serious reaction that can occur with intrathecal drug delivery—particularly opioids.

11. **What is a catheter-tip-associated inflammatory mass or granuloma, and what is their clinical presentation?**
Granulomas are an inflammatory mass that can develop on the catheter tip as a result of intrathecal drug administration. They are most commonly associated with continuous infusion of high concentrations of opioid medications—particularly morphine. The problems created by granuloma formation are twofold: they are highly vascular, resulting in rapid clearance of administered medications, and can form space-occupying lesions within the spinal canal, impinging upon neural structures and resulting in neurologic deficits. Consequently, practitioners should have a high clinical suspicion for granuloma formation if a patient reports diminished efficacy of intrathecal therapy, despite the escalation of therapy and/or if they report new neurologic symptoms and signs.

12. **How can a diagnosis of granuloma be confirmed, and what is the treatment for it?**
The primary method to confirm the presence of a granuloma is with imaging, either magnetic resonance imaging (MRI) or computed tomography myelography, focusing on the area around the catheter tip that can reveal a mass or filling defect, respectively, confirming the diagnosis. Treatment of a granuloma will depend upon the clinical symptoms of the patient. For those patients who present with new neurologic deficits attributable to the granuloma, emergent surgical decompression is warranted. If neurologic deficits are not present on exam, the intrathecal catheter can be revised on an urgent basis. The best method to prevent granulomas from forming is to avoid the use of highly concentrated intrathecal analgesics, particularly opioids, beyond recommended limits. Revisions should be performed with a surgeon familiar with granuloma management.

13. **Does intrathecal analgesic drug delivery place patients at higher risk of serious adverse events than other interventional pain procedures?**
Recent observational studies suggest that patients who undergo permanent implantation of intrathecal drug delivery systems for the treatment of pain have a significantly higher risk of mortality than patients who receive other invasive interventions for their pain (e.g., spinal cord stimulator implantation). This elevated risk was most evident within the first few days after implantation, but remained elevated at all time points studied, including up to 1 year after implantation. There are many factors that likely contribute to this phenomenon, including patient comorbidities, surgical anesthetic, initiation of intrathecal therapy, priming bolus of highly concentrated drug, and concomitant medications. High-risk patients receiving intrathecal therapy should be closely monitored for serious side effects, especially during the initial postimplant period.

14. **What type of complications can occur with intrathecal therapy?**
Aside from drug side effects and surgical complications, intrathecal drug delivery systems are complicated devices that can fail in several ways. The pump itself can break free from securing sutures and flip within the pump pocket such that the reservoir cannot be accessed to be refilled. The internal mechanism of the pump can corrode over time, resulting in a motor stall and cessation

of drug delivery. Battery-powered pumps will eventually run out and require replacement. The intrathecal catheter can become kinked or fracture, again resulting in cessation of drug delivery. Drug mixing errors can occur, resulting in overdose. Lastly, refilling of intrathecal pumps can result in advertant injection of highly concentrated drugs into the subcutaneous tissues of the pump pocket, rather than the intrathecal pump itself resulting in overdose.

15. **What effect does a magnetic resonance imaging have on an intrathecal pump?**
Except for the Codman3000 system, the intense magnetic field produced by an MRI can have profound effects on intrathecal drug delivery systems. For example, the Medtronic Synchromed II system will temporarily suspend drug delivery until the patient is removed from the MRI's magnetic field, at which point the system will spontaneously restart. On occasion this does not occur; therefore the pump should be interrogated after all MRIs to ensure proper functioning. In contrast, the magnetic field of an MRI will result in an opening of the flow restriction mechanism of the Flowonix Prometra pump, leading to an increase in intrathecal drug delivery and potential overdose. The new generation of the Flowonix pump prevents this complication with a shutoff valve that will engage if the delivery valve remains open. If the shut-off valve is engaged, the pump requires reprogramming to restart.

KEY POINTS

1. FDA-approved intrathecal medications in the United States for pain include morphine and ziconotide.
2. There is no consensus on which trialing method is most appropriate or accurate, and all have advantages and disadvantages. Further, a negative trial does not necessarily predict a negative treatment response to intrathecal drug delivery, while conversely placebo effect may produce a false positive trial.
3. Conservative dosing regimens should be used for patients with multiple and/or severe comorbidities.
4. Practitioners should have a high clinical suspicion for granuloma formation if patients report diminished efficacy of intrathecal therapy, especially with escalation of therapy and/or if they report new neurologic signs and symptoms.

BIBLIOGRAPHY

1. Ahmed SU, Martin NM, Chang Y. Patient selection and trial methods for intraspinal drug delivery for chronic pain: a national survey. *Neuromodulation.* 2005;8:112-120.
2. Brinker T, Stopa E, Morrison J, Klinge P. A new look at cerebrospinal fluid circulation. *Fluids Barriers CNS.* 2014;11:10.
3. Brogan SE, Winter NB, Abiodun A, Safarpour R. A cost utilization analysis of intrathecal therapy for refractory cancer pain: identifying factors associated with cost benefit. *Pain Med.* 2013;14:478-486.
4. Coffey RJ, Owens ML, Broste SK, et al. Mortality associated with implantation and management of intrathecal opioid drug infusion systems to treat noncancer pain. *Anesthesiology.* 2009;111:881-891.
5. Deer TR, Prager J, Levy R, et al. Polyanalgesic Consensus Conference 2012: recommendations for the management of pain by intrathecal (intraspinal) drug delivery: report of an interdisciplinary expert panel. *Neuromodulation.* 2012;15:436-466.
6. Deer TR, Prager J, Levy R, et al. Polyanalgesic Consensus Conference 2012: consensus on diagnosis, detection, and treatment of catheter-tip granulomas (inflammatory masses). *Neuromodulation.* 2012;15:483-495.
7. Deer TR, Smith HS, Cousins M, et al. Consensus guidelines for the selection and implantation of patients with noncancer pain for intrathecal drug delivery. *Pain Physician.* 2010;13:E175-E213.
8. Knight KH, Brand FM, Mchaourab AS, Veneziano G. Implantable intrathecal pumps for chronic pain: highlights and updates. *Croat Med J.* 2007;48:22-34.
9. Kumar K, Hunter G, Demeria DD. Treatment of chronic pain by using intrathecal drug therapy compared with conventional pain therapies: a cost-effectiveness analysis. *J Neurosurg.* 2002;97:803-810.
10. West SJ, Bannister K, Dickenson AH, Bennett DL. Circuitry and plasticity of the dorsal horn—toward a better understanding of neuropathic pain. *Neuroscience.* 2015;300:254-275.

CHAPTER 46

NEUROSTIMULATION: BRAIN

Alon Y. Mogilner

1. **What is spinal cord stimulation?**
   Spinal cord stimulation (SCS), also known as dorsal column stimulation, is a technique that can provide pain relief for a variety of chronic pain syndromes, via electrical stimulation of the dorsal columns of the spinal cord. Stimulation is delivered through permanently implanted electrodes placed in the epidural space of the spinal cord, which are connected to an implantable pulse generator (IPG) placed under the skin, similar to a cardiac pacemaker. Prior to permanent implantation, a trial is performed using externalized electrodes to assess efficacy. If the trial is successful, the patient is then a candidate for a permanent SCS implant.

2. **List the criteria for choosing patients who may benefit from spinal cord stimulation for treatment of pain.**
   - Chronic pain refractory to conventional medical management
   - Those having a trial of SCS showing greater than 50% pain relief
   - Patients with reasonable expectations that this device only will treat up to 50% of their pain and will not rid them of chronic pain
   - Patients with a psychological profile free of untreated severe depression, psychosis, or personality disorders

3. **Which conditions traditionally respond to spinal cord stimulation?**
   SCS has been used to successfully treat a variety of neuropathic pain conditions, including:
   - Radicular pain from failed spine surgery
     - While pain following lumbar spine surgery ("failed back surgery syndrome" or FBSS) is a very common indication for SCS, SCS has traditionally been shown to be most effective for radicular pain and less effective for axial back pain.
   - Ischemic pain from peripheral vascular disease
   - Complex regional pain syndrome (reflex sympathetic dystrophy, causalgia)
   - Angina pectoris
   - Pain from peripheral nerve injury
   - Phantom limb pain

4. **What is the mechanism of action of spinal cord stimulation?**
   The exact mechanism of pain relief via SCS remains unclear. A common proposed mechanism is the "gate control theory." Specifically, the larger Aα/Aβ fibers are activated and prohibit pain signals from smaller fibers from being appreciated. Recent work utilizing novel stimulation waveforms ("burst stimulation") suggest that different SCS waveforms may effect pain relief by activating a secondary ascending pain pathway known as the medial pathway.

5. **What does the patient feel during spinal cord stimulation?**
   During traditional paresthesia-producing SCS, the patient feels paresthesias—a tingling sensation that should overlap with the distribution of the pain. Recently, two new forms of SCS have been introduced: *high-frequency stimulation* and *burst stimulation*. These forms of stimulation do not generate paresthesias but can provide pain relief.

6. **What types of electrodes and generators are used for spinal cord stimulation and where are the electrodes placed?**
   There are two basic types of electrodes used for SCS. Percutaneous electrodes are thin cylindrical electrodes that can be placed through an epidural needle with a minor surgical procedure. Paddle electrodes are larger and wider, and require a more invasive procedure—laminectomy and bone removal—for placement. While paddle electrodes require a more invasive procedure, they are associated with a lower risk of lead migration and lower current requirements. Generators can be

either primary cell or rechargeable. Rechargeable generators last longer but require the patient to comply with recharging at fixed intervals, and thus may not be appropriate for all patients.

7. Where in the spine are the electrodes placed?
The most common location for SCS electrodes is over the mid-lower thoracic spinal cord, approximately T8 to T10. Lower placements can be indicated for pain in the distal leg and foot. Cervical placement is used for upper extremity pain. Recently, stimulation of the dorsal root ganglion has been reported to be effective for treating focal regions of pain that may not be covered by traditional SCS. When dorsal root ganglion stimulation is used, the usual targets are in the lumbar region, from L1-L5.

8. What are some of the complications of spinal cord stimulation for treatment of chronic pain?
The most common surgical complications are device-related, including device infection, which usually requires complete system removal, lead migration, and lead fracture. Permanent neurologic deficit such as paralysis is a rare but devastating complication of SCS.

9. What is occipital nerve stimulation?
Occipital nerve stimulation (ONS) is a neurostimulation technique that is used to treat a variety of pain and headache syndromes. Electrodes are placed percutaneously over the distribution of the occipital nerves and connected to an IPG analogous to SCS. Although currently not FDA-approved, studies have demonstrated efficacy of ONS for occipital neuralgia, migraine, and cluster headache.

10. What is the most common indication for delivery of pain medication via implantable pumps?
Intrathecal pumps are most commonly used to treat chronic pain of both nociceptive and neuropathic origin in patients who cannot achieve adequate pain relief via an oral medication regimen due to adverse side effects. They are also used, albeit less commonly, in patients with pain associated with malignancy who cannot obtain adequate pain relief with systemic opioid delivery via the oral or transdermal route.

11. What is the dorsal root entry zone operation?
The most common indication for dorsal root entry zone (DREZ) is the treatment of pain associated with brachial plexus avulsion. This procedure consists of making small lesions in the dorsal horn along the nerve rootlets that relate to the avulsions. It may be performed in the lumbar spine, less commonly.

12. Can neurostimulation be used to treat trigeminal neuralgia?
While stimulation of the trigeminal nerve has been attempted to treat classic trigeminal neuralgia (TN), there is little evidence to suggest it is effective. Subcutaneous stimulation of TN branches such as the infraorbital and supraorbital nerves is used to treat facial neuropathic pain, but it is not effective for the intermittent electrical shooting pain associated with TN.

KEY POINTS

1. Prior to permanent spinal cord stimulator implantation, pain relief should be demonstrated with a temporary externalized trial.
2. Radicular, constant neuropathic pain is more likely to respond to SCS than nonradicular, movement-related pain.
3. Nondestructive procedures such as neurostimulation are associated with low risk and may be preferred in many cases over ablative procedures. However, ablative procedures remain an appropriate intervention for a variety of indications, including pain associated with malignancy as well as trigeminal neuralgia.

BIBLIOGRAPHY

1. Belverud S, Mogilner A, Schulder M. Intrathecal pumps. *Neurother.* 2008;5:114-122.
2. Deer TR, Grigsby E, Weiner RL, Wilcosky B, Kramer JM. A prospective study of dorsal root ganglion stimulation for the relief of chronic pain. *Neuromodulation.* 2013;16:67-71, discussion 71-62.
3. Kanpolat Y, Ugur HC, Ayten M, Elhan AH. Computed tomography-guided percutaneous cordotomy for intractable pain in malignancy. *Neurosurgery.* 2009;64(suppl 3):187-193, discussion ons193-184.

4. Kinfe TM, Pintea B, Link C, et al. High frequency (10 kHz) or burst spinal cord stimulation in failed back surgery syndrome patients with predominant back pain: preliminary data from a prospective observational study. *Neuromodulation.* 2016;19:268-275.
5. Konrad P. Dorsal root entry zone lesion, midline myelotomy and anterolateral cordotomy. *Neurosurg Clin N Am.* 2014;25:699-722.
6. Kumar K, Taylor RS, Jacques L, et al. Spinal cord stimulation versus conventional medical management for neuropathic pain: a multicentre randomised controlled trial in patients with failed back surgery syndrome. *Pain.* 2007;132:179-188.
7. Mammis A, Agarwal N, Mogilner AY. Occipital nerve stimulation. *Adv Tech Stand Neurosurg.* 2015;42:23-32.
8. Mammis A, Sinclair GL 3rd, Mogilner AY. Peripheral neuromodulation for headache and craniofacial pain: indications, outcomes, and complications from a single center. *Clin Neurosurg.* 2012;59:114-117.

SPINAL CORD STIMULATION IN TREATMENT OF PAIN

Vignessh Kumar, Sara Gannon and Julie G. Pilitsis

CHAPTER 47

1. **What is spinal cord stimulation?**
   Spinal cord stimulation (SCS) is a surgical treatment option for patients with chronic pain. Since the inception of SCS in 1971, research and advances in technology have established spinal cord stimulation as an effective method of treating various manifestations of pain.

2. **How many patients use spinal cord stimulation?**
   A majority of the 50,000 neuromodulation devices implanted every year are spinal cord stimulators. SCS has proven to effectively treat chronic pain in the majority of cases (50% to 70%).

3. **What kinds of pain does spinal cord stimulation treat?**
   SCS is used for treatment of chronic pain that has failed multimodal therapy. Neuropathic pain tends to be more responsive than other forms of pain, and radicular symptoms tend to respond better than axial symptoms. Conditions most commonly treated by SCS include complex regional pain syndrome type 1, failed back surgery syndrome, and neuropathic pain.

4. **Who is a candidate for spinal cord stimulation therapy?**
   Patients who undergo SCS therapy typically (a) have been afflicted with chronic pain that has persisted for more than 6 months, (b) have exhausted conventional pain therapy, and (c) have undergone a trial period of stimulation lasting 5 to 7 days, which has demonstrated efficacy in relieving pain. Patients who undergo SCS therapy complete a psychological evaluation and magnetic resonance imaging, where the lead will be placed prior to SCS implantation.

5. **What does trial stimulation involve?**
   A trial stimulator is implanted prior to implantation of a permanent stimulator to ensure that SCS adequately covers the patient's area of pain. The trial SCS pulse generator is carried outside of the body. A permanent SCS device is implanted only if pain relief efficacy of trial stimulation is greater than 50%.

6. **How are spinal cord stimulation devices implanted?**
   The three components of SCS devices are the implantable pulse generator (IPG), connecting wires, and electrodes.
   The IPG is a battery-powered generator responsible for creating the electrical impulses that stimulate the spinal cord. The IPG can be controlled through a remote control and may be rechargeable or nonrechargeable. SCS may be percutaneous or paddle leads.
   Percutaneous electrodes are rod-shaped leads, and thus exhibit a cylindrical energy distribution vector. As a result, percutaneous electrodes exhibit multidirectional energy distribution, meaning that energy delivery of percutaneous electrodes is less effective than paddle electrodes. The size and shape of percutaneous leads allow placement through a needle. Paddle electrodes exhibit a unidirectional energy distribution vector, epidurally only, and are implanted through a laminotomy. Which type of lead is placed is variable depending on patient and implanter.

7. **What is the mechanism of spinal cord stimulation action?**
   Although the mechanism of SCS action has not been fully understood, the Melzack-Wall gate control theory of pain provides a partial explanation of how SCS stimulation can decrease pain perception. Electrical stimulation of Aβ afferent fibers works to downregulate the anterolateral pain perception tract, resulting in the analgesic effects characteristic of SCS. A consequence of electrical stimulation of Aβ afferent fibers is the sensation of paresthesia, a tingling sensation in stimulated dermatomes.
   Although the Melzack-Wall gate control theory of pain partially explains the analgesic mechanisms of SCS, this theory does not fully explain SCS mechanism of action. Specifically, high-frequency stimulation (HFS), a stimulation pattern characterized by frequency of stimulation of

1000–10,000 Hz, does not induce paresthesia characteristic of traditional SCS. Loss of paresthesia sensation in HFS indicates that the Melzack-Wall gate control theory of pain does not fully account for SCS mechanism of action.

8. **Spinal cord stimulation electrical impulses have qualities such as amplitude, frequency, and pulse width. What do these mean?**
Amplitude, frequency, and pulse width are characteristics of any form of electric current. These parameters can be adjusted to best optimize pain relief (Fig. 47.1).

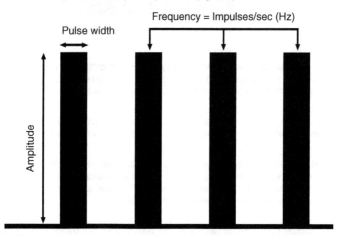

Figure 47.1. SCS current dynamics. Three aspects of SCS current dynamics include amplitude, pulse width, and frequency. Amplitude, pulse width, and frequency collectively contribute to stimulation intensity. These three aspects of SCS current dynamics can be individually customized to suit patient needs.

Amplitude refers to the magnitude of electrical stimulation, and is measured in volts. Frequency refers to number of impulses per second, and is measured in hertz. Pulse width refers to duration of the electrical impulse, and is measured in microseconds. Amplitude, frequency, and pulse width can be increased to increase intensity of stimulation.

KEY POINTS

1. Candidates for SCS should be patients with chronic pain who have tried conventional pain therapy but have not experienced adequate pain relief.
2. Where possible, pain relief with temporary stimulation should be demonstrated before more permanent implantation.
3. 50% to 70% of patients experience short-term relief with SCS. At 2 years, SCS was shown to provide superior pain relief, improve quality of life, and improve functional capacity as compared to conventional medical management alone. (At 2 years, 93% of patients reported satisfaction with SCS treatment. At 2 years, patients showed statistically significant improvements in pain and disability measures, as measured by visual analogue scale and Oswestry disability index. At 2 years, 47% of patients showed >50% improvement in leg pain.)

BIBLIOGRAPHY

1. Shimoji K, Higashi H, Kano T, Asai S, Morioka T. Electrical management of intractable pain. *Masui.* 1971;20(5):444-447.
2. Kunnumpurath S, Srinivasagopalan R, Vadivelu N. Spinal cord stimulation: principles of past, present and future practice: a review. *J Clin Monit Comput.* 2009;23(5):333-339.
3. Melzack R, Wall PD. Pain mechanisms: a new theory. *Science.* 1965;150(3699):971-979.
4. Benzon H, Rathmell JP, Wu CL, et al. *Practical Management of Pain.* 5th ed. Philadelphia: Elsevier Health Sciences; 2013.
5. Kumar K, North R, Taylor R, et al. Spinal cord stimulation vs. conventional medical management: a prospective, randomized, controlled, multicenter study of patients with failed back surgery syndrome (PROCESS study). *Neuromodulation.* 2005;8(4):213-218.

CHAPTER 48

NEUROABLATIVE PROCEDURES

Gaddum Duemani Reddy and Ashwin Viswanathan

1. **What are neuroablative procedures and some pain-associated conditions that are treated by neuroablative procedures?**
   Neuroablative procedures are destructive procedures that are used to interrupt the transmission of pathological pain pathways. Pain-associated conditions that can be treated with neuroablative procedures include cancer pain, trigeminal neuralgia, and spasticity. Given the permanency of these procedures in contrast to medication or stimulation procedures, patient selection is critical.

2. **What are some types of neuroablative procedures for cancer pain?**
   - **Anterolateral cordotomy**—This procedure focuses on lesioning the lateral spinothalamic tract in the anterolateral part of the spinal cord. It is ideally suited for a patient with unilateral cancer-related nociceptive pain involving a dermatome lower than C5. Bilateral high cervical cordotomies risk inducing Ondine's curse, which is characterized by suppression of the spontaneous respiratory drive. Neuropathic pain may be more difficult to treat with cordotomy. Techniques include open, fluoroscopic guided, and CT-guided percutaneous approaches.
   - **Dorsal root entry zone (DREZ) lesioning**—DREZ lesioning involves ablating hyperactive neurons in the dorsal horn of the spinal cord and the excitatory portion of Lissauer's tract. Ideal patients have segmental pain associated with lesions in the nerve, root, or spinal cord, and the most successful results have been in treating brachial plexus avulsions, where it has been shown to provide relief in over 75% of patients. Techniques for inducing the lesion include microsurgical, radiofrequency, ultrasound, or laser.
   - **Myelotomy**—This procedure interrupts the ascending posterior visceral pain pathway. It is ideally suited for patients with midline abdominal or pelvic pain, and may be performed using an open surgical technique or percutaneously. A commissural myelotomy which interrupts the crossing fibers of the spinothalamic tract may be useful for bilateral leg pain or sacral pain.
   - **Cingulotomy**—Lesioning of the cingulate gyrus has been used in the treatment of pain as well as psychiatric disorders. The exact mechanisms for pain reductions are unknown, but ideal candidates have multiples sites of pain secondary to widely metastatic disease. This procedure can be performed using either stereotactic radiofrequency thermocoagulation or laser interstitial thermal therapy.

3. **What are some types of ablative procedures for trigeminal neuralgia and their associated complications?**
   - **Glycerol rhizotomy**—This procedure involves injection of glycerol into the trigeminal cistern. The volume injected is determined by the division of the nerve that is to be affected. Possible complications for all of the percutaneous procedures include damage to the surrounding structures, in particular the surrounding cranial nerves or carotid artery.
   - **Percutaneous balloon compression (PBC) rhizotomy**—PBC is a procedure that involves inflation of a radiopaque balloon under fluoroscopic guidance in the proximal region of the trigeminal fossa. Unlike other ablative procedures, it can be performed under general anesthesia. Due to a trigeminal depressor response, patients may become acutely and severely bradycardic during balloon inflation. Though a useful marker of an adequate compression, the anesthesia team must be prepared to treat this bradycardia.
   - **Radiofrequency (RF) rhizotomy**—RF rhizotomy involves thermocoagulation of the trigeminal ganglion. Patients are awake and stimulation of the segments of the ganglion is done prior to ablation to ensure selective ablation of the target trigeminal divisions. Possible complications of this procedure include corneal numbness, keratitis, anesthesia dolorosa, and dysthesias.
   - **Stereotactic radiosurgery (SRS)**—SRS can be used to target the trigeminal ganglion. Complications are similar to the percutaneous procedures and include sensory dysfunction, and a very low risk of anesthesia dolorosa.

4. **What is a dorsal rhizotomy, what does it treat, and what is its mechanism of action?**

Dorsal rhizotomy is an ablative technique designed to reduce spasticity, particularly in children with cerebral palsy. It works by eliminating a pathologically hyperactive reflex arc between sensory and motor fibers from the same muscle group.

5. **How is a dorsal rhizotomy performed and what are some possible complications?**

   - While the procedure has evolved over the last century, the current technique, which is known as a selective dorsal rhizotomy, involves performing a laminectomy over the conus, isolating the dorsal/sensory nerve roots from L1 to the sacrum, dividing these roots into rootlets, recording EMG responses to tetanic stimulation from these rootlets, and sectioning rootlets that have diffuse responses that extend beyond their distribution. Approximately 60% to 70% of the sensory nerve roots are divided in this fashion. Possible complications of a modern dorsal rhizotomy include transient dysesthesias, with a low risk of permanent hypoesthesia, as well as transient urinary retention with a low risk of incontinence.

KEY POINTS

1. Neuroablative techniques are destructive procedures that when used in the appropriate circumstances help reduce pain in several conditions, including metastatic cancer, trigeminal neuralgia, and spasticity.
2. Cordotomy is ideal for unilateral pain below the C5 dermatome.
3. Midline myelotomy can be performed open or percutaneously to facilitate treatment in patients with advanced cancer.

BIBLIOGRAPHY

1. Harsh V, Viswanathan A. Surgical/radiological interventions for cancer pain. *Curr Pain Headache Rep.* 2013;17(5):331.
2. Bender MT, Bettegowda C. Percutaneous procedures for the treatment of trigeminal neuralgia. *Neurosurg Clin N Am.* 2016;27(3):277-295.
3. Lopez BC, Hamlyn PJ, Zakrzewska JM. Systematic review of ablative neurosurgical techniques for the treatment of trigeminal neuralgia. *Neurosurgery.* 2004;54(4):973-982.
4. Aquilina K, Graham D, Wimalasundera N. Selective dorsal rhizotomy: an old treatment re-emerging. *Arch Dis Child.* 2015;100(8):798-802.

PAIN PSYCHOLOGY

Marilyn S. Jacobs and Lekeisha A. Sumner

CHAPTER 49

1. What is pain psychology?

   Pain psychology is the subdiscipline of clinical psychology and clinical health psychology investigating science and clinical practice of pain medicine. The foundational paradigm for pain psychology is the interaction of neurological sensitization from tissue damage with affective/emotional and cognitive/discriminatory factors resulting in the pain experience. This model is based upon the definition of pain adopted by the International Association for the Study of Pain (IASP, 1979): pain is "an unpleasant sensory and emotional experience." The literature has demonstrated there are connections between sensory, emotional and cognitive regions of the brain in the final integration of pain phenomena into consciousness. Pain psychology includes protocols for the psychological assessment (including testing) and treatment of patients with pain.

2. How is psychological treatment relevant to pain management?

   Evolving best practice pain medicine guidelines are now largely based upon a multidisciplinary model including psychological evaluation and treatment. Treatment based upon scientific pain medicine findings is insufficient for comprehensive patient care. Psychological factors are understood to be both etiological and consequential to the pain experience. Given the severity of suffering from pain and the "chronification" that may occur, pain psychology is very beneficial.

3. What is the history of pain psychology?

   There is a vast literature on the history of pain and its psychological aspects. Historians studying pain through the ages have emphasized that each generation creates its own narrative for the psychology of pain. The formal inclusion of clinical psychology as a component of the pain field took hold in the mid-20th century with the advent of the Gate Control Theory. This disciplinary integration was deepened by later theoretical explanations of pain perception (such as the Neuromatrix Theory and the Ensemble Theory). It was established that descending neural tracts from emotional and cognitive centers in the brain influenced transmission of pain signals from peripheral areas of tissue damage, establishing a biological relationship between sensation, emotion, and cognition. Prior to this reconceptualization, pain was mostly viewed according to Cartesian dualism with the mind and body believed to be separate entities. Therefore, psychosocial inputs were not considered. Developments in clinical medicine with the advent of the biopsychosocial model for medical care also had a decisive influence. With this paradigm shift, research into the psychological aspects of the pain experience expanded significantly, such that now there is a wide basis of validation to support pain psychology. Inclusion of behavioral science in pain medicine was codified in 2011 by the Institute of Medicine.

4. What are the qualifications of a psychologist or other mental health professional to be able to work with pain medicine?

   Ideally a clinical psychologist in the pain field would have training in clinical medicine and health psychology. Training can occur formally with a doctorate specialization or through professional development. Other mental health professionals can become involved with pain management with training in clinical medicine and the psychological evaluation of medical patients. Psychiatrists are well suited to this application of mental health care due to their education and training, although these professionals would also need to have an understanding of pain medicine. Presently a specialty training credential in pain psychology has not been formalized. Mental health professionals working with pain patients generally have diverse backgrounds of training and experience. At a minimum, the mental health practitioner would benefit from participation in a pain medicine board review and study of the pain medicine literature. Several training sites for clinical psychology have recently established pain psychology internships and fellowships. A listing of related training programs is available through the American Psychological Association, and their Division of Health Psychology of that organization has a listing of trained psychologists.

5. **Are there different psychological symptoms and/or disorders with the different types of pain?**
Psychological reactions to pain involve a range of emotional distress and dysfunction. Neuropathic, visceral, and somatic pain can all cause psychological symptoms (such as depression or anxiety) and/or disorders (such as major depression or generalized anxiety). It is difficult to tie a specific type of emotional distress to a specific type of pain. However, acute pain generally leads to anxiety, while chronic pain generally leads to depression. Likely, it is not the type of pain but the duration and severity that correlate with more or less severe psychological disturbance. Further, the extent to which pain interferes with functioning is an important factor.

6. **What is the risk of not including psychological treatment in pain management?**
Pain patients have significant psychological comorbidity. Psychological syndromes found in the pain patient population include depression, anxiety, fear, sleep, appetite and sexual dysfunction, cognitive impairment, somatization, alexithymia, and negative emotions such as anger, hostility, and guilt. Occasionally, more severe psychological problems will develop, such as psychosis, dissociation, abuse of substances, addiction, eating disorders, or suicidal ideation. Psychological trauma is a frequent component of the chronic pain condition. People arrive at a pain state after a medical illness or a physical injury. These events are usually highly stressful, aversive, and can cause personality deterioration. Chronic illness can cause psychological trauma due to the burden of disruption of life goals and functioning. It is an established fact that a significant percentage of patients with pain disorders have had a history of psychological trauma. Often, one finds a significant history of childhood abuse (emotional, physical, and/or sexual), workplace harassment, domestic violence, and human rights abuses. Therefore, to omit a psychological perspective in evaluation and treatment of the person with pain is to neglect an essential etiological data point. If the psychological trauma is not treated, there is a risk the condition may worsen and the chronic nature may become intractable. This can lead to higher utilization costs and iatrogenic complications. It is important to understand there is a distinction between posttraumatic stress disorder and complex trauma. The former is usually a defined experience of a catastrophic event, while the latter indicates a more global deterioration in personality functioning. These can co-occur.

7. **At what stage in pain management should psychological treatment (and/or other mental health treatment) be introduced?**
The basis for referral of a patient for a pain psychology evaluation is the clinician's judgment that psychological factors are implicated in the presentation of the pain and the suffering. It should be emphasized that not all patients with pain have psychological comorbidity and so the determination by the pain practitioner is individual and on a case-by-case basis. If a patient does not seem to be benefiting from pain medicine treatment, if there are questions about serious emotional distress, if there are concerns about medication abuse, or if a history of trauma is known or suspected, a psychological referral is in order. Additionally, third-party insurers require certain invasive pain therapies—such as spinal cord stimulation—provide psychological clearance as to the patient's suitability for the procedure.

8. **Is psychological evaluation and treatment recognized by third-party payers?**
Under the Mental Health Parity and Addiction Equity Act of 2008 and Affordable Care Act of 2010, all health insurance plans are required to provide mental health treatment benefits. However, not all mental health professionals are members of all available health insurance networks. Third-party payers are varied in scope and operate under diverse administrative guidelines. In some cases, preauthorization may be necessary. In that instance, the referring physician will need to make a request for approval through medical utilization for this service.

9. **What is the biopsychosocial model, and how does it inform pain treatment?**
The biopsychosocial model of health care is a theory and guide which holds that disease, illness, pain, and suffering are constituted by interacting dimensions, and scientific data is only one of these. It recommends a holistic approach to medical care that transcends objectivism. All medical conditions are created by biological phenomena, psychological experience, and social context. One can provide expert medical care yet fail to alleviate pain and suffering if the patient's relationships in his/her life and society are not also considered. Further, the relationship between the patient and the practitioner is essential to consider. This paradigm is often overlooked, given the rapid advances in pain scientific research and technology over the past two decades.

10. **What are operant learning and social learning, and how do these models of behavior relate to pain?**

Operant learning in pain management is based on the idea that pain behaviors arise along with a pain condition, and these presentations can be altered, as they are reinforced by environmental influences. The person in pain will act in pain; these actions represent a distinct domain from the actual pain condition. The patient learns how to be in pain and can therefore learn how to not be in as much pain. Operant conditioning as a therapy is a method designed to increase a pain patient's awareness of how their pain causes them to behave. Social learning is a theory that is based on the idea that social contexts can increase or decrease the perception of pain due to the reinforcement of interpersonal and social influences. The treatment method is directed at increasing the patient's awareness of these processes. Both of these models rely upon conscious awareness of pain perception and control of the outcome of behaviors related to this perception.

11. **What can psychoanalysis contribute to pain psychology?**

Sigmund Freud created psychoanalysis from his work as a neurologist with patients who had "pain without lesion"—a concern of 19th century physicians. Psychoanalytic theory has much to offer pain psychology. Unconscious factors in emotional life—such as repressed memories or traumas, unresolved conflicts, unprocessed emotions, or ineffective mechanisms of defense against negative emotions—may all influence pain perception. The patient's relational style may impact their interactions with medical practitioners. Attachment in early life influences emotional regulation and management of distress. Mental schemas are used to manage distress; these develop from interactions with caregivers. These "attachment styles" may determine the response to stress. Research has substantiated that people with insecure attachment styles may influence pain outcomes due to a more realistic assessment of threat and a more positive outlook.

12. **How does culture play a role in the experience of pain?**

A person's cultural background—that is, their ethnicity, religion, nationality, sexual orientation, and social practices—will influence how they experience pain. Pain may be thought of differently in differing social contexts. It may be regarded as a necessary aspect of human life or a punishment for wrongs committed. It may be seen as an experience to be borne with courage, or one for which therapeutic means are required. Western medicine may be eschewed for traditional healing practices. It may also be the case that many scientifically based treatments are not optimal for nonwhite populations. Health care professionals should apply a sociocultural approach to all patients, keeping in mind the divergence of values, behaviors, expectations, and beliefs. The pain medicine evaluation should include multicultural awareness. This perspective is especially relevant given the pluralistic nature of most Western societies in the 21st century.

13. **What are the differences in the psychology of acute versus chronic pain?**

Acute pain involves an evolutionary-based survival mechanism to repair damaged tissue through sympathetic nervous system activity and inflammatory processes. The emotions generated in acute pain are anxiety, fear, disorganization, and uncertainty. Acute pain is self-limited, and the underlying condition most often responds fully to treatment. Chronic pain is determined after a period of acute pain that fails to resolve with treatment. There is no survival value in chronic pain. The person becomes depressed, withdrawn, and vegetative. The attitude may be one of giving up and hopeless despair. There is an overall parasympathetic response that results in a decrease in vital functions, including psychological ones. Often with chronic pain the underlying condition is insufficient to explain the extent of debilitation and suffering—hence psychosocial factors may impinge. There is a growing realization among pain practitioners that timely multidisciplinary intervention (including psychological care) can decrease the frequency and/or severity of the transition from acute to chronic pain.

14. **How does a person adjust to pain, and how can psychotherapy help this process?**

Once pain becomes chronic and medical treatment has been maximized, the patient will need to develop an acceptance of their condition and reorient their identity to include the experience of pain. Over-reliance upon medical treatments in lieu of a psychological adaptation process (which would include the development of coping skills and a realistic appraisal of the condition) may prolong or lessen treatment gains. If there are significant psychosocial losses, the patient would need to understand the meaning of the pain experience as it relates to their life situation, and find ways to reframe and restructure their thinking. If the pain condition has exacerbated psychological vulnerability, these aspects would benefit from review and understanding. Most patients with chronic pain experience a wide-range of losses and thus will need to reorganize expectations. They need to understand their emotional and cognitive reaction to the changed circumstances and find a means to create new meaning structures. Psychotherapy can assist with this process by the identification and transformation of painful emotions, negative thinking, difficulties in relationships with family and society, reduction of stress, encouragement of functioning, and supportive advocacy that life will continue for the person in new and rewarding ways. The evidence for the improvement of pain with this process has been well established in the pain psychology literature. There can be a value in overcoming difficult circumstances that can enhance personal growth and evolve consciousness. Positive life change may occur after a pain-related condition if the patient is given the tools to move forward in altered circumstances. They are alienated from the life they once knew.

15. **What is the difference between pain and suffering, and what is the role of suffering in pain?**
Suffering is a high level of distress that poses a danger to the patient's view of their life. Pain almost always creates suffering. Each person's conception of suffering is unique and relates to personal history, relationships, ideals, experiences, and life goals. Most patients with pain will have a feeling of loss—at times profound—at how their life has been changed by the burden of illness and the restrictions on how they wish to live. The suffering index is the degree to which the person is apart from the world that they once inhabited. Regaining a connection to the world and de-emphasis upon the body as the primary means of knowing and valuing the self can reduce suffering. The development of the ability to think about experience and understand it (in psychotherapy) can enlarge the patient's ability to cope with pain.

16. **How does a history of abuse and trauma contribute to the onset, course, and treatment of pain?**
For all humans, stressful and traumatic experiences are maintained in memory, even with adaptation and growth. With an injury or illness that causes tissue damage, repressed traumatic experiences can be revived. This process is an amplification of past exposure—the lifting of a defensive barrier. People with a history of developmental intrusions (such as neglect and deprivation as well as violence and instability) may be more vulnerable to a less optimal outcome when they become medically ill with pain, and may be more likely to develop complicated health problems. Circumstances in early development such as psychiatric or substance-use disorders in caregivers, violence, poverty, social dislocation, marginalization due to minority status, early loss of close relationships, neglect, insufficient attachment relationships, untreated medical conditions, academic difficulties, as well as emotional, physical, or sexual abuse will create vulnerability in the person that may lead to chronic pain. Some patients with such a background tend to not respond well to pain treatments unless some form of psychological intervention is included with the medical treatment. The experiences that come to consciousness which were previously repressed can be managed with psychotherapy.

17. **What is somatization, and how does it relate to pain?**
Somatization is the process whereby emotional stress and/or adversity are converted into physical symptoms. Somatization occurs when a physical experience cannot be fully processed in the mind. It is important to appreciate that somatization may be a normal process in response to an unexpected situation where the person is overloaded with stress. A patient may develop somatic expression of mental distress if a social context to convey the narrative of unhappiness, loss, or other types of psychological suffering is absent. Empathy and compassion goes a long way to decrease somatic reactions. A concerned health care practitioner can alleviate a patient's mental pain and thereby decrease somatization, which may include pain. Pain may develop in individuals who cannot bear emotions and feelings. They may then retreat to the physical expression of mental distress, short-circuiting their mental sorrow. This phenomenon has recently been termed "medically unexplained symptoms." People who lack supportive relationships in their lives may develop somatization and pain. For these individuals, medical treatments are insufficient.

18. **What is alexithymia, and how does it relate to pain?**
Alexithymia is a personality trait whereby the person has a diminished capacity to process emotions. These individuals may not have the ability to describe feelings with language. They may not recognize how they feel in response to experiences. They may attribute their response to external factors. Patients with this type of psychological organization are less competent in the identification

of feelings and differentiation of feelings from body sensations. Alexithymia is not a mental disorder; however, it is a risk factor for medical and psychological conditions, including pain. Research has substantiated that many patients with pain also have alexithymic personality traits.

19. **What is the diathesis-stress model, and how does it relate to pain?**
The diathesis-stress model is a psychological theory which posits that a predisposition of biological and/or emotional vulnerability in the context of exposure to life stress will determine the outcome for the person. As a psychological theory, diathesis-stress has been used to explain the etiology and onset of many mental disorders. It has also been applied to the understanding of why some patients with pain will become disabled after trauma induced tissue damage, while others will be more resilient and be able to return to functionality. Referral of pain patients with this presentation and referral for mental health evaluation and treatment can improve pain treatment outcomes.

20. **What is the diagnostic classification system used for mental disorder diagnoses of pain patients?**
Pain patients with mental disorders are classified according to the DSM-5 and ICD-10 nosological systems. Pain can result in any mental disorder listed in these classification systems.

21. **How does a mental disorder interact with chronic pain?**
Persons with a premorbid mental disorder (such as depression or anxiety) are likely to have limitations in their stress management and coping abilities. Therefore, the stress of chronic pain may be too difficult of a load to integrate and lead to a worsening of their overall condition.

22. **What are some of the mental disorders which pain patients develop?**
The comorbidity of mental disorders among pain populations is considered to be high, although precise prevalence rates vary by the pain condition and demographics of the populations (e.g., age, educational attainment, gender). Among the most common found are disorders of depression, anxiety (including posttraumatic stress disorder, panic, and generalized anxiety disorder), alcohol abuse/dependence, and somatization. Sleep and substance use disorders are also common. Despite the large body of evidence demonstrating the presence of mental disorders, they are not usually evaluated, identified, or treated. The difficulty detecting mental disorders, especially depression, in pain populations is complicated by overlap of psychiatric symptoms and pain symptoms. For example, sleep disturbance is often due to both medical and psychiatric factors, such as depression. Moreover, research has substantiated a relationship of reciprocity with psychiatric distress, the pain experience and pain outcomes, in part because they share many biological pathways. Psychiatric distress has been shown to worsen severity, frequency, and duration of pain. Conversely, as the severity of pain increases, so does the severity of psychiatric distress. Although the prevalence rates of mental disorders vary by pain condition, empirical evidence demonstrates high comorbidity. Depression appears to be the most prevalent mental disorder seen in pain populations.

23. **What is the difference between psychological treatments of noncancer versus cancer pain?**
Many aspects of cancer treatment may cause the development of psychological symptoms. These etiologies include stress from procedures, chemotherapy, radiation treatment injuries, changes in physical appearance and loss of functioning, fear of suffering and death, loss of social role, and alienation from social network and family problems. Therefore, it is important to keep in mind that patients with cancer-pain can also develop secondary pain and psychological problems.

24. **What are the limitations of medical treatments for chronic pain?**
Medical treatments alone do not target the pathways and mechanisms responsible for pain processing, perception, and management. Also, chronic pain can usually not be cured but managed.

25. **How can psychological therapies be useful in chronic pain and affect medical utilization?**
Psychological treatments can reduce the perception of pain intensity, medication use, and pain disability and improve overall functioning. Pain patients experience changes in their autonomy and identity and over time deplete internal and external psychosocial resources. Many life domains (e.g., ability to work, changes in marital and relational roles, sexual functioning) are severely impaired, which further perpetuates chronic strain, emotional pain, and psychiatric distress. Psychological therapies can benefit pain patients by restoring, strengthening, and harnessing their resources, self-image, coping styles, and ability to engage in self-care. Treatments also identify and shape environmental reinforcements of sickness and other maladaptive behaviors, help adjustment and

management of pain and stress, construct meaning from the condition and interpretation of pain experience, discriminate between negative affective states and psychical pain, and alleviate emotional distress. All of these can improve emotional functioning. Treatments also promote treatment adherence, foster health lifestyle behaviors, challenge maladaptive patient beliefs about pain and fear-avoidance activity, enhance coping efforts, and increase self-efficacy. Once psychiatric distress has been reduced and positive emotions and adaptive coping strategies are employed, patients may reduce overutilization of health care, decrease medication usage, report reductions in pain and sleep disturbance, become more active, and overall have an improvement in their quality of life.

26. **How can presurgical psychological screening be helpful for medical practitioners?**
Emotional, behavioral, cognitive, and social factors contribute considerably to treatment outcomes, and the pain experience varies greatly among individuals with even the same pain conditions. Presurgical psychological evaluations can optimize treatment outcomes and are an essential component of the medical decision when determining patient eligibility for surgery. Poor surgical outcomes are not only costly and time-consuming for patients and providers but can be tragic for the patient. Not uncommonly, patients report having their hopes dashed when they experience limited benefit from yet another treatment that they believed would be providing substantial pain relief. Presurgical psychological evaluation, which relies on an empirical approach to make recommendations based on psychodiagnostic assessment and medical information, will help ensure that patients possess the basic knowledge and cognitive capacity necessary to understand the mechanisms involved in the proposed procedure, including the risks and benefits, and are able to provide consent for surgery. The evaluation and delivery of psychoeducation can also prepare patients psychologically for the surgery, assess motivation, and help develop feasible and realistic expectations for pain reduction with the outcome of the intervention. In addition to the psychoeducation component, presurgical psychological evaluation can assess and quantify the extent to which psychological, social, cultural, and behavioral factors may contribute to surgical outcomes. For example, it can identify patients at heightened probability to experience poor outcomes, overutilize health care and prescription medications, adhere to postsurgical recommendations, decompensate or improve psychologically, and engage in litigation or make extreme requests to the medical treatment team. Moreover, the patient's psychosocial and behavioral strengths and vulnerabilities can be identified and considered in treatment planning to optimize outcomes. The information obtained from the presurgical psychological evaluation can inform individualized treatment planning for each patient and provide information to determine if the patient is suitable for the surgery or if a decision should be made to delay the surgery until after the provision of psychological treatment and reduction of psychiatric distress. This approach has been found to improve surgical outcomes.

27. **What is the benefit of psychotherapy provided as part of a multidisciplinary team?**
Pain is best conceptualized and treated using the biopsychosocial model of care. Multiple life domains are influenced by emotional functioning and psychosocial factors. Thus psychotherapy as part of a multidisciplinary team targets an important aspect in treating a complex condition. Psychotherapy can potentially alter the pain experience and response to treatment. It also addresses factors that influence patient engagement and burnout among health professionals. The information obtained from treatment can help inform health care through the consideration of each patient's unique risk and protective factors in managing pain effectively.

28. **How common is substance misuse, pharmaceutical overuse, and dependence among pain populations?**
Prescription misuse and substance dependence has been described as an epidemic in some nations and has sparked considerable debate on how to best use these agents for management of pain conditions. Subsequently, substance abuse poses challenges in the treatment of pain. When medications are monitored and taken as prescribed, risk of abuse is low. As patients experience unrelenting and unremitting pain that does not adequately respond to medical treatments, their levels of psychological distress and suffering increase. Over time, their ability to effectively cope with pain and discriminate between emotional distress and physical pain becomes strained, making it easier to use medication to reduce physical pain intensity, alleviate psychiatric distress, and cope

with suffering. Although not effective, patients may use alcohol to promote relaxation and sleep disruptions. Risks of using opiates and analgesics in the long-term treatment of pain include changes in drug tolerance, pain sensitivity, and risk of medication misuse. Not surprisingly, many patients express concern of becoming addicted to their medications and are reluctant to take it altogether. Several factors contribute to one's vulnerability of developing medication dependence, including the type and duration of the condition and treatments, and psychological and familial risk factors. Notably some people do not respond well to non-opioid medications.

29. How common is cognitive impairment among pain populations, and what are some of the causes?

Decrements in cognitive functioning are common among pain populations, although the severity varies greatly by the type of pain condition, developmental stage of the patient, types of treatments they have received, and their age and gender. Cognitive impairments often manifest and can include difficulties in attention, problem solving, perception, working memory, learning, and psychomotor ability. Although the precise mechanisms responsible are not fully known, it is known that the brain's circuitry changes with chronic pain and cognitive impairments can influence the processing and sensitivity to pain, decision-making, and experience of emotion, and impact daily functioning. There is some research that implicates medications, overlapping brain regions, and neurochemical substrates of pain and cognition, and changes in grey matter over time. Research has recently found that patients with long-standing pain disorders may show decreases in cerebral volume—a change that has also been found to remit when the pain is under control.

30. What types of psychological treatments are available for chronic pain treatment?

Acceptance and commitment therapy (ACT), cognitive-behavioral therapy (CBT), dialectical behavioral therapy (DBT), emotionally focused therapy (EFT), somatic experiencing psychotherapy (SE), and psychodynamic psychotherapy (PDT) have shown effectiveness in treating chronic pain populations. These modalities can be provided in the settings of individual therapy, group therapy, and family and couples therapy. Furthermore, behavioral treatments such as biofeedback, hypnosis, meditation, neurofeedback, and relaxation therapy have been shown to be useful aspects of mental health care for pain patients. Many therapies may be augmented, having the patient participate in exercises organized around engaging in artwork, creative writing and music appreciation, as well as a wide variety of other modalities that are directed at the promotion of emotional expression and self-regulation. It is important to tie the therapy choice to the patient's presentation and establish a good fit based on the patient's capacities.

31. How do you determine a patient's suitability for a particular type of psychotherapy?

Several considerations are made in determining patient suitability for a particular type of psychotherapy. Ideally evidence-based treatments that are tailored for pain populations should be considered. Other considerations focus on the patient's primary presenting complaints and psychiatric diagnosis, level of insight and motivation, preference of the patient style and goals, and the training and expertise of the psychotherapist. Time and financial resources are also necessary to consider.

32. What is the difference between short-term and long-term psychotherapy?

Manualized treatments are usually considered short-term, as they may consist of a specified number of therapy sessions. These treatments generally focus on one or two problem areas and not global personality functioning. Both short-term and long-term psychotherapies focus on the reduction of emotional (e.g., stress) and social distress (e.g., isolation) and psychiatric symptoms (e.g., depression). In addition to symptom reduction and fostering more adaptive health beliefs about pain and coping strategies, longer-term therapies may be more intensively focused on past developmental traumas and disruptions. A patient with a history of trauma will usually require a longer-term treatment model. For these patients, it is not only symptoms of distress but also patterns of behavior and adjustment that are the focus. In addition, conscious and unconscious conflicts that may underlie patient motivation, levels of medical engagement, psychiatric and personality structures that influence the trajectory of the pain condition, and meaning of suffering are areas of focus for longer therapies. There is some evidence that suggests short-term treatments are more effective in improving work ability in a shorter time span relative to longer-term therapies, but lacking the long-term effectiveness of long-term therapies.

33. **What is the difference between a psychotherapist and a psychiatrist?**

Psychiatrists are physicians who have attended medical school and had extensive training specific to the psychological and biological mechanisms involved in mental health. As physicians, they are licensed to prescribe medications to treat mental disorders and can also provide psychotherapy. Many studies have demonstrated that psychiatric medications alone are insufficient to adequately treat and manage mental disorders. Similar to psychiatrists, other mental health professionals (e.g., psychologists, marriage and family therapists, social workers) have received extensive training in the provision of psychotherapy and delivery of evidence-based psychotherapeutic interventions, although in general they are not licensed to prescribe medications. In addition to training in the diagnosis and treatment of psychiatric disorders, doctoral-level psychologists also receive significant training in administering psychodiagnostic assessment.

34. **What are the ethical issues involved in providing psychotherapy for pain populations?**

Patients who are referred for pain psychology evaluation and treatment by their health care practitioner may not appreciate that the referring party will confer with the mental health professional about their psychological condition. The way in which information is communicated needs to be discussed and understood by the patient. In addition, in cases where the patient has ongoing litigation, they should be made aware that they may have waived the privilege of confidentiality due to the legal case, and that therefore all of their psychological records may be subject to discovery and open to subpoena. The potential for harm in these circumstances requires a thoughtful informed consent, patient education, consultation with the patient's attorney if permission is granted, and an understanding of the implications of the release of sensitive personal information. Another area of ethical concern is that patients and providers may request professional opinions that are outside the psychotherapist's scope of expertise, such as providing legal or medical recommendations. Psychotherapists, especially psychologists, are often asked to conduct psychological evaluations for pain populations. An important ethical consideration with these evaluations is the selection of tests and measures appropriate for pain populations, and the use of standardized normative data based on these populations for the interpretation of test data (i.e., not only relying on psychological tests standardized on psychiatric patient populations but including those standardized on medical patient populations to avoid inflation of scales due to incorrect norms).

35. **What is the concept of multimodal psychotherapy?**

Multimodal psychotherapy (developed by Lazarus) asserts that psychological problems are multifaceted and result from interactive processes. Accordingly, patients should be assessed and treated with consideration of seven dimensions or modalities of the human experience. Known by their acronym, BASIC ID, the modalities include: behavior, affect, sensation, imagery, cognition, interpersonal relationships, and drugs/biology. In this approach, a variety of psychotherapy orientations can be integrated (such as CBT, ACT, DBT and PDT).

36. **What are the objectives of psychotherapeutic treatment?**

The objectives of psychotherapeutic treatment are tailored to the referral requests and patient emotional and physical needs. All treatments strive to enhance quality of life through improved emotional and physical functioning, and include the following goals:
a. Improve adjustment and management of the pain condition.
b. Alleviate emotional distress.
c. Increase self-efficacy.
d. Increase motivation for change.
e. Foster development of effective coping strategies, including pain-specific coping.
f. Increase social ties and decrease isolation.
g. Strengthen social support.
h. Improve patient-provider communication.
i. Improve problem solving and pain-beliefs.
j. Decrease psychological dependence on pain medications.
k. Assess and modify potentially health behaviors that contribute to the pain experience and quality of life (e.g., sleep disruptions, nicotine, high-fat diets, sexual functioning, treatment adherence).
l. Provide psychoeducation on the rationale of mental health treatment, its utility, and value the therapeutic alliance.
m. Prevent relapse and prepare for maintenance.

KEY POINTS

1. Pain is best understood according to the biopsychosocial model—that is, it is a perceptual experience that involves sensation (tissue damage due to illness or injury), emotion (feelings), and cognition (thoughts).
2. Patients with pain disorders may have premorbid psychological vulnerabilities and also can develop psychological symptoms due to the stress of pain.
3. Treatment of the psychological components of pain will improve the physical components of pain and may reduce medical utilization.
4. It is important to consider sociocultural factors when assessing pain patients.
5. Pain is most effectively treated with the approach of a multidisciplinary team.

BIBLIOGRAPHY

1. *International Association for the Study of Pain.* Pain taxonomy. http://www.iasp-pain.org/Taxonomy?navItemNumber=576. Accessed 7 March 2017.
2. Eccleston C. Role of psychology in pain management. *Br J Anaesth.* 2001;87(1):144-152.
3. Roy R. *Psychosocial Interventions for Chronic Pain: In Search of Evidence.* New York, NY: Springer; 2008.
4. Bourke J. *The Story of Pain: From Prayer to Painkillers.* Oxford, UK: Oxford University Press; 2014.
5. Mayer EA, Bushnell MC, eds. *Functional Pain Syndromes: Presentation and Pathophysiology.* Seattle, WA: IASP Press; 2009.
6. Flor H, Turk DC. *Chronic Pain: An Integrated Biobehavioral Approach.* Seattle, WA: IASP Press; 2011.
7. *Institute of Medicine.* Relieving pain in America: a blueprint for transforming prevention, care, education, and research. http://www.nationalacademies.org/hmd/Reports/2011/Relieving-Pain-in-America-A-Blueprint-for-Transforming-Prevention-Care-Education-Research/Report-Brief.aspx#sthash.oWZoyxkT.dpuf. Accessed 7 March 2017.
8. Bruns D A step-by-step guide to obtaining reimbursement for services provided under the health and behavior codes. http://www.healthpsych.com/tools/resolving_h_and_b_problems.pdf. Accessed 7 March 2017.
9. Tait RC, Chibnall JT. Racial/ethnic disparities in the assessment and treatment of pain: psychosocial perspectives. *Am Psychol.* 2014;69(2):131-141.
10. Gatchel RJ. *Clinical Essentials of Pain Management.* Washington, DC: The American Psychological Association; 2005.
11. Bullington J, Nordemar R, Nordemar K, Sjostrom-Flanagan C. Meaning out of chaos: a way to understand chronic pain. *Scand J Caring Sci.* 2003;17:325-331.
12. Francis DM. *The psychomatrix: a deeper understanding of our relationship with pain.* London: Karnac Books; 2015.
13. Grzesiak RC, Ciccone DS, eds. *Psychological vulnerability to chronic pain.* New York, NY: Springer; 1994.
14. Gustin SM, McKay JG, Peterse ET, et al. Subtle alterations in brain anatomy may change an individual's personality in chronic pain. *PLoS ONE.* 2014;9:e109664. doi:10.1371/journal.pone.0109664.
15. Jacobs M. Psychological factors influencing chronic pain and the impact of litigation. *Curr Phys Med Rehabil Rep.* 2013;1:135-141. doi:10.1007/s40141-013-0015-0.

CHAPTER 50

INTEGRATED APPROACHES TO PAIN MANAGEMENT

Sarah Narayan and Andrew Dubin

Those with chronic pain may be frustrated as their pain complaints may prevail, refractory to allopathic or Western medicine techniques. There is a certain population of sufferers who actively seek a mind-body or spiritual means of coping with chronic disease. It provides them individual empowerment in coping with their pain. Most medical professionals value evidence-based research to back up conventional treatments. This is something that complementary medicine may lack. When patients seek out alternative treatments, some may expect a certain degree of hesitancy physicians may have in supporting patients' desire to seek alternative therapy. This is likely one of the reasons why patients are less inclined to fully enumerate the treatment they are receiving. This may take away from the trust and mutual understanding that are important building blocks for a doctor-patient relationship. It is important that physicians be open and patients be honest in order to avoid certain drug interactions or techniques that may cause harm when combining treatments. Proper communication lines must be present in order to integrate complementary with allopathic medicine.

How can exercise help with pain?

When it comes to chronic pain the objective of exercise is to make once painful though benign movements be more tolerable. In order to do this, the pain sufferer must change neuronal function by repeatedly simulating movement despite firing of the brain's pain centers. Exercise may be able to alter the sensitivity to pain, the more persistently an activity is performed. It most certainly is advised that the patient receive clearance to perform certain exercises by their treating physician before engaging in exercise. Walking can be a good initial activity, as well as slowly reintegrating back into daily activities during the acute phase of a back spasm, for example. Exercise has also been proven to increase the likelihood that back pain sufferers will return to work faster. Randomized trials suggest that many exercises, such as Zumba, Pilates, yoga, and so on, are shown to be beneficial in some way for back pain sufferers. The objective of exercise is to create postural awareness in order to limit stresses on nerve, disc, and soft tissue structures that are prone to injury. In addition, exercise will improve circulation to promote healing. Exercise will strengthen the supportive framework around major musculoskeletal structures (such as the spine and joints). Exercise also reduces the fear of movement, often plaguing pain sufferers. It has been proven to assist in the management of depression associated with chronic pain. It may also improve cardiovascular health, improve flexibility, and promote restful sleep.

What are the benefits of chiropractic treatment and massage for pain?

These are the most common alternative treatment options sought out for chronic pain. The chiropractic treatment aims to improve physiologic alignment of the body through manual treatments, modalities, and manipulation. Massage treatment uses direct manual treatment of muscle and soft tissue, in order alleviate pains and ailments in these areas. Research does not strongly back up these treatments, although the US Agency of Health Policy and Research indicates that chiropractic care may have some benefits for acute pain, although there is no supportive data backing this treatment for chronic pain. There may be some utility involving massage in the treatment for rheumatic and low back pain.

Tell me about how mind-body treatments can help chronic pain?

Although stress does not cause back pain to occur, it can exacerbate chronic pain. Cognitive behavioral therapy can decrease the amplified signal of pain that is brought on by stress and fear-avoidance of activity. Fear and avoidance of activity is a common response found in chronic pain sufferers. Nonetheless avoiding activity can limit daily life and social and occupational experiences long term. Functional restoration programs are multidisciplinary programs that incorporate cognitive behavioral therapy. This technique is used to empower the patient to be able to perform tasks by modifying their pain levels. Cognitive behavioral therapy is a way to educate and reframe perception and attitudes toward chronic pain. This therapy can be taught by trained psychiatrists, psychologists or other mental health professionals. It has been proven that the combination of physical activity and cognitive behavioral therapy can improve one's perception of pain. Biofeedback and relaxation techniques have shown promising improvements in those with migraines.

Tell me about acupuncture for pain?

Acupuncture has shown some benefits in certain chronic pain conditions. This treatment is most beneficial for dental issues or temporomandibular joint pain. Acupuncture may be beneficial in the management of osteoarthritis, fibromyalgia, and some headaches. There is less convincing support that acupuncture will help manage chronic pain syndromes or back pain. Studying efficacy is challenging, given the varying degree of practitioner style and technique, as well as the limited quality and quantity of current research available.

KEY POINTS

1. Cognitive behavior therapy has been proven effective in modifying pain.
2. Cognitive behavior therapy in combination with physical therapy can be cumulatively more beneficial for the management of chronic back pain.
3. It is important that patients are comfortable enough to discuss complementary treatments with their physician(s).

BIBLIOGRAPHY

1. Astin JA. Why patients use alternative medicine: results of a national study. *JAMA*. 1998;279:1548-1553.
2. Eisenberg DM, Davis RB, Ettner SL, et al. Trends in alternative medicine use in the United States, 1990–1997: results of a follow-up national survey. *JAMA*. 1998;280:1569-1575.
3. Sherman KJ, Cherkin DC, Wellman RD, et al. A randomized trial comparing yoga, stretching, and a self-care book for chronic low back pain. *Arch Intern Med*. 2011;171:2019-2026.
4. Hall AM, Maher C, Lam P, Ferreira M, Latimer J. Tai Chi exercise for treatment of pain and disability in people with persistent low back pain: a randomized controlled trial. *Arthritis Care Res*. 2011;63:1576-1583.
5. Cramer H, Lauche R, Haller H, Dobos G. A systematic review and meta-anaysis of yoga for low back pain. *Clin J Pain*. 2013;29:450-460.
6. Woodman JP, Moore NR. Evidence for the effectiveness of Alexander Technique lessons in medical and health-related conditions. A systematic review. *Int J Clin Pract*. 2012;66:98-112.
7. Marshall PWM, Kennedy S, Brooks C, Lonsdale C. Pilates exercise or stationary cycling for chronic nonspecific low back pain: does it matter? A randomized controlled trial with 6-month follow-up. *Spine*. 2013;38:E952-E959.
8. Choi BKL, Verbeek JH, Tam WWS, Jiang JY. Exercises for prevention of recurrences of low-back pain. *Cochrane Database Syst Rev*. 2010;(1):CD006555.
9. Mannion AF, Muntener M, Taimela S, Divorak J. Volvo award winner in clinical studies: a randomized clinical trial of three active therapies for chronic low back pain. *Spine*. 1999;24:2435-2448.
10. Mannion AF, Caporaso F, Pulkovski N, Sprott H. Spine stabilization exercises in the treatment of chronic low back pain: a good clinical outcome is not associated with improved abdominal muscle function. *Eur Spine J*. 2012;21:1301-1310.
11. Bigos SJ, Bowyer OR, Braen GR, et al. Acute low back problems in adults. Clinical practice guideline no. 14. Rockville, MD: Agency for Health Care Policy and Research, Public Health Service, US Department of Health and Human Services; 1994.
12. Ernst E. Massage treatment for back pain. *BMJ*. 2003;326:562-563.
13. Gatchel RJ, Rollings KH. Evidence-informed management of chronic low back pain with cognitive behavioral therapy. *Spine J*. 2008;8:40-44.
14. Henschke N, Ostelo RWJG, van Tulder MW, et al. Behavioral treatment for chronic low back pain. *Cochrane Database Syst Rev*. 2010;(7):CD002014.
15. Monticone M, Ferrante S, Rocca B, et al. Effects of a long-lasting multidisciplinary program on disability and fear-avoidance behaviors in patients with chronic low back pain: results of a randomized controlled trial. *Clin J Pain*. 2013;29:929-938.
16. Nicholas MK, Asghari A, Blyth FM, et al. Self-management intervention for chronic pain in older adults: a randomized controlled trial. *Pain*. 2013;154:824-835.

17. Vong SK, Cheing GL, Chan F, So EM, Chan CC. Motivational enhancement therapy in addition to physical therapy improves motivational factors and treatment outcomes in people with low back pain: a randomized controlled trial. *Arch Phys Med Rehabil*. 2011;92:176-183.
18. Haddock CK, Rowan AB, Andrasik F, et al. Home-based behavioral treatments for chronic benign headache: a meta-analysis of controlled trials. *Cephalalgia*. 1997;17:113-118.
19. Gauthier JG, Ivers H, Carrier S. Nonpharmacological approaches in the management of recurrent headache disorders and their comparison and combination with pharmacotherapy. *Clin Psychol Rev*. 1996;16:543-571.
20. Legget Tait P, Brooks L, Harstall C. *Acupuncture: Evidence From Systematic Reviews and Meta-Analysis*. Edmonton: Alberta Heritage Foundation for Medical Research; 2002.

CHAPTER 51

PAIN CLINICS

Sarah Narayan

How must one evaluate acute low back pain? And how about chronic low back pain?

Acute versus chronic low back pain represent two separate and distinct issues. Acute pain, regardless of location, is typically associated with tissue damage and serves a protective function. Chronic pain, in contradistinction, is typically thought of as pain that has outlived its purpose or protective function. In the case of chronic low back pain, the persistence of pain actually negatively impacts on the patient's ability to participate in activities of daily living, as well as vocational and avocational activities.

Initial assessment of the patient with low back pain, regardless of acuity versus chronicity, should entail observation. Patients should be observed while they ambulate to the examining room. Significant data can be gleaned during this period of the physical exam, as the patient does not appreciate that the exam has already started, and as such more objective data may be obtained than during the formal exam. This is particularly true in the patient with chronic low back pain issues. Many maladaptive movements may be delineated during the initial observation period.

Once in the room, observation should continue during the history taking. Does the patient prefer to sit as opposed to stand? A patient who is comfortable sitting and prefers to sit and does not change position from sit to stand may well have lumbar stenosis, or posterior column issues, such as facet joint arthropathy. Patients who prefer to stand may well have anterior and middle column dysfunction related to lumbar vertebral disc issues. Patients who constantly change position during the interview may have underlying degenerative changes in their lumbar spine, but may be primarily symptomatic with reactive muscle spasm and dysfunction secondary to the underlying degenerative changes in the lumbar spine. A classic case would be the patient who notes limited sitting tolerance with marked low back pain and stiffness noted after arising from prolonged sitting, such as going to the movies. In this instance, reactive psoas muscle spasm secondary to chronic muscle shortening may well be the problem, and a physical therapy program designed to address this issue may work quite well.

Acute low back pain is typically associated with a distinct event specific inciting event. Lifting and twisting mechanisms are most common causes of acute low back pain. They may result in acute disc herniation, muscle strain, or possibly even compression fracture. The risk for compression fracture increases with age. Additionally, female gender ethnicity and slender body habitus also increase risk for compression fracture. In the patient with the correct demographics, acute low back pain that is localized to the back and worsened with sitting or bending forward is highly concerning for a compression fracture and does warrant immediate radiographic assessment. Correlative findings on x-ray confirm the clinical diagnosis and help guide treatment. In the acutely symptomatic lumbar compression, fracture management with a lumbosacral orthosis to limit flexion will be very helpful for managing pain and restoring patient mobility. Those patients experiencing frequent fractures should receive a workup for osteoporosis by their primary care physician or referred to an endocrinologist or rheumatologist.

Evaluation of the patient with acute low back pain should initially focus on mechanism in injury. Twisting type activities or twisting with lifting are common causes of acute disc herniation. Pertinent parts of the history should include what positions or activities intensify as well as relieve symptoms. Is there a pattern or distribution of pain? Does the patient note any weakness in the leg? What tasks are problematic? And lastly what is the status of bladder function? Typically in a patient where there is concern for a cauda equine spinal cord syndrome secondary to massive low lumbar disc extrusion, bladder incontinence will be more quickly noted than bowel dysfunction if for no other reason than it is more difficult to control liquids than solids. As such, careful questioning regarding bladder function is imperative when trying to determine if a patient may have a cauda equine syndrome. Alteration in saddle distribution sensation is also helpful, but less reliable. When truly present on physical examination, it is highly correlative, but as a subjective complaint much less so.

How must one approach the management of acute pain?

Along with the previously listed items, the patient should also be questioned about what they have tried to relieve the pain, over-the-counter nonsteroidal antiinflammatory drugs (NSAIDs), brief activity modification, and what has been the response to these interventions. Treatment objective for acute injury is to manage pain while promoting self-healing to jump-start activity. Pain management may be in the form of NSAID use, neuro-modulating agents (Neurontin, Lyrica), muscle relaxants, steroids, or narcotic pain medications. Interventional pain management in the form of steroid epidural injections, nerve blocks, or steroid joint injections may also be used. One must also encourage patients to reintegrate back into daily routine and work-related activities. Physical therapy may help encourage movement and functional reintegration. Should the patient experience red flags such as bowel/bladder changes, focal extremity weakness, signs or symptoms of myelopathy or other emergent central nervous system damage, immediate attention should be made to treat the issue seriously (beyond the standard conservative management stated earlier).

What are some ways of managing chronic pain?

Treatment for chronic pain has certainly evolved over the course of many years. The objective of chronic pain management is to manage, not treat, the pain syndrome in order to provide pain patients the ability to function and become active members of society. Functional goals can be executed solely through a single pain practitioner or through a multidisciplinary team approach. Single chronic pain providers may work on interventional pain management in combination with medication management with routine, long-term follow-up. The multidisciplinary approach will include multiple providers of different specialties with the same treatment objective—of assisting in the management of chronic pain. Providers may include a chronic pain specialist as well as a pharmacist to incorporate pharmacotherapies. Pain psychologists or psychiatrists can address behavioral issues that may modify the patient's pain level. They may also address associated mood disorders such as anxiety, posttraumatic stress disorder, or depression. Physical therapists or occupational therapists may incorporate therapeutic exercise and conditioning. This will help empower the patient to be able to move and function despite their pain or fear/avoidance of activity.

What is an addiction clinic?

Addiction is a chronic disease that should be treated as such. It is a complex illness marked by uncontrolled drug seeking behavior despite adverse health risks. This is quite frequently a relapsing illness. Those afflicted with addiction require long-term, repeated care. Treatment objectives in addiction clinics would be to eventually discontinue drug use, promote long-term cessation, and advise patients to return to their roles as active members of society. The most effective drug addiction clinics are multidisciplinary. They incorporate members of different specialties to address different facets of recovery. Addiction medicine treatment involves detoxification of the medication from the patients' system. Alternative methods under an outpatient clinic setting occur through a slow process of weaning. This typically occurs with a long-acting narcotic such as suboxone or methadone. Medication management helps suppress withdrawal symptoms. Use of medication is incorporated in close to 80% of addiction clinics. It is also important to incorporate mental health experts, incorporating behavior counseling. Behavioral counseling will help modify any dysfunctional behaviors and attitudes toward drug use. Cognitive behavioral therapy, peer counseling, group therapy, or family therapy are different means of behavioral counseling. Identifying and treating anxiety and depression should also be incorporated in a well-rounded treatment plan, since mental health disorders are often co-occurring conditions affiliated with addiction. Necessary steps should be made to ensure patients participate in long-term follow-up in order to prevent relapse. Inpatient or residential programs as well as outpatient clinics are available for those suffering drug or alcohol addiction. In 2014 22.5 million people ages 12 years or older needed treatment for addiction. Only 4.2 million received treatment for addiction that year.

What is a Functional Restoration Program?

Functional restoration programs use a biopsychosocial approach to chronic pain. One must understand that there are physiologic, psychologic, and social factors that perpetuate the presentation of pain. This program aims to empower the patient to take control of these factors that could negatively modify pain. The treatment objective is to decrease pain, restore functions, allow patients to return to work, improve strength and conditioning, and limit unnecessary health care utilization (frequent emergency room visits for severe pain). Typically those with chronic pain will have deconditioning syndromes marked by 4- to 6-month periods of very limited activity. They will present with decreased mobility, strength, and endurance, as well as anxiety and depression. Anxiety related to activity may also be present in this population. Candidates for enrollment include those who present with pain focused behaviors; those who do not progress with conventional rehabilitation; those with pain disproportionate to injury; and those with disruption of daily life, social interaction, work participation, and family responsibility. A functional restoration program is an extensive outpatient program lasting several weeks. The program typically includes individual and group sessions. Programs will include rigorous physical therapy to improve strength and flexibility. Physical therapy will help allay fear that activity will worsen or exacerbate pain. Occupational therapy will assist in performing activities of daily living and ergonomic training. Social work will assist participants to reintegrate back into the workforce. Psychiatry or psychology will work on behavioral strategies to cope with pain, including cognitive behavioral therapy and therapy for related anxiety or depression. Physicians may work on detox to minimize medication management. Clinicians will also work with the patients on any associated medical or musculoskeletal complaints that arise. Functional restoration programs have been proven beneficial for low back pain sufferers.

KEY POINTS

1. Acute pain is typically associated with tissue damage and serves a protective function.
2. Chronic pain is typically thought of as pain that has outlived its purpose or protective function.
3. Barring and emergent red flag signs and symptoms, acute pain treatment is geared to improve comfort while encouraging reintegration back into activity as soon as possible.
4. Addiction should be considered and treated as a chronic disease. It is a complex illness marked by uncontrolled drug-seeking behavior despite adverse health risks.
5. Chronic pain management is more complex and may require a multidisciplinary approach either through an established pain clinic or functional restoration program.

BIBLIOGRAPHY

1. Newman RI, Seres JL, Yospe LP, Garlington B. Multidisciplinary treatment of chronic pain: long-term follow-up of low-back pain patients. *Pain.* 1978;4:283-292.
2. Center for Behavioral Health Statistics and Quality (CBSHQ). *2014 National Survey on Drug Use and Health: Detailed Tables.* Rockville, MD: Substance Abuse and Mental Health Services Administration; 2015.
3. Substance Abuse and Mental Health Services Administration (SAMHSA). *National Survey of Substance Abuse Treatment Services (N-SSATS): 2013. Data on Substance Abuse Treatment Facilities.* Rockville, MD: Substance Abuse and Mental Health Services Administration; 2014. HHS Publication No. (SMA) 14-489. BHSIS Series S-73.
4. Hazard RG, Fenwick JW, Kalisch SM, et al. Functional restoration with behavioral support: a one-year prospective study of patients with chronic low-back pain. *Spine.* 1989;14(2):157-161.
5. Jousset N, Fanello S, Bontoux L, et al. Effects of functional restoration versus 3 hours per week physical therapy: a randomized controlled study. *Spine.* 2004;29(5):487-599.
6. Caby I, Olivier N, Mendelek F, et al. Functional restoration of the spine: effect of initial pain level on the performance of subjects with chronic low back pain. *Pain Res Manag.* 2014;19(5):133-138.

CHAPTER 52

COMPLEMENTARY AND ALTERNATIVE MEDICINE

Ian Walling, Meghan Wilock and Julie G. Pilitsis

1. **Can we define complementary and alternative medical treatment?**
   Pinning down what constitutes the field of complementary or alternative medicine (CAM) is complicated by the constantly shifting nature of the field; therapies evolve and change over time, and some become incorporated into mainstream medicine. The integration of what has once been considered alternative or complementary can be seen in the adoption of practices such as chiropractic or acupuncture therapies as the efficacy of the treatments becomes better documented and supported via study. A good working definition for alternative therapies would be that the methods are often taught in medical schools while not seeing widespread use in conventional treatment regimens.

2. **What is the prevalence and usage of complementary or alternative medicine therapies in the United States?**
   The National Center for Complementary and Investigative Health (NCCIH), which functions as a subsidiary of the NIH, had conducted surveys in 2002, 2007, and 2012 as to the prevalence of different CAM therapies and the usage of CAM by different population groups in the United States. In 2012, 32.2% of adults age 18 to 44, 36.5% of adults age 45 to 64, and 29.4% of adults over 65 reported using at least one CAM over the past year. The survey additionally indicated that populations with higher levels of education demonstrate increased utilization of CAM therapies, with the largest difference being between 15.6% of non-high-school educated adults and 42.6% of adults with college degrees choosing to utilize CAM.

3. **What are the primary divisions of complementary or alternative medicine therapies?**
   The NCCIH splits CAM therapies into five general categories as follows:
   a. Alternative medicine systems
   b. Mind-body interventions
   c. Biologically based techniques
   d. Manipulative and body-based methods
   e. Energy therapies

4. **What is the philosophy of traditional Chinese medicine, and what are its major components?**
   One of the most popular forms of alternative medicine systems in the United States is traditional Chinese medicine (TCM). TCM attacks the concepts of treatment and health from a holistic angle, viewing "healthy" and "diseased" not as a distinct dichotomy, but rather as parts of a spectrum. TCM focuses on the flow of energy called "qi" or "chi" (pronounced as "chee") through the body between the vital organs along paths called "meridians." TCM focuses on balancing the flow of qi throughout the body and physiological functions (such as breathing or digestion), which are grouped together into "concepts" rather than anatomical components. The formulation of diagnoses in TCM is based on determining how the symptoms fit into the idea of the eight principles, which express fundamental disease qualities through paired concepts, such as heat/cold, internal/external, yin/yang, and vacuity/repletion (deficiency/excess).

5. **What are the primary methods and therapies of traditional Chinese medicine?**
   TCM places a strong focus on living healthfully through correct dietary nutrition as well as exercise based around the movements of tai chi or qigong. Practitioners also often utilize variations of acupuncture needles, consumption of Chinese herbal or mineral-based supplements, and tui na massage therapy.

6. **How is acupuncture applied?**
   The goal of acupuncture is to obtain a desired physiological effect via the insertion of needles into the skin at specified points on the body, which are chosen based on the desired effect and the pathology of the patient. At its most basic level, acupuncture involves the piercing of the skin with metallic needles along the body's meridians, as well as at points known as ah shi. Further therapies can be performed using mechanical stimulation, electrical stimulation, applying heated needles, using moxa made of mugwort and other plants, or applying a laser. While evidence is lacking for determining which forms of acupuncture provide superior treatment when compared to the others, some anecdotal evidence indicates that electroacupuncture demonstrates potential for myofacial pain applications.

7. **How does acupuncture act to induce analgesia in patients?**
   Traditionally, TCM has viewed acupuncture's method for improving patient status by altering the flow of qi to different areas via needling along meridians for increasing, suppressing, or otherwise changing the behavior of the patient's qi. One currently suggested method for acupuncture's analgesia is that the needles increase blood flow throughout the body, while also reducing prostaglandin, histamine, and other inflammatory agents at a local level. Electrical stimulation in combination with acupuncture has been indicated in several studies to affect the central nervous system, with special focus falling on the spinal cord, pituitary, and midbrain; insertion of acupuncture needles results in elevated levels of enkephalin, endorphins, and possibly gamma-aminobutyric acid released at the spinal cord, enkephalin, norepinephrine, and serotonin at the midbrain, and endorphins at the pituitary. The opioid antagonist naloxene has been demonstrated to be capable of partially inhibiting or reversing the analgesia induced by acupuncture, pointing to the involvement of endogenous opioids as a possible mechanism for analgesia. Another proposed mechanism for acupuncture is the inhibition of spinal microglia, which studies say perform a role in inflammatory responses and the pain induction process.

8. **What is the stance of the National Institute of Health on the use of acupuncture?**
   In 1997 the National Institute of Health's Acupuncture Consensus Panel issued a statement that, based on research conducted at the time, there was evidence for the use of acupuncture in management of postoperative dental pain for adult patients, as well as postoperative and chemotherapy-related nausea. Some studies indicated acupuncture demonstrated potential as an alternative therapy or as an adjunct to standard treatments for managing lower back pain, myofacial pain, fibromyalgia, lateral epicondylitis (tennis elbow), migraine headache, carpal tunnel syndrome, osteoarthritis, and menstrual cramps, though some of these uses were based on single studies at the time.

9. **Is there a consensus on acupuncture as an effective treatment of fibromyalgia?**
   In 2013 a review of nine trials indicated that while moderate evidence existed for acupuncture improving pain and stiffness when compared to standard therapies, evidence indicated that sham acupuncture was capable of achieving the same results, though the review noted the absence of standardized, ideal sham acupuncture methods weakened these conclusions. The review also indicated that electroacupuncture showed greater potential for treating both pain and stiffness than manual acupuncture, but that the duration for improvements was less than 6 months.

10. **Does evidence support the use of acupuncture for other chronic pain conditions?**
    Migraine headaches have been shown to be attenuated via the use of acupuncture. A 2015 review of 22 trials comparing acupuncture's effects versus standard care, sham therapy, and/or prophylactic pharmaceuticals found evidence that acupuncture was beneficial in treating acute migraine attacks and in reducing the frequency of migraines. Additionally, though no evidence indicated a difference between acupuncture and sham treatment, when compared with prophylactic drugs, acupuncture produced slightly better outcomes and minimized adverse side effects from treatment.

11. **What concerns and contraindications should be considered when conducting acupuncture?**
    Proper training for handling and placement of needles is critical for preventing complications with acupuncture, such as causing pneumothorax with poorly positioned needles at the chest.

Practitioners should be cautious when working with patients on anticoagulants, so as to minimize side-effect severity. Electroacupuncture should similarly not be administered to patients with implanted pacemakers, due to possibly interfering with their function. Patients may experience an increased sense of euphoria, sedation, or pain for up to 24 hours following treatment. Acupuncture should be practiced using disposable, sterile needles to minimize the possible transmission of blood borne pathogens such as HIV or hepatitis B and C.

12. What constitutes bioenergetic therapy?

Bioenergetic therapies aim to balance the energy of the body through a mixture of exercise, energy manipulation, and diet based on the teachings of TCM, Western medical practices, and Ayurveda. Some methods involve practitioners directly manipulating the energy of their patients, such as therapeutic touch, which transfers energy from caregiver to patient without direct contact. Another bioenergy manipulation therapy is Reiki, developed in 1922 by Mikao Usui, which has practitioners send energy through their palms to patients over different targets on their body. A 2008 analysis of nine randomized clinical trials for Reiki's efficacy for different medical conditions failed to demonstrate any effects for diabetic neuropathy or recovery from ischaemic stroke, but one trial showed differences between Reiki and sham treatment for pain and anxiety. The analysis found evidence insufficient to support Reiki as a treatment for any condition used in the trials, due to issues such as poor study designs and small study populations.

13. What is Ayurveda?

A Sanskrit term that translates into "knowledge (veda) of life (ayur)," Ayurveda is primarily a doctrine focused on healthy living and preventing illness rather than fighting disease. Texts dealing with the concepts of Ayurveda have been found from between 1000 BC and 1500 BC, and have addressed a range of conditions that include rheumatism, arthritis, and nervous-system disorders. Taking a holistic view of health, Ayurveda deals with spiritual elements in addition to the diet, exercise, and herbal medicines for addressing ailments. Ayurveda has a focus on balancing influences and the cleansing or removal of toxins.

14. Which bioenergy therapies are common in Western medicine?

When working with bioenergies, Western medicine generally applies external energy sources to patients to enact a change, the most common forms being electrical or thermal. The application of heat via thermal therapy or cold via cryotherapy is very popular in spite of a lack of evidence in the literature to support their use. One therapy that has seen growing popularity is transcutaneous electrical nerve stimulation (TENS), which is similar to electroacupuncture in that it utilizes electricity towards a therapeutic end. A 2016 analysis of nine studies on TENS for lower back pain found patients saw improvements in VAS scores, with a standardized mean difference of 0.844 between pre- and posttreatment testing. Another study on complex regional pain syndrome (CRPS) showed that TENS, when added to physical therapy, significantly improved the recovery in CRPS, with improvements noted in spontaneous and neuropathic pain scores. Additionally, the application of ultrasound for therapeutic purposes is being researched as a noninvasive energy delivery mechanism for pain treatment, is seeing positive results for both improving pain and function of osteoarthritis in knees, and has phase 1 trials studying its potential for use with Parkinson's disease and other chronic pain conditions.

15. How is spinal manipulation involved in the treatment of headache and back pain?

Spinal manipulation has been shown in several studies to positively impact pain related to tension-type headaches, and the severity of side effects patients experienced was reported to be less than those who underwent pharmaceutical treatment with amitriptyline; there is also some evidence that spinal manipulation can improve outcomes for cervicogenic headaches as well. Much of the benefit from spinal manipulation is gained in acute headache pain relief—the benefits and mechanisms for the therapy are less understood in chronic pain models.

16. Which "mind-body" modalities are seeing use for treatment of pain?

The use of biofeedback, cognitive behavioral feedback, or being mindful of and regulating bodily functions that are typically involuntary has frequently been taught as a tool for controlling pain; patients are taught to rethink pain and view it as something manageable, while also teaching how to regulate the changes which occur with onset of pain using relaxation techniques. There is some evidence indicating that biofeedback has use as a method for controlling chronic pain. Similarly, recent studies have shown the potential for "mindfulness," and using meditation or yoga to change how one interprets pain have similar potential for dealing with pain. It is possible that, through meditation, the activity of the regions of the brain dealing with attention experience changes in activity, resulting in decreased activity in the part of the brain receiving pain signals from the body. Additional mind-body techniques, such as progressive muscle relaxation, deep breathing, and music therapy, can also be used to relieve pain.

17. Can headache pain be treated using vitamins or supplements?
A study in 1998 has shown that, when compared to a control group receiving placebos, 400 mg daily doses of riboflavin (as opposed to the recommended 1.8 mg daily value) were more effective at relieving pain from tension-type headaches and migraines over a 3-month period. While the study found significant differences between groups, a double-blind trial conducted in 2004 failed to replicate these findings and found no difference between control and riboflavin rats. While riboflavin has shown potential for preventing headache, in the case of acute migraine headache, administration of magnesium via intravenous means can work as an abortive agent. While studies of magnesium's potential as a prophylactic agent have started, the results have been mixed.

18. Are there uses for feverfew and butterbur in treating headache?
Some traditional folk remedies, such as plants or minerals that have been believed to treat various conditions, have come under new interest with the growth of studies in CAM. Grown throughout the United States and Europe, *Tanacetum parthenium* (feverfew) is a plant that produces parthenolide, a compound believed to inhibit proinflammatory agents. This potential to prevent inflammation has resulted in studies to assess whether it can attenuate or prevent headaches, but results so far have been mixed. Another plant of interest in headache treatment is *Petasites hybridus* root (butterbur). In 2004 two studies were conducted looking at different doses of butterbur (one looking at daily 50 or 75 mg doses, the other using 50 mg doses twice a day) versus placebos, and both found significant reductions in headache frequency following butterbur treatment for 12 weeks for daily 75 mg and two daily 50 mg doses. There are concerns about butterbur use due to possible hepatic toxicity.

19. Create a partial list of drug-herb interactions to be aware of.
    a. NSAIDS—ginger, willowbark, feverfew, horse chestnut
    b. Opioids—valerian root, kava, chamomile

20. To what scientific standard should complementary or alternative medicine therapies be held?
It is worth considering that there are many current, mainstream medical practices that have never undergone truly rigorous scientific examination: the best practices for preventing stroke other than lowering blood pressure are still being tinkered with, the use of epidural steroid injections for pain relief is still not fully accepted, and much of the work with lower back surgeries has been conducted without properly randomized trials. It is also important to remember that while many forms of CAM are not commonly accepted in Western society and the West is working to incorporate them into its understanding of health and medicine, the same can be said for Western practices in China and other regions where medical practices differ. Just because something is currently the standard does not necessarily make it correct or the best, and what is standard in one area may be an alternative treatment in another.

21. How can clinicians best minimize patient exposure to risk from complementary or alternative medicine and their exposure to legal risk by treating using complementary or alternative medicine?
Categorization of CAM therapies based on the evidence for the treatment's effectiveness and also for its safety to the patient has been proposed by Cohen and Eisenberg. Clinicians should assess the relative risk for the treatment to the patient compared with other therapies, keep clear documentation of the logic and arguments supporting the use of the CAM, and also explicitly inform the patient as to risks, the nature of the treatment, and other alternatives for consent purposes. Once starting a CAM, patients should be monitored conventionally. Practitioners should also inquire about the confidence of others who utilize the particular treatment modality.

KEY POINTS

1. CAM, while differing greatly in method of implementation, generally shares the ideas of focusing on the body's ability for self-recovery and the importance of preventative measures in health care.
2. A broad range of CAM are currently implemented with varying degrees of evidence to back up their efficacy for treating different conditions, and as studies improve in quantity and quality, these practices will either be further refined and introduced into mainstream medicine or fall into disuse if shown inefficacious.
3. Due to the potential for a drug-herb/supplement interaction having potential deleterious consequences, it is crucial that practitioners, both mainstream and alternative, conduct thorough medication history checks in order to prevent such interactions.

BIBLIOGRAPHY

1. Allais G, DeLorenzo C. Acupuncture as a prophylactic treatment of migraine without aura: a comparison with flunarizine. *Headache*. 2002;44(9):855-861.
2. Berman BM, Lao L, Langenberg P, et al. The effectiveness of acupuncture as an adjunctive therapy in OA of the knee. *Ann Intern Med*. 2005;141(12):901-910.
3. Birch S, Hesselink JK. Clinical research on acupuncture. Part 1. What have the reviews on the efficacy and safety of acupuncture told us so far? *J Altern Complement Med*. 2004;10(3):468-480.
4. Chopra A, Doiphode VV. Ayurvedic medicine: core concept, therapeutic principles, and current relevance. *Med Clin North Am*. 2002;86(1):75-89.
5. Cohen MH, Eisenberg DM. Potential physical malpractice liability associated with complementary and integrative medical therapies. *Ann Intern Med*. 2002;136:596-603.
6. Cohen MH, Hrbek A, Davis RB, et al. Emerging credentialing practices, malpractice liability policies, and guidelines governing complementary and alternative practices and dietary supplement recommendations. *Arch Intern Med*. 2005;165(3):289-295.
7. Eccles NK. A critical review of randomized controlled trials of static magnets for pain relief. *J Altern Complement Med*. 2005;11(3):495-509.
8. Ernst E, Pittler MH. The efficacy and safety of feverfew (*Tenacetum parthenium* L.): an update of a systemic review. *Public Health Nutr*. 2000;3(4A):509-514.
9. Kaptchuk TJ, Eisenberg DM. Varieties of healing. 2: a taxonomy of unconventional healing practices. *Ann Intern Med*. 2001;135(3):196-204.
10. Khadilkar A, Milne S, Brosseau L, et al. Transcutaneous electrical nerve stimulation (TENS) for chronic low back pain. *Cochrane Database Syst Rev*. 2005;(3):CD003008.
11. Lipton RB, Gobel H. *Petasites hybridus* root (butterbur) is an effective preventative treatment for migraine. *Neurology*. 2004;63(12):2240-2244.
12. Maizels M, Blumenfeld A, Burchette R. A combination of riboflavin, magnesium feverfew for migraine prophylaxis: a randomized controlled trial. *Headache*. 2004;44(9):885-890.
13. Mazzata G, Sarchielli P, Alberti A, Gallai V. Electromyographical ischemic test and intracellular and extracellular magnesium concentration in migraine and tension type headache patients. *Headache*. 1996;36(6):357-361.
14. Montazeri K, Farahnakian M. The effect of acupuncture on the acute withdrawal symptoms from rapid detoxification. *Acta Anaesthesiol Sin*. 2002;40(4):173-175.
15. Nestler G. Traditional Chinese medicine. *Med Clin North Am*. 2002;86(1):63-73.
16. Park J, Ernst E. Ayurvedic medicine for rheumatoid arthritis. *Semin Arthritis Rheum*. 2005;34(5):705-713.
17. Schoenen J, Jacquy J, Lenaerts M. Effectiveness of high dose riboflavin in migraine prophylaxis. *Neurology*. 1998;50(2):466-470.
18. Tindle HA, Davis RB, Phillips RS, Eisenberg DM. Trends in the use of complementary and alternative medicine by US adults: 1997–2002. *Altern Ther Health Med*. 2005;11(1):42-49.
19. Tsui MLK, Cheing GLY. The effectiveness of electroacupuncture in the management of chronic low back pain. *J Altern Complement Med*. 2004;10:803-809.
20. Vickers AJ. Statistical reanalysis of four recent randomized trials of acupuncture for pain using analysis of covariance. *Clin J Pain*. 2004;20:319-323.

INDEX

Page numbers followed by "*f*" indicate figures, "*t*" indicate tables, and "*b*" indicate boxes.